THERAPEUTIC MODALITIES

THERAPEUTIC MODALITIES

Second Edition

Chad Starkey, PhD, ATC
Athletic Training Program Director
Bouvé College of Health Professions
Northeastern University
Boston, Massachusetts

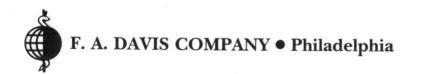

F. A. DAVIS COMPANY • Philadelphia

F. A. Davis Company
1915 Arch Street
Philadelphia, PA 19103

Printed in the United States of America

Last digit indicates print number: 10 9 8 7 6 5 4 3 2 1

Publisher: Jean-François Vilain
Developmental Editor: Crystal R. Spraggins
Production Editor: Jessica Howie Martin
Cover Designer: Louis J. Forgione

As new scientific information becomes available through basic and clinical research, recommended treatments and drug therapies undergo changes. The author and publisher have done everything possible to make this book accurate, up to date, and in accord with accepted standards at the time of publication. The author, editors, and publisher are not responsible for errors or omissions or for consequences from application of the book, and make no warranty, expressed or implied, in regard to the contents of the book. Any practice described in this book should be applied by the reader in accordance with professional standards of care used in regard to the unique circumstances that may apply in each situation. The reader is advised always to check product information (package inserts) for changes and new information regarding dose and contraindications before administering any drug. Caution is especially urged when using new or infrequently ordered drugs.

Library of Congress Cataloging-in-Publication Data

Starkey, Chad, 1959–
  Therapeutic modalities / Chad Starkey. — 2nd ed.
    p.   cm.
  Rev. ed. of: Therapeutic modalities for athletic trainers. c1993.
  Includes bibliographical references and index.
  ISBN 0-8036-0354-1
  1. Sports medicine.   2. Athletic trainers.   3. Athletes—
Rehabilitation.   4. Sports injuries—Treatment.   I. Starkey, Chad,
1959– Therapeutic modalities for athletic trainers.   II. Title.
  [DNLM: 1. Athletic Injuries—therapy.   QT   261   S795t   1999]
RC1210.S785   1999
617.1'027—dc21
DNLM/DLC
for Library of Congress   98-6340
                                                                    CIP

Dedication for the Second Edition

I'm just about glad that I knew you once and it was more than just a passing acquaintance.
I'm just about glad that it was a memory that doesn't need constant maintenance.
There are a few things that I regret,
But nothing that I need to forget.
For all of the courage that you never had
I'm just about glad.

Once again, these words mean so much more than they might.
And so the cycle continues:

Dedication for the First Edition

A statement of resiliency more than despair:

I never wanted to hear that song you dedicated tonight.
Because, you see, I heard that song so long before we met,
That it means so much more than it might.

Preface to the Second Edition

When rewriting this book, I attempted to adhere to my original philosophy of writing an entry-level therapeutic modalities text that was understandable and easy to read. I have also attempted to develop an equal balance between theory and application without creating a protocol "cookbook."

Chapter 1 provides an overview of the body's physiological response to trauma. Chapter 2 is new, describing the physiology and psychology of pain. These two chapters are the focal point for the text, with each subsequent chapter referring back to this information. Based on the availability of several new administration texts, administration has been de-emphasized in the second edition, with the relevant aspects being incorporated into Chapter 3, "Development and Delivery of Treatment Protocol," or into other appropriate chapters. Likewise, the principles of physics found in Chapter 2 of the first edition have been blended into the applicable chapter, with general principles found in Appendix B.

Chapter 4 covers thermal agents and Chapter 5 electrical modalities. Ultrasound is now covered in its own chapter, Chapter 6. Finally, Chapter 7 describes mechanical agents. As with the first edition, the modality or modality type is described in terms of its physics and its physiological effects on the injury response process and pain. Where applicable, different delivery mechanisms for the modality are discussed as well, followed by instrumentation, setup, application, precautions, indications, and contraindications.

The most noticeable change in this text, other than perhaps its cover, is its title. After much internal debate and soul-searching, I elected to change the book's original title, *Therapeutic Modalities for Athletic Trainers,* to simply *Therapeutic Modalities.* References to "the athlete" have been changed, in most cases, to read "the patient."

Although some may think that these changes were made to expand the text's market, this was not the motivation for the change. Ultimately, physics was the deciding factor. Three megahertz is 3,000,000 cycles per second, regardless of what profession is using it. The old name of this text somehow suggested that therapeutic modalities were different among the professions that use them, a perception that I feel personally responsible for helping to change. The change from "athlete" to "patient" was made to reinforce the fact that, although they may run, jump, score touchdowns, or shoot baskets, once athletes are injured, they become patients.

I encourage feedback from both instructors and students who use this text. Contact me directly using e-mail at chadstar@aol.com.

Chad Starkey

Preface to First Edition

This is an introductory text designed to fill the void between the baseline knowledge of undergraduate student athletic trainers and the information presented in existing therapeutic modality texts. Its scope and content are written in a style that will accommodate a wide range of students with varying educational backgrounds. The presentation of these modalities has a strong slant toward their application but not at the expense of theory and research. Traditional application techniques are supported or refuted based on current literature.

The aim was to write this text to the students in a manner that facilitates their comprehension of the material. The information in this text is presented in a sequential manner. Each chapter begins with the "basics" and progresses to higher levels of information. Terms that may be new to the student are defined on the same page for quick reference, and the text also includes a complete glossary. Chapters conclude with a short quiz to measure the student's learning.

The focal point of this text is Chapter 1, which presents the body's physiological and psychological response to trauma. Each subsequent chapter relates how individual modalities affect the injury response process. Chapter 2 discusses the basic physics involved in the transfer of energy.

Specific modalities are categorized by the manner in which they deliver their energy to the body. Chapter 3 presents thermal agents and the diathermies. Chapter 4 covers the principles, effects, and application of electricity. Chapter 5 deals with mechanical agents. Each modality is prefaced by an introductory section that is followed by the specific effects that the energy has on the injury response process. The unit then progresses to the modalities' instrumentation, set-up, and application and concludes with the indications, contraindications, and precautions of its use.

Chapter 6 introduces clinical decision making through the use of the problem solving approach and is supplemented through the use of case studies. The text concludes with a chapter addressing organizational and administrative concerns in the use of therapeutic modalities.

Chad Starkey

Acknowledgments

Many people contributed to the completion of the second edition of this text. A sincere "thank you" goes out to the reviewers:

Sara Brown, MS, ATC
Barton P. Buxton, EdD, ATC
David O. Draper, PhD, ATC
Susan Foreman, PT, ATC
Peter Koehneke, MS, ATC
Sheri Martin, PT, ATC
Paula Sue Randall, PT
Robert Sikes, PhD

My sincere thanks are also extended to Kim Terrell, who first read over each chapter and provided valuable input before the reviewers saw it. Jeff Ryan again contributed the material for the treatment planning section of Chapter 3 and the subsequent case study information at the end of the following chapters. Barton P. Buxton wrote the chapter on pain, provided the basis for some of the figures in Chapter 3, and provided input on the pain-control techniques described in Chapter 5. And, of course, no Acknowledgments section would be complete without thanking the staff at F. A. Davis Publishers, without whom this work would not be possible. My contractual arrangements require that I provide an extra level of thanks to Jean-François Vilain, but this time with no cheap shots thrown in.

Either by coincidence or fate, the writing of each of the editions of this text has coincided with some of the lowlights of my life. The support I received from my friends and acquaintances helped me pull through the darkness and complete the manuscript, although both took longer than I would have liked. Needless to say, at this rate I'm not looking forward to the third edition.

Lastly, Rusty (see my dedication in the Starkey and Ryan text), you will be missed. Thanks for always believing in me. I'm just about sad that others didn't feel the same.

OK, now go and try to figure out the Dedication.

Contributors

Barton P. Buxton, EdD, **ATC**
Executive Director
Tulane Institute of Sports Medicine
New Orleans, Louisiana

Jeff Ryan, PT, **ATC**
Director of Rehabilitation
Temple University
Department of Orthopedics and Sports Medicine
Adjunct Professor, Temple University
Undergraduate Athletic Training Curriculum
Philadelphia, Pennsylvania

Contents

CHAPTER 5
Electrical Agents 170

CHAPTER 1

The Injury Response Process

This chapter provides an overview of the body's physical and psychological reactions to stress and injury. It also introduces many of the terms and concepts used throughout the text. The physiological effects of the therapeutic modalities described in this book relate back to the events described in this chapter. The other primary component of the injury response, pain, is presented in Chapter 2.

Why does a text dealing with therapeutic modalities focus its initial attention on the cell? To understand the purpose and effects of therapeutic modalities, we must first gain a basic knowledge of the body's response to injury. We will see that when therapeutic modalities are applied to living tissue, we are more than simply treating an ankle or a knee. We are applying *stress* to the cells that will influence their metabolic function.

No modality can accelerate the healing of an injury. The body heals the injury at its own rate. However, by treating an injury with thermal, electrical, or mechanical energy, we attempt to provide the best environment for the healing process to take place. Thus, we do not speed the healing of an injury but rather prevent the healing process from being hindered by regulating the environment and the function of the cells. As an illustration of this concept, consider a lacerated finger. If we allow dirt and grime to enter the cut, an *infection* occurs and delays the healing process by hindering the normal physiological healing response. If we clean the area, apply an antibiotic, and cover the wound with a dressing, healing is relatively unhindered.

Stress: A force that disrupts the normal homeostasis of a system.
Infection: A disease state produced by the invasion of a contaminating organism.

STRESSES PLACED ON THE CELL

Any type of physical, chemical, or emotional force placed on the body and its cells may be regarded as stress. For example, consider the various types of stressors encountered by an athlete: the cardiovascular benefits associated with conditioning, the physical contact associated with sports such as football, the repeated pounding of the feet when running, and the emotional elation or anguish related to the outcome of an athletic contest. If stress, regardless of its nature, is applied at a sufficient magnitude, the body will undergo several physiological changes at both the cellular and *systemic* levels.

When a stress is placed on a cell, it reacts in one of three ways:

- It adapts to the stress.
- It becomes injured, but recovers.
- It dies.

Despite the negative connotations, all stresses do not have negative effects on the body. Indeed, researchers have noted that to be without stress is to be without life.[1] Both positive and negative stressors are commonplace in athletics. Contact sports, by their very nature, deliver *acute,* traumatic forces to the body. Athletes in sports such as baseball, tennis, and track are exposed to repetitive stresses whose trauma accumulates and results in an overuse injury.

Cardiovascular conditioning programs, *acclimatization,* strength training, and the actual practice of the sport are considered positive stressors. These activities prepare the participants for the forces they will be exposed to during their activity.

The General Adaptation Syndrome

The way in which humans respond to stress has been the topic of many studies since the early 1900s. One early researcher, Hans Selye, observed that hospitalized patients, no matter what their underlying *pathology,* shared a common set of symptoms. These symptoms included diffuse aches and pains in the joints, loss of muscular strength, loss of appetite, and an elevated body temperature. These striking similarities led him to conclude that the body's systems had a common mechanism for coping with stress. Selye termed this phenomenon the **general adaptation syndrome** (GAS) and outlined three stages of stress response:[1]

1. alarm stage
2. stage of resistance
3. stage of exhaustion

The **alarm stage,** best exemplified by the "flight-or-fight response," is the body's initial reaction to a change in *homeostasis.* The body's systems spring to life,

---

Systemic: Affecting the body as a whole.

Acute: Of recent onset. The period after an injury when the local inflammatory response is still active.

Acclimatization: The process of becoming physiologically adapted to an environment.

Pathology: Deviations from the normal that characterize disease or injury.

Homeostasis: State of equilibrium in the body and its systems that provides a stable internal environment.

mobilizing its resources to thwart the effects of the stressor by readying its defensive systems. Increased blood supplies are routed to those areas needing the resources by elevating the heart rate, cardiac stroke volume, and the force of *myocardial* contractions. The blood supply to nonessential areas is decreased by *vasoconstriction* of the superficial and abdominal arteries. *Cortisol* is released into the bloodstream, stimulating many "animalistic" responses. Proteins are broken down into *amino acids* in preparation for long fasting periods to provide a potential energy source in the event that injury does occur.

After the alarm stage, there is a plateau in the body's adaptation to the stress, the **resistance stage.** The body continues to adapt to the stressor by using its homeostatic resources to maintain its integrity. This is the longest phase of GAS, lasting many days, months, or years. During this stage of stress response, the individual achieves physiological resistance or, as it is commonly referred to in athletics, "physical fitness."[2]

When the body can no longer withstand the applied stresses, it reaches the **exhaustion stage.** At this point, one of the body's systems cannot tolerate the stress and therefore fails. This exhaustion may manifest itself in the form of traumatic injuries, overuse injuries, or, in the most severe case, cardiac failure. This stage may also be referred to as the point of distress, at which the stressors being placed on the body produce a negative effect.

The General Adaptation Syndrome and Its Relationship to Trauma

It should now be apparent that all people experience stresses that may be either beneficial or harmful to the body. Harmful stresses may take the form of an acute injury such as a *sprain, strain,* or fracture. In these types of injuries, the body is overwhelmed by too much force in too short a time (macrotrauma). Distresses may also result from repeated, relatively low-intensity forces, as exemplified by stress fractures or *chronic* inflammatory conditions (microtrauma). These are the types of harmful stresses that healthcare professionals spend most of their time preventing, treating, and rehabilitating.

The amount of stress applied to the body must be of a proper intensity and duration for the body to develop physiological resistance. Therefore, if the stimulus is too intense or of too great a duration, the body reacts negatively to the stress and injury occurs. In the context of athletics, little (if any) physiological resistance occurs if an athlete trains at an insufficient intensity. Conversely, if the intensity of the workout is too great, the body is placed in the stage of exhaustion and injury occurs.

Myocardial: Pertaining to the middle layer of the heart walls.
Vasoconstriction: Reduction in a blood vessel's diameter. This results in a decrease in blood flow.
Cortisol: A cortisonelike substance produced in the body.
Amino acids: Building blocks of protein.
Sprain: A stretching or tearing of ligaments.
Strain: A stretching or tearing of tendons or muscles.
Chronic: Continuing for a long period; with injury, extending past the primary hemorrhage and inflammation cycle.

BOX 1-1   **Wolff's Law**

> **Bones remodel and adapt to the forces placed on them** by increasing their strength along the lines of mechanical stress. Based on changes in the intrinsic electrical current of bones, the osteoblastic and osteoclastic activity changes in response to the presence or absence of functional stress. Bone is removed from sites of little or no stress and is formed along the sites of new stress.
>
> Most commonly, these stresses are caused by compressive forces associated with running, throwing, and so on. However, the removal of these stresses can also result in the bone's remodeling itself. If a limb is immobilized, the daily stresses placed on its bones are removed. As a result, the body adapts to the lack of stress by removing bone.

The body has certain mechanisms to balance the effects of positive and negative stressors. As stated by Wolff's law, bone adapts to the forces placed on it (Box 1-1). This remodeling may be exemplified by the deposition of *collagen* fibers and inorganic salts in response to prolonged presence of stressors. This adaptation is based on the balance between the activities of *osteoblasts* and *osteoclasts*. For example, the repeated physical stresses associated with running increase the rate of osteoblastic activity along the lines of stress. This increased osteoblastic remodeling results in new areas of structural strength and increased bone density. If this stress is applied too rapidly, osteoclastic activity outweighs osteoblastic activity, resulting in a stress fracture. In contrast, a femur immobilized for 20 days can lose up to 30 percent of its mineral deposits, which causes it to become porous and fragile.[2]

The principles presented in the GAS and Wolff's law also apply to the use of therapeutic modalities. If the magnitude of the modality is too low, little or no benefit is gained. Likewise, if the magnitude of the modality is too great—or applied at the wrong point in the healing process—further injury occurs.

TYPES OF TISSUES FOUND IN THE BODY

The body is comprised of five different types of tissues with which we will concern ourselves in this text: (1) epithelial, (2) adipose, (3) muscular, (4) nervous, and (5) connective. Each of these tissue types has unique properties that allow it to reproduce after trauma, depending on its cellular structures (Table 1-1). When an injury occurs, the scope and severity of the trauma are generally in direct proportion to the number and type of cells that have been damaged. Another important consideration when applying therapeutic modalities is the ability of each of these tissues to transmit or absorb various forms of energy.

Epithelial Tissues

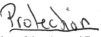

Epithelial tissues line the skin (stratified squamous epithelium), heart and blood vessels (simple squamous epithelium), hollow organs (transitional epithelium),

---

Collagen: A protein-based connective tissue.
Osteoblast: A cell concerned with the formation of new bone.
Osteoclast: A cell that absorbs and removes unwanted bone.

TABLE 1-1   **Types of Cells Found in the Body**

Type	Location	Ability to Regenerate
Labile cells	Skin, intestinal tract, blood	Good
Stabile cells	Bone	Some
Permanent cells	Peripheral nervous system	Some
	Central nervous system	None

glands, external openings, and other organs. This type of tissue is able to secrete and absorb various substances and has the distinction of being devoid of blood vessels. Fortunately, epithelial tissue has a high potential to regenerate because it is the most commonly injured type of tissue. Imagine what our bodies would look like if our skin failed to regenerate each time we suffered a cut.

The skin's outer layer is formed by the *stratum corneum,* a layer of flat, densely packed dead cells. Unlike living cells, which are filled with cytoplasm, the stratum corneum cells are filled with **keratin,** a dry, fibrous protein. This structure forms a barrier that prevents many external substances, such as germs, from entering the body and assists in keeping the body's fluids inside.

Most of the forms of energy produced by the therapeutic modalities discussed in this text must pass through the stratum corneum and the remainder of the epidermis to affect the target tissues. Thermal agents initially heat or cool this layer, and the underlying tissues lose or gain heat through *conduction.* Ultrasonic energy passes relatively easily through this layer. Because the cells of the stratum corneum are dead and dry, this tissue layer resists electrical stimulating currents and prevents them from affecting the underlying tissues. *Transdermally* applied medications must pass through the stratum corneum by finding portals surrounding hair follicles and sweat glands.

Adipose Tissue

Immediately underlying the epidermis is a layer of adipose tissue that stores fat cells and, in areas such as the heel and palm, protects the underlying structures from hard blows. The high water content of adipose tissue makes it an ideal medium for ultrasound to pass through and is selectively heated during diathermy. However, because the body's fat layering also serves as insulation against cold, the effectiveness of thermal agents is reduced when they are applied over thick layers of adipose tissue.

Stratum corneum: The outermost, nonliving portion of the epidermis.
Conduction: The transfer of heat from a high temperature to a low temperature between two objects that are touching each other.
Transdermal (Transdermally): Introduction of medication to the subcutaneous tissues through unbroken skin.

TABLE 1–2 **Types of Connective Tissue and Their Function**

Tissue Type	Function
Fibroblasts	Secrete extracellular matrix components
Chondrocytes	Produce extracellular matrix components in cartilage
Myofibroblasts	Produce extracellular matrix components with contractile properties
Adipocytes	Store *lipids*

Connective Tissue

Connective tissue (also known as "support cells") is the most abundant type of tissue in the body. It serves as a cement that supports and connects the other tissue types.[3] This tissue provides strength, support, nutrition, and defense for the other tissues. The fundamental types of connective tissue and their function are presented in Table 1–2.

Collagen is found in high density in fascia, tendons, ligaments, cartilage, muscle, and bone. Eleven types of collagen are found in the body and, with the exception of meniscal cartilage, are located in highly vascular areas (Table 1–3).

The connective tissue's elasticity is determined by the ratio of inelastic collagen fibers to elastic yellow **elastin fibers.** To illustrate the effect of collagen density and elasticity, consider the difference between muscle and tendon. Muscles are highly elastic and contain a much higher percentage of elastin fibers than collagen fibers. Tendons, in contrast to muscles, have very little elasticity because 86 percent of their dry weight is collagen.[4] Collagen is also found in other inelastic tissues such as ligaments, fascia, and cartilage.

Collagen can be elongated through stretching, especially when it is heated, and it can be selectively heated by ultrasonic energy. Collagen located in the superficial tissues can also be heated through moist heat.

TABLE 1–3 **Collagen Fiber Types**

Type	Location
I	Skin, fascia, tendons, ligaments, bone, fibrous cartilage
II	Hyaline cartilage, elastic cartilage, vertebral disks
III	Smooth muscles, nerves, bone marrow, blood vessels
IV	*Basement membranes*
V	Smooth muscle, skeletal muscle
VI	Found in most, if not all, of the body's structures
VII	Basement membranes of skin
VIII	Endothelium
IX	Cartilage
X	Mineralizing cartilage
XI	Cartilage

Lipid: A broad category of fatlike substances.

Basement membrane: Extracellular material that separates the base of epithelial cells from connective tissue.

Muscular Tissues

Muscular tissues possess the ability to actively shorten and passively lengthen and are classified by the function they serve. **Smooth muscle,** which is not under voluntary control, is associated with the hollow organs of the body. **Cardiac muscle** is responsible for the pumping of blood. **Skeletal muscle** is responsible for the movement of the body's joints. Muscular tissue possesses little or no ability to regenerate duplicates of lost cells.

Skeletal muscle fiber is classified by the intensity and duration of the contraction it can produce. **Type I** (slow-twitch) **muscle fibers** produce a low-intensity contraction, but because they use the *aerobic* energy system, the contractions can be sustained for a long time. Being slow to fatigue, these fibers are prevalent in postural muscles (e.g., the spinal erector muscles and the quadriceps femoris group). **Type II** (fast-twitch) **muscle fibers** primarily use the *anaerobic* energy system and produce a high-intensity, short-duration contraction. Capable of generating a high amount of force in a short time, these fibers are predominant in explosive muscle contractions. Type II fibers are subcategorized as type II-B, which is totally anaerobic, and type II-A, which has traits of both type I and type II fibers.

Muscular tissues are heated or cooled through conduction with the overlying tissues. The flow of warm blood and increased cell *metabolism,* such as that experienced during exercise, also increases the temperature of muscles. In some circumstances, a direct electrical current can cause muscle fibers to shorten, but stimulating *motor nerves* most commonly produces therapeutic muscle contractions.

Nervous Tissue

Nervous tissue has the ability to conduct *afferent* and *efferent* impulses (Box 1–2). Individual nerve cells, or neurons, form the basic functional unit of the nervous system. Two distinct segments form each neuron: (1) dendrites, which transmit impulses toward a cell body, and (2) the axon, which transmits impulses away from the cell body (Fig. 1–1). Nerves that transmit information toward a *synapse* are termed **presynaptic** neurons; those that transmit the impulse away from the synapse are **postsynaptic** neurons. As shown in Figure 1–1, a nerve may be both presynaptic and postsynaptic.

Aerobic: Requiring the presence of oxygen.
Anaerobic: Able to survive in the absence of oxygen. Anaerobic systems derive their energy through the breakdown of adenosine triphosphate (ATP) into adenosine diphosphate (ADP).
Metabolism: The sum of physical and chemical reactions taking place within the body.
Motor nerve: A nerve that provides impulses to muscles.
Afferent: Carrying impulses toward a central structure, for example, the brain.
Efferent: Carrying impulses away from a central structure. Nerves leaving the central nervous system are efferent nerves.
Synapse: The junction where two nerves communicate.

BOX 1–2   Propagation of Nerve Impulses

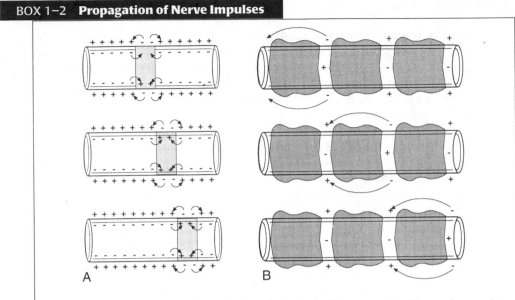

A

B

Nerve impulses are created by the depolarization of the nerve's cell membrane. At rest, the outside of the nerve membrane has a positive charge, and the inside has a negative charge. When a stimulus that exceeds the nerve's threshold is received, the nerve depolarizes and the sodium ions (Na^+) rush inside, causing a sequential reversal of the membrane's polarity. This sequence repeats throughout the length of the nerve until the impulse reaches the synapse.

All excitable cell membranes have a different electrical charge between the inside and the outside of the membrane, the **resting potential.** Transmission of impulses in unmyelinated nerves involves depolarization along the length of the axon, a slower and less efficient mechanism than the saltatory conduction mechanism associated with myelinated nerves (*A*). The axons of myelinated nerves are covered by a fatty myelin sheath that is interrupted by the nodes of Ranvier, gaps where the cell membrane is exposed. Depolarization occurs only at the nodes of Ranvier, jumping from one node to the next. Because only selected areas of the axon are depolarized, **transmission along myelinated nerves is faster, more efficient, and requires less metabolic activity than unmyelinated fibers** (*B*).

In addition to the nerve's myelin sheath, the nerve's diameter also affects the speed at which the impulse is transmitted. Wider-diameter nerves transmit impulses faster than nerves having a smaller diameter, although small-diameter myelinated nerves have a faster conduction velocity than larger unmyelinated nerves.

Each impulse is followed by a refractory period, during which the nerve repolarizes. Corresponding to the change in sodium permeability, the absolute refractory period represents the period of time during which no additional stimulus, regardless of its magnitude, will trigger another *action potential*. The absolute refractory period ensures that the nerve can completely recharge before the next action potential is initiated, and the length of this period determines the frequency at which the nerve can depolarize in a given length of time. Following the absolute refractory period, there is a brief relative refractory period during which a stronger-than-normal stimulus can initiate another action potential.

Action potential: The change in the electrical potential of a nerve or muscle fiber when stimulated.

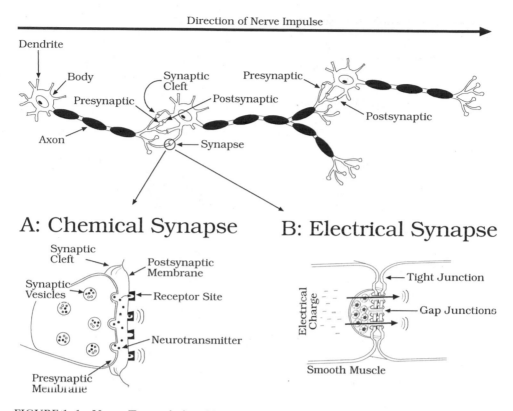

FIGURE 1–1 **Nerve Transmission.** Nerve impulses originate at the dendrite, pass through the body, and are transmitted along the axon (see Box 1–2 for a discussion of the propagation of nerve impulses). The junctions between two nerves are termed the synapses. Inset A depicts a chemical synapse in which the impulse is continued by the release of a neurotransmitter from the presynaptic nerve that crosses the synaptic cleft and binds to a postsynaptic receptor site. Inset B portrays an electrical synapse in which the depolarization of the presynaptic nerve continues directly to the postsynaptic nerve.

Synaptic junctions are classified as either electrical or chemical. **Electrical synapses** are characterized by a **gap junction** that allows the nerve impulse to be transferred directly to the next nerve in sequence. Most of the body's synapses are **chemical synapses.** Here a small gap, the **synaptic cleft,** separates the presynaptic and postsynaptic nerves. A chemical neurotransmitter is released from the presynaptic nerve, diffuses across the synaptic cleft, and binds into a receptor site on the postsynaptic neuron (Table 1–4). At an **excitatory synapse,** the neurotransmitter release tends to activate the postsynaptic nerve via an **excitatory postsynaptic potential.** Activation of an **inhibitory synapse** increases the postsynaptic nerve's resting polarity, potentially stopping the *propagation* of the impulse.

Cells damaged in the central nervous system are not replaced and their functions are lost. Nerve cells damaged in the peripheral nervous system possess some ability to regenerate. Their functions may also be restored by a collateral system in which intact nerves migrate toward the damaged tissues.

Given the proper intensity, electrical stimulation units can result in the activation of sensory, motor, and pain nerves. The electrical stimulus causes a depo-

---

Propagation: Transmission through a medium.

TABLE 1-4   **Common Neurotransmitters and Their Functions**

Neurotransmitter	Location	Functions
Acetylcholine	Motor nerves Central nervous system	Transmits motor impulses
Dopamine	Brain stem	Absence results in motor dysfunction Increases blood pressure Increases cardiac output Produces vasoconstriction
Epinephrine	Brain stem	Behavior Bronchial dilation Emotions Mood Vasoconstriction
Norepinephrine	Autonomic nervous system	Arousal (flight-or-fight response) Dreams Mood regulation Vasoconstriction
Serotonin	Platelets Mast cells	Sensory perception Sleep Temperature regulation Vasoconstriction
Substance P	Pain-transmitting nerve fibers	Transmits *noxious* impulses Produces inflammationlike responses in local tissues

larization of these nerves in an orderly, predictable manner. Thermal agents and ultrasound influence nerve function by altering their conduction velocities.

THE INJURY PROCESS

The body's reaction to injury may be divided into two distinct parts. The primary response to injury is the tissue destruction directly associated with the traumatic force. Secondary damage occurs from cell death caused by a blockage of the oxygen supply to the injured area. The damage done during the primary stage is irreversible, and the treatment efforts used after trauma attempt to contain the effects and limit the amount of secondary injury.

Dead and damaged cells release their contents into the area adjacent to the injured site. The presence of these substances causes an inflammatory reaction from the body's tissues. As a result of both the primary trauma and the inflammatory mediators, *hemorrhage* and *edema* occur. The buildup of fluids results in both mechanical pressure on and chemical irritation of the nerve receptors in the area. Because of the clogging of the vasculature, further cell death results from a lack of oxygen

---

Noxious: Harmful, injurious.
Hemorrhage: Bleeding from veins, arteries, or capillaries.
Edema: An excessive accumulation of serous fluids.

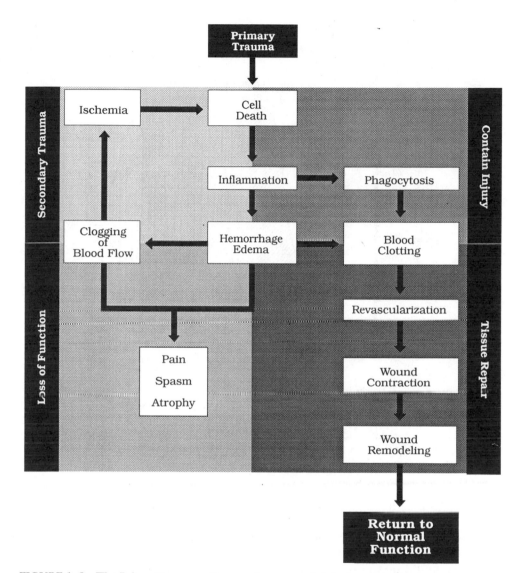

FIGURE 1–2 **The Injury Response Process.** In traumatic injuries, the primary trauma stems from an outside force and the physical damage inflicted is irreversible. Secondary injury occurs from deprivation of oxygen to the tissues. This, combined with pain, spasm, and/or atrophy, leads to the tissues or body parts losing the ability to function normally. The body begins its road to repair by first containing the injury and then rebuilding the damaged tissue.

in the surviving tissues. A subcycle occurs as a result of pain and *ischemia,* causing muscle spasm and increasing the possibility of atrophy over time (Fig. 1–2).

This sequence of events, commonly referred to as the injury response cycle, the pain-spasm pain cycle, or the vicious cycle, leads to a self-perpetuating sequence of events. For the injury to resolve in the least time, this cycle must be controlled so that healing may occur.

Ischemia: Local and temporary deficiency of blood supply caused by obstruction of circulation to a part.

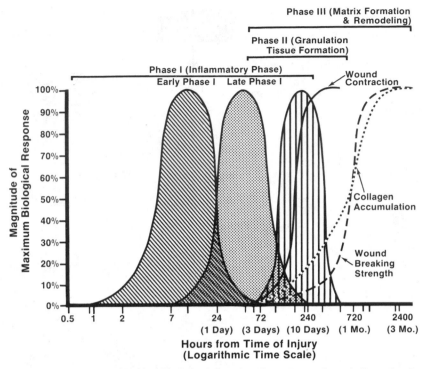

FIGURE 1–3   **Overlapping Stages of Wound Repair.** There is no clear delineation between the end of one stage of healing and the beginning of the next stage; it is possible for portions of all three stages to overlap. Phase I is the acute inflammatory response stage, phase II is the revascularization stage, and phase III is the remodeling stage. (From McCulloch, JM, et al (eds): Wound Healing: Alternatives in Management, ed 2. FA Davis, Philadelphia, 1995, p 33, with permission.)

The course of healing is described in three phases: (1) the acute inflammatory response, (2) the proliferation phase, and (3) the remodeling (maturation) phase. Although the central events of each of these phases are marked by distinct responses within a theoretical time frame, an overlap of these stages can, and does, occur (Fig. 1–3). The acute **inflammatory** response involves the delivery of phagocytes, specifically fibroblasts, to the area and the formation of *granulation tissue* in an attempt to isolate and localize the trauma. During this time, *histamine* released from the traumatized cells increases capillary permeability, resulting in swelling as the proteins follow water out into the tissues. During the **proliferation** phase, the number and size of fibroblasts increase, causing *ground substance* and collagen to collect in the traumatized area in preparation

***

Granulation tissue: Delicate tissue composed of fibroblasts, collagen, and capillaries formed during the revascularization phase of wound healing.

Histamine: A blood-thinning chemical released from damaged tissue during the inflammatory process.

Ground substance: Material occupying the intercellular spaces in fibrous connective tissue, cartilage, or bone (also known as matrix).

to rebuild the damaged tissues. The injury process is completed during the **maturation** phase, when collagen and fibroblasts align themselves and attempt to adapt to the original tissue orientation and function, although this does not always occur.[5]

Acute Inflammatory Response

The natural physiological reaction to any form of injury is the acute inflammatory response or **inflammation,** the process that mobilizes the body's defensive systems. Although inflammation is not a pathological condition, it represents the sum of the body's tissue reactions to cell injury or cell death and may be triggered by factors such as chemical irritation, heat, mechanical trauma, or bacterial invasion.[6] The purpose of inflammation is to control the effects of the injurious agent and to return the tissue to its normal state. This process destroys, dilutes, or contains the injurious agents in an attempt to protect the area from further insult. This response occurs at two levels: (1) changes in local blood flow (hemodynamic) and (2) changes in cellular functioning. The effects of inflammation are needed in the healing process. However, if the duration or intensity of the inflammation is excessive, the process becomes detrimental and chronic inflammation itself becomes a debilitating event.

Inflammation has a poor reputation as an unwanted and unneeded part of the body's response to injury. Nothing could be further from the truth. Inflammation is essential to the healing process. Only when inflammation runs amuck is it detrimental to healing. Through the application of therapeutic modalities, we can influence the duration and magnitude of the inflammatory response and deter its unwanted effects.

The inflammatory process may be divided into three distinct phases: (1) acute inflammation associated with the body's initial reaction to injury, (2) the subacute phase when symptoms begin to decrease (2 weeks to 1 month from onset), and (3) chronic inflammation, when the reaction persists for longer than 1 month (Table 1–5).[7]

When the body first receives a stress (in this context, "stress" refers to a traumatic injury) of sufficient magnitude, the cells undergo a primary reaction. This primary phase, also known as the reactive or inflammatory phase, is characteristic of the first 3 or 4 days after the injury.

One of the body's initial responses to trauma is the release of norepinephrine in the traumatized area, causing vasoconstriction of local vessels to prevent blood loss in the affected area.[8] While the vessels are in the state of vasoconstriction, the

TABLE 1–5 Stages of Inflammation after Injury

Stage	Process	Elapsed Time since Injury (Days)
Acute	Reaction to the injury	0–14
Subacute	Symptoms diminish	14–31
Chronic	Unwarranted inflammation	>31

coagulation process begins to repair the primary damage. This initial vasoconstriction is transitory, and in as little as 10 minutes after the injury, the vessels begin to dilate, increasing the volume of blood being delivered to the area.

Gaps form between the *endothelial cells* in the capillary beds, increasing their permeability to fluids and proteins. As the volume of blood being delivered to the area increases, a protein-rich *exudate* is formed in the tissues. The prostaglandin PGE_1 increases vascular permeability, and prostaglandin PGE_2 attracts *leukocytes* to the area.[9] The fluids and proteins leak into the tissue through the newly formed gaps in the capillaries, depositing leukocytes along the site of the injury to localize and remove any harmful substances.

Swelling occurs as a result of the presence of fluids, proteins, and cell debris in the area. As the amount of swelling increases, vascular flow to and from the area is decreased. The venous and lymphatic networks are blocked, causing further clogging of blood flow to the area and perpetuating the process.

Prolonged inflammation damages the connective tissue and thickens the synovial membrane. When unchecked, this condition may lead to the development of adhesions within a joint, affecting its functional range of motion. The release of cortisol, as described in the GAS, is effective in reducing the effects of chronic inflammation because of its cortisonelike anti-inflammatory effects.[10]

Cardinal Signs of Inflammation

Five cardinal signs mark the inflammation process (Table 1–6). Heat and redness (**hyperemia**) are present secondary to the increased blood flow in the area and the increase in the rate of cell metabolism. **Swelling** occurs as a result of the various inflammatory agents in the area and is further promoted by the high concentration of proteins, *gamma globulins,* and *fibrinogen.* **Pain** is caused by the release of chemical irritants—bradykinin, histamine, prostaglandin, and other substances—in the inflamed area and increased tissue pressure. The long-term result of inflammation is the **loss of normal function.**

The magnitude of the patient's inflammation can be clinically quantified based on the amount of swelling, point tenderness, and loss of joint motion.[11] The amount of swelling and loss of range of motion can be measured relative to the uninvolved extremity. Tenderness can be loosely quantified by slight or severe discomfort during palpation, the inability to palpate because of pain, and pain caused by mild stimulation (e.g., blowing on the skin, clothing touching the area). Various blood tests can also accurately determine the biophysical stage of inflammation.

Coagulation: The process of blood clotting.
Endothelial cells: Flat cells lining the blood and lymphatic vessels and the heart.
Exudate: Fluid that collects in a cavity and has a high concentration of cells, protein, and other solid matter.
Leukocytes: White blood cells that serve as scavengers.
Gamma globulin: An infection-fighting blood protein.
Fibrinogen: A protein present in the blood plasma and essential for the clotting of blood.

TABLE 1–6 Cardinal Signs of Inflammation

Sign	Associated Inflammatory Events
Heat	Increased blood flow, increased metabolic rate
Redness	Increased blood flow, increased metabolic rate, histamine release
Swelling	Leakage of inflammatory mediators into the surrounding tissues, hemorrhage, blockage of the venous return mechanism
Pain	Mechanical pressure on and/or chemical irritation of nerves
Loss of function	Primary tissue damage, the sum of preceding signs, *muscle guarding*

Mediators of Inflammation

Chemicals released into the area control the inflammatory process. Collectively known as **mediators,** these chemicals are responsible for a wide range of cellular and vascular events (Table 1–7). Some of these chemicals are directly released by the damaged cells; others are attracted to the area by *chemotaxis.* Some mediators cause *vasodilation* of the vessels, increasing both the amount of blood, plasma proteins, and phagocytic leukocytes and the speed with which these products are delivered to the area. Other mediators increase the permeability of the vessels, allowing the movement of blood proteins and blood cells out of the vessels into the surrounding tissues.

The presence of proteins changes the osmotic relationship between the blood and the adjacent tissues. During the inflammatory response, the protein content of the plasma decreases while the protein content of the *interstitial* fluid increases.[12] Water tends to follow the blood proteins out of the vessel via osmosis, resulting in edema. Edema, in turn, increases the tissue pressure, irritating the nerve receptors and blocking capillary flow.

Hemorrhage

For hemorrhage to take place, one of two prerequisites must be met: the vessel must (1) lose its continuity (be ruptured) or (2) have a marked increase in permeability so that cells and fluids can escape, or a gradient must be present in which the pressure inside the vessel is greater than the external pressure.[13] For hemorrhage to cease, the reverse of the two conditions must be met: the vessel must be repaired and/or the pressure gradient must be equalized.

Muscle guarding: A voluntary or subconscious contraction of a muscle to protect an injured area.

Chemotaxis: Movement of living protoplasm toward or away from a chemical stimulus.

Vasodilation: Increase in a blood vessel's diameter. This results in an increase in blood flow.

Interstitial: Between the tissues.

TABLE 1-7 Selected Inflammatory Mediators

Heparin: Inhibits coagulation by preventing the conversion of prothrombin into thrombin.
Histamine: Located in mast cells, basophils, and platelets. Its primary function is vasodilation of *arterioles* and increased vascular permeability in venules.
Kinins: A group of polypeptides that dilate arterioles, serve as strong chemotactics, and produce pain. They are primarily involved in the inflammatory process in the early stages of vascular response.
Prostaglandins: Comprised of many different types and are responsible for vasodilation and increased vascular permeability. These are synthesized locally in the injured tissues and influence the duration and intensity of the inflammatory process
Serotonin: Causes local vasodilation and increased permeability of the capillaries.
Leukotrienes: Fatty acids that cause smooth muscle contraction, increase vascular permeability, and attract neutrophils.

Subcutaneous hemorrhage is easily recognized by the *ecchymosis* of the skin associated with bruising. When the hemorrhage occurs deeper in the tissues, a *hematoma* may result. In the short term, hematomas assist the healing process by equalizing the pressure gradient between the inside and the outside of the injured vessels, thus limiting the amount of blood loss. However, the long-term presence of a hematoma in a muscle can result in a restriction and will hinder the repair process by perpetuating the inflammatory response.

Even in the best possible scenario, the treatment provided immediately after an injury does not affect primary hemorrhaging. By the time the injured athlete is removed from competition; the shoe, sock, and pads are removed; the initial evaluation is performed; and ice is applied, several minutes have passed. In most instances, this time is sufficient for the coagulation process to seal the injured vasculature.[8] Application of cold treatments in this time frame helps to limit the amount of secondary hypoxic injury and to decrease pain, and the application of an external wrap helps to equalize the pressures inside and outside the vessel.

Edema

Edema is the buildup of excessive fluid in the interstitial space as a result of the imbalance between the pressures inside and outside the cell membrane, or of an obstruction to *lymphatic return* and venous return. This collection of fluids causes the tissues to expand. The amount of edema that accumulates in the injured area is proportional to:

Arteriole: A small artery leading to a capillary at its distal end.
Subcutaneous: Beneath the skin.
Ecchymosis: A blue-black discoloration of the skin caused by movement of blood into the tissues. In the latter stages, the color may appear greenish brown or yellow.
Hematoma: A mass of blood confined to a limited area, resulting from the subcutaneous leakage of blood.
Lymphatic return: A return process similar to that of the venous network, but specializing in the removal of interstitial fluids.

- The severity of the injury (the number and type of cells damaged)
- Changes in vascular permeability
- The amount of primary and secondary hemorrhaging
- The presence of chemical inflammatory mediators

Although interrelated, these factors function independently to cause the release of proteins that attract fluids to the injured area.[12]

The movement of fluids across the capillary membrane is contingent on three basic forces[14]: (1) the **vascular hydrostatic pressure** that forces the contents from the capillary outward to the tissues, (2) the **plasma colloid osmotic pressure** that moves fluids from the tissues into the capillaries, and (3) **limb hydrostatic pressure.** The limb's hydrostatic pressure is independently altered by changes in the position of the limb.

The formation and removal of edema are based on the relationship among these pressures. Normally, the vascular hydrostatic pressure and the plasma colloid pressure are approximately even, keeping the inflow and outflow equal (a small percentage of normal venous return occurs through the lymphatic system). Capillary permeability increases after injury, making it easier for fluids and solid matter to leave the vessels (Fig. 1–4). If the vascular hydrostatic pressure exceeds the plasma colloid osmotic pressure, excessive fluids are forced out of the capillaries into the tissues, and edema results. Likewise, if the plasma colloid osmotic pressure exceeds the vascular hydrostatic pressure, fluids are forced back into the vessels and may then be removed from the area.

The limb's hydrostatic pressure is dependent on the position of the body part. When your arm is hanging at your side, the limb's hydrostatic pressure is increased because gravity is pulling the blood in your vessels downward. The pressure exerted tends to force fluids back out into the interstitial space. When your arm is lifted above your head, the limb hydrostatic pressure decreases. The limb hydrostatic pressure is used to help control and reduce swelling in the extremities. This mechanism is discussed in the following sections.

Lymphatic flow is disrupted by edema when the tissues become so expanded that the flap valves between the endothelial cells in the capillaries become separated. This parting of the valves renders them ineffective, thus allowing the fluids to "slosh" back into the injured area. The expansion of tissues causes further hypoxic injury by clogging the vascular pathways. When the limb is placed in a gravity-*dependent position,* interstitial pressure increases to the point where the lymphatic vessels collapse, further obstructing flow in the area.[15] These events not only prevent the delivery of fresh blood and oxygen to the injured structures but also inhibit venous and lymphatic return from the site, causing perpetuation of the cycle. In addition, the pressure caused by the fluid buildup produces mechanical pain by stimulating mechanical nerve receptors in the area and causes chemically induced pain by depriving the tissues of oxygen.

Edema is not only a sign that an injury has occurred but also a contributing factor in the injury cycle. The edema clogs the vascular and cellular spaces, increasing tissue pressure and preventing oxygen from reaching the tissues and causing further cell death, pain, and decreased motion.[16] The healing process itself is slowed by de-

---

Dependent position: An arrangement in which the body part is placed lower than the heart, increasing the intravascular pressure.

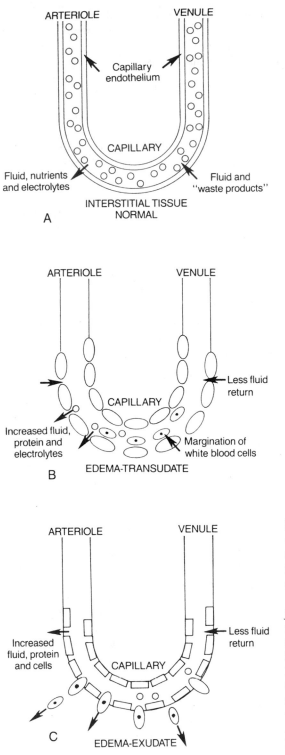

FIGURE 1–4 **The Formation of Edema.**
(*A*) The normal pressure inside and outside the vessel causes an outward flow of fluids and nutrients at the arteriole end and absorption of wastes at the venule end. (*B*) **The Transudate Stage.** Following an injury, inflammatory mediators cause the arterioles to dilate. The increased capillary filtration pressure moves proteins and fluids into the tissues. (*C*) **The Exudate Stage.** Increased inflammation forces neutrophils and other blood cells out to the tissues, resulting in a thick, edematous fluid formation. (From Michlovitz, SL [ed]: Thermal Agents in Rehabilitation, ed 2. FA Davis, Philadelphia, 1990, p 7, with permission.)

layed cellular regeneration and improper collagen formation.[17] Collagen deposition is increased in the edematous area and, when uncontrolled, leads to *fibrosis* and joint *contractures*. These factors lead to a decrease in joint range of motion, loss of normal function, and eventually, atrophy and fibrosis in the afflicted body part.[16]

A primary goal during the early treatment and rehabilitation phase is to reduce the amount of edema that is formed and remove it from the injury site. Removal of edema can occur through increased venous return, increased lymphatic flow, or increased blood circulation. The only mechanism for removing protein from the interstitial space is through the lymphatic system.[18]

Venous and/or Lymphatic Return

Swelling and edema are reduced only by transporting the fluid and solid wastes away from the area through the venous and lymphatic system, with the contents of the lymphatic system eventually returning to the venous network via the *thoracic duct*. Because the mechanisms of these systems are similar, the function of the venous return system is used to describe the process of returning the contents of the lymphatic system from the extremities to the thorax.

In contrast to its influence on arterial blood flow, blood pressure has little effect on returning venous blood to the heart, exerting a pressure of approximately 15 mm Hg on the venous system.[13] Once the blood passes through the capillaries, the body must rely on other mechanisms to return blood to the heart. During **skeletal muscle contraction,** the veins are compressed, reducing their diameter. Because of the function of one-way valves, the blood is forced to move out of the extremity toward the heart. As the force of the contraction is reduced, the one-way valves close, preventing the blood from moving back to its original position (Fig. 1–5). During walking, for instance, contraction of the calf muscles increases the local venous pressure to as high as 200 mm Hg.[19] Although voluntary muscle contractions provide the most efficient method of increasing venous return, gravity, electrically induced contractions, passive motion, mechanical pressure, and massage can also increase venous flow.[20]

The **respiratory process** serves to enhance venous return during both inspiration and expiration. When we take a breath of air, the diaphragm descends and places pressure on the abdominal organs. This pressure is then placed on the veins, partially compressing them and forcing the blood toward the heart. During expiration, a negative pressure gradient is created between the thorax and the abdomen, causing a siphonlike effect that pulls the blood up the venous system, much like sucking on a straw.

Last, **gravity** serves to return the blood to the heart. The fluids within the venous return system are affected by gravity. Placing the extremity in a dependent position increases the limb's hydrostatic pressure within the peripheral blood vessels and forces fluids into the tissues. When an extremity is placed in a nondependent position (elevated), the venous return system becomes a passive process in

---

Fibrosis: An abnormally large formation of inelastic fibrous tissue.
Contracture: A condition resulting from the loss of a tissue's ability to lengthen.
Thoracic duct: A central collection point for the lymphatic system. The contents of the thoracic duct are routed into the left subclavian vein, where it returns to the blood system.

(A) (B) (C)

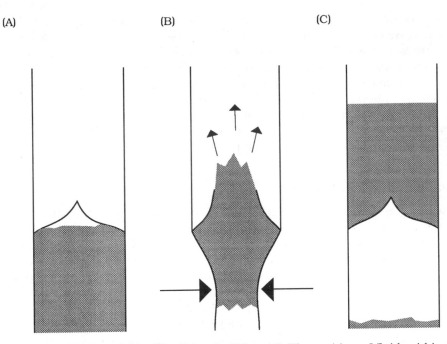

FIGURE 1–5 **Function of One-Way Valves in Veins.** (*A*) The position of fluids within the vein when the muscle is relaxed. (*B*) As the muscle contracts, pressure causes the distal portion of the vein to collapse, opening the one-way valves and forcing blood toward the heart. (*C*) As the muscle relaxes, the valves close, preventing blood from moving back into the area.

which there is a natural downward flow of the fluids in the vessels. The effectiveness of gravity in returning blood to the heart is based on the angle of the extremity relative to the ground, the diameter of the veins, and the *viscosity* of the blood.

The maximal effect of gravity on venous return occurs when the limb is perpendicular (90°) to the heart and least effective when the limb is horizontal. The effect that the limb's position has on gravity influencing venous return can be calculated using trigonometric sine function (Fig. 1–6).

The resistance to blood flow is inversely proportional to the diameter of the vessel. As the cross-sectional size of the vessel decreases, the resistance to flow increases to the fourth power of the radius (radius × radius × radius × radius)[13] (Fig. 1–7). Consequently, small changes in the vessel's diameter result in great changes in its resistance to flow. *Venules* have a smaller diameter than veins; therefore, greater resistance to flow occurs closer to the capillary-venule interface, but the rate of blood flow to the tissues cannot exceed the rate of exchange at this interface.

Viscosity is a fluid's resistance to flow. Normally the viscosity of blood remains constant. However, after injury, the viscosity of blood increases because of the loss of plasma into the surrounding tissues, and the ratio of liquids to solids decreases.

Viscosity: The resistance of a fluid to flow.
Venule: A small vein exiting from a capillary.

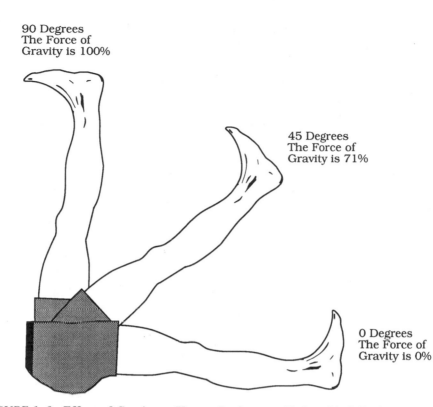

90 Degrees
The Force of
Gravity is 100%

45 Degrees
The Force of
Gravity is 71%

0 Degrees
The Force of
Gravity is 0%

FIGURE 1–6 **Effect of Gravity on Venous Drainage at Various Limb Positions.** Gravity is most effective when the limb is at 90° and least effective when the limb is parallel to the ground. A compromise between comfort and function is found when the limb is elevated at a 45° angle.

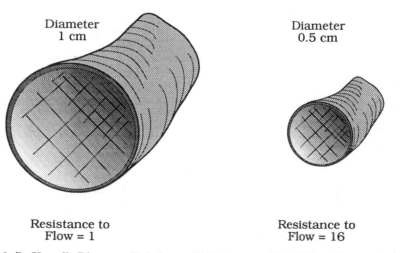

Diameter
1 cm

Diameter
0.5 cm

Resistance to
Flow = 1

Resistance to
Flow = 16

FIGURE 1–7 **Vessel's Diameter Relative to Resistance to Blood Flow.** Decreasing the diameter of a vessel by one-half increases the resistance to blood flow 16 times.

Although this change in viscosity is not large enough to affect the systemic flow of blood, it may be sufficient to clog the area adjacent to the injury.

Hypoxia

In the primary stage of injury, cell death is the result of physical trauma. After this stage, further cell death is a result of ischemia, a decreased oxygen supply to the area, which essentially suffocates the cells. Once an injury occurs, several vascular changes take place that block the supply of fresh blood and result in ischemia. Capillaries in the adjacent areas rupture as a result of swelling in the interstitial space, perpetuating the cycle by obstructing the oxygen supply and killing additional cells. Subsequent cell death continues to block more vascular structures, preventing even more blood and oxygen from being delivered to the site.

This phenomenon, known as **secondary hypoxic injury,** may be limited by decreasing the amount of blockage and decreasing the need for oxygen in the area. The blockage of the vasculature may be reduced by limiting the amount of fluids that collect in the area via the use of compression and elevation. The need for oxygen may be reduced by decreasing the rate of cellular metabolism through the use of cold application (see Chap. 4, pp. 110–121).

Muscle Spasm

Muscle spasm, the involuntary shortening of muscle fibers, is regarded as the body's intrinsic mechanism for splinting and protecting the injured area and can result from direct trauma or a decreased oxygen supply.[21] Muscle spasm causes pain by stimulating mechanical and chemical pain receptors. The tension produced by the shortened fibers stimulates mechanical pain fibers. The effects of a decreased oxygen supply irritate chemical pain fibers. If the muscle spasm persists, irritation of the associated ligaments and tendons occurs.[22] As a result, the amount of muscle spasm increases in an attempt to protect the structures. This becomes a self-perpetuating cycle that is continued by pain, decreased oxygen supply, and a decreased amount of positive stress (in the form of movement).

Atrophy

When a muscle is immobilized or has lost its nerve supply, its fibers become progressively smaller and its *actin* and *myosin* contents are decreased. Disuse atrophy results when a body part is immobilized by an external splint or when the individual consciously or unconsciously refuses to use the extremity because of pain. Denervation atrophy occurs when there is no intact nerve supply to the muscle group. In either case, the resultant changes are similar.

Actin: A contractile muscle protein.
Myosin: Noncontractile muscle protein.

BOX 1–3   **Misguided Intentions**

Golgi tendon organs (GTOs) function closely with **muscle spindles** in monitoring the amount of tension placed on a muscle and its tendon. Located within the muscle belly, projections from the spindle twine around individual muscle fibers. When the muscle contracts, the spindles monitor the rate and magnitude of tension produced.

Golgi tendon organs divide into many branches, with the highest density being located at the muscle-tendon junction. When the muscle contracts, it places varying amounts of force on the tendon. The GTOs monitor the amount of strain placed on the tendon to prevent damage resulting from too much tension. If the rate of stimulation of GTOs or muscle spindles becomes too great, a nerve impulse is generated that inhibits the muscle contraction.

During the process of injury response these nerves can be mechanically stimulated by pressure resulting from muscle spasm and/or edema, or they can be chemically stimulated by inflammatory mediators. **Regardless of the nature of the stimulation, an inhibitory influence is placed on the muscle. If this process is allowed to perpetuate, atrophy of the muscle group occurs.**

Muscle fibers begin to show physiological changes in as little as 24 hours after immobilization. The size and function of the cells decrease in response to a lack of physical stress and afferent information sent from the injured area.[23] Accordingly, synthesis of protein, energy production, and contractility of the tissues begin to dwindle to the point of **degeneration,** at which the muscle's ability to generate force decreases. The postural muscles, composed of slow-twitch (type I) fibers, are the first to show clinical and laboratory signs of atrophy.[24]

The injury response process accelerates the rate of atrophy. Edema and inflammation stimulate *Golgi tendon organs,* increasing the rate of atrophy (Box 1–3). As a muscle atrophies, the blood supply to the remaining fibers decreases, and the innervation of the muscle is hindered.[25] The continuing process of atrophy leads to reflex inhibition, in which the effusion and painful impulses create an inhibitory loop that essentially causes the person to "forget" how to contract the muscle.

Rest is a double-edged sword in the treatment and rehabilitation of athletic and orthopedic injuries. Immobilization is necessary to protect the injured structures, but the lack of physical stress can inhibit proper remodeling of the tissues.[26] If you have ever seen an arm or leg that has been immobilized for a long time, you know that the adverse effects of immobilization are readily apparent.

The atrophy process may be deterred by several methods. Muscles immobilized in a lengthened position are more resistant to atrophy than those immobilized in a shortened position.[27] However, depending on the body part, the structures involved, and the type of injury, it is not always practical to immobilize the muscle in a lengthened position. Isometric exercise and/or electrical muscle stimulation have also been shown to be effective in delaying the atrophy process (see Chap. 5, p. 206).

Golgi tendon organ: A sensory nerve ending found in tendons and aponeuroses.

Blood Clotting

The body's return to normal function begins with the inflammatory process. This process encourages the removal of debris and toxic substances from the injured area and protects the tissues from further damage. *Phagocytosis,* the body's cellular defense system, involves ingestion of toxic organisms and other foreign particles and their removal via the lymphatic system. These wastes, known as exudate, are commonly visible in the form of pus. During this process, scavenger cells, *monocytes, macrophages,* and leukocytes debride the area, devouring toxic and dead tissues by trapping them with armlike appendages and engulfing them (Fig. 1–8). This entrapment occurs by random chance, and the use of pain-free range-of-motion exercises may increase the level of phagocytic activity.

The repair of the vascular bodies in the injured area consists of the formation of a *platelet* plug and the transformation of fibrinogen into *fibrin.* This is a complex process and is presented in this text only in its basic form.

When disruption occurs in a vessel, an initial seal is formed by platelets. **Margination** occurs where the platelets and neutrophilic leukocytes flowing in the bloodstream begin to tumble along the walls of the vessel. Eventually, these substances adhere to collagen exposed by the trauma through the process of **pavementing.** Because platelets cannot adhere to each other, they must release adenosine diphosphate, which "glues" one layer of platelets to the other.[7] This series of platelet depositions forms an unsteady and leaky patch over the injured site. Further events must occur to form a permanent repair.

The ruptured vessel releases an enzyme that acts as a distress signal to the body, alerting it that an injury has occurred. A subsequent set of reactions, combined with the platelet deposition, results in formation of a permanent seal. *Prothrombin,* a free-floating element found in the bloodstream, reacts with the enzyme factor X, converting prothrombin into *thrombin.* The presence of thrombin in the area then stimulates fibrinogen to unwind into its individual fibrin elements (Fig. 1–9).

Single, activated fibrin filaments, fibrin monomers, are split from fibrinogen and group together with fibronectin and collagen to form a "fibrin lattice" around the injured area. During this process, the fibrin threads trap red and white blood cells, along with platelets. As these threads contract, they remove the plasma and compress the platelets, forming a "patch" to repair the damaged vessel.

Inflammation serves as both an aid and a deterrent to the coagulation process. In general, the inflammatory process encourages the delivery of prothrombin to the injured area by increasing blood flow. However, one of the chemical

---

Phagocytosis: The ingestion and digestion of bacteria and particles by phagocytes.
Monocyte: A white blood cell that matures to become a macrophage.
Macrophage: A cell having the ability to devour particles; a phagocyte.
Platelet: A free-flowing cell fragment in the bloodstream.
Fibrin: A filamentous protein formed by the action of thrombin on fibrinogen.
Prothrombin: A chemical found in the blood that reacts with an enzyme to produce thrombin.
Thrombin: An enzyme formed in the blood of a damaged area.

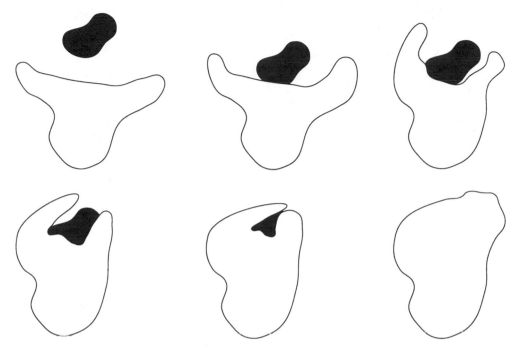

FIGURE 1–8 **The Process of Phagocytosis.** Scavenger cells randomly collide with vascular debris. Using armlike appendages, the phagocytes surround, devour, and subsequently remove the waste.

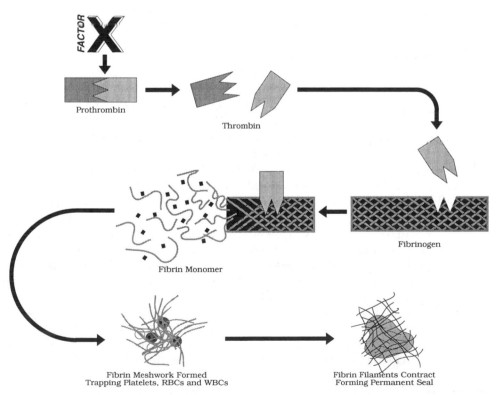

FIGURE 1–9 **The Process of Blood Clotting.** Activated by the presence of factor X, prothrombin is broken down into thrombin. In turn, the presence of thrombin causes fibrinogen to unwind into individual fibrin elements. The fibrin monomer deposits itself over the site in the damaged vessel, trapping platelets, red blood cells, and white blood cells. After contraction of the fibrin filaments, a permanent seal is formed.

TABLE 1–8   **Phases of Wound Healing**

Phase	Events
Inflammatory phase	Platelet accumulation, coagulation, leukocyte migration
Proliferation phase	Growth of new tissue (re-epithelization), development of new blood vessels (angiogenesis), development of fibrous tissue (fibroplasia), wound contraction, formation of collagen matrix
Maturation phase	Resolution of matrix, deposition of permanent tissues, return to function

Source: Adapted from Kirsner, RS, and Eaglstein, WH: The wound healing process. Dermatol Clin 11:629, 1993.

mediators, *heparin,* hinders the coagulation process by preventing prothrombin from being converted to thrombin. A proper balance must be maintained between heparin and the other mediators. Too much heparin could completely inhibit blood coagulation; too little heparin could result in unwanted blood clots.

Proliferation Phase

The proliferation phase is marked by removal of the debris and temporary repair tissue formed during the inflammation stage and by the development of new, permanent replacement tissues (Table 1–8). The exact length of transition from acute inflammatory response to proliferation is unclear, but it is thought to begin approximately 72 hours after the onset of trauma and may last 3 weeks.[28]

Repair of an injured structure involves the interaction between two types of cells: (1) the cells belonging to the injured structure and (2) connective tissue. Inflammation is needed for tissue repair. However, too much inflammation is detrimental to the process. Athletic trainers, physical therapists, physicians, and other healthcare professionals attempt to regulate the inflammatory process through the application of therapeutic modalities, the use of immobilization devices, exercise, the administration of anti-inflammatory medication, and so on. In acute trauma, inflammation is considered an active process in which the rate is controlled by the body's metabolism. In chronic situations, inflammation is a passive process in which the body forms new, and possibly unwanted, connective tissues.

Regeneration of tissues occurs when the new cells are of the same type and can perform the same function as the original structure. **Replacement** of tissues results when a different type of cell replaces the damaged cells. When uncontrolled, this process leads to scar tissue and eventual decrease or loss of function.

The quality of the repair process is related to the number and type of cells that have been damaged. Labile cells (see Table 1–1), such as those found in the skin, have the greatest ability to produce a "clone" of the original tissues. In the case of skeletal muscles, the process involves the deposition of fibrous scar tissue

---

Heparin: An inflammatory mediator produced by the mast cells of the liver. It inhibits the clotting process by preventing the transformation of prothrombin into thrombin.

that does not replicate the original structure. Evidence suggests that microregeneration can occur following minor skeletal muscle strains and microscopic meniscal tears.[28]

Adenosine triphosphate (ATP) is a critical factor that regulates the rate and quality of healing. Serving as the cell's primary source of energy, ATP is required to provide the metabolism needed to restore the cell's membrane properties by moving sodium and potassium into and out of the cell, to build new proteins, and to synthesize proteins.

Soft-tissue repair occurs through the proliferation of granulation tissue, requiring four separate but related processes[4]: (1) fibroblast formation, (2) synthesis of collagen, (3) tissue remodeling, and (4) tissue alignment. The growth of granulation tissue requires the presence of fibroblasts, *myofibroblasts,* and endothelial cells and is regulated by *growth factors* produced by platelets and macrophages.

Revascularization

The process of repair begins at the periphery, where macrophages and *polymorphs,* both of which can withstand the low-oxygen environment, produce new capillary beds, and form granulation tissue. This process gradually works its way toward the center of the injured area, forming a scaffold around which new tissue will be formed. Dermal wound repair involves the presence of mast cells. These cells release agents that stimulate fibroblasts and are involved in the remodeling of the extracellular matrix.[29]

Fibroblasts are attracted to the area indirectly by the presence of macrophages. Once in the area, fibroblasts begin laying down collagen to form a seal over the injured structure and creating the wound's *extracellular* matrix.[30] This deposition of collagen is random, with little order in the fibrous arrangement (Fig. 1–10). Stresses, in the form of gentle joint movements, may cause these fibers to arrange themselves rapidly in a more orderly fashion.[31]

Wound Contraction

Wound contraction occurs following the revascularization of the injured area and is marked by a decrease in size of the original fibrin clot. Myofibroblasts accumulate at the margins of the wound and begin to move toward the center. Possessing a high actin filament content, each new myofibroblast shortens to pull the ends of the damaged tissues closer together (Fig. 1–11).[29] Fibroblasts produce weak type III collagen, making the area vulnerable to tensile forces. Water is drawn to the area of repair, and blood vessels, proprioceptive nerves, and sensory nerves begin to develop. In superficial wounds, these events form the characteristic "scar."

As the scar tissue matures, its continuity begins to resemble that of the tissue it is replacing. With time, the strength of the scar is increased by the replacement of the old collagen with a newer, stronger type. Wound contraction should not be confused with a contracture, which results in the limitation of a joint's range of

---

Myofibroblasts: Fibroblasts that have contractile properties.
Growth factors: Substances that stimulate the production of specific types of cells.
Polymorph: A type of white blood cell; a granulocyte.
Extracellular: Outside the cell membrane.

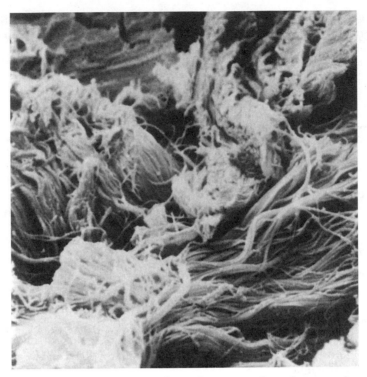

FIGURE 1–10   **Collagen Replacement.** Shown by means of an electron microscope, new, unorganized collagen can be seen interlacing with older, more densely packed collagen. (From Hunt, TK and Dunphy, JE [eds]: Fundamentals of Wound Management. Appleton-Century-Crofts, New York, 1979, p 38, with permission.)

motion and strength. With proper remodeling of the collagen, contractures may be avoided.

Wound Remodeling

The purpose of the remodeling stage is to develop order in the previously deposited scar tissue. The presence of external stress causes the alignment of the fibers to remodel the wound. Approximately 5 to 11 days following the injury, type III collagen begins to be replaced by stronger type I collagen, resulting in improved *tensile strength*.[32,33]

The use of early range-of-motion exercises has been shown to increase the tensile strength of healing ligaments.[34] Initially, the collagen is laid down in a random matrix, causing the scar to be fragile. During remodeling, the fibers form a more organized matrix, thus increasing their strength. However, scar tissue is never as functional as the tissue it replaces.[3] Consider a tear of one of the hamstring muscles. After a small tear, there is usually no residual deficit in strength or range of motion. After a massive tear in which a large amount of scar tissue is needed for repair, the muscle tends to produce less strength and have a decreased range of motion.

Tensile strength: The ability of a structure to withstand a pulling force along its length; resistance to tear.

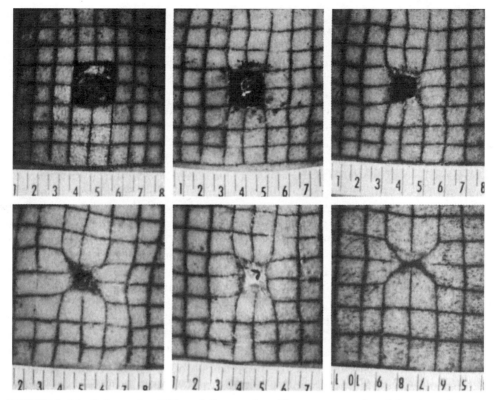

FIGURE 1–11 **Schematic of Wound Contraction.** The outer margin of the wound moves toward the center, drawing the ends together. (From Fitzpatrick, TB: Dermatology in General Medicine. McGraw-Hill, New York, 1987, p 330, with permission.)

Because scar tissue is inelastic, it is more similar in structure and function to ligaments and tendons than it is to muscle. Repair of muscular tissue may be enhanced through a mechanism similar to that which occurs when muscle hypertrophies in response to strength training. Muscle fiber contains **satellite cells** that remain dormant in certain muscular tissues. These cells lack the cytoplasm and proteins found in other muscle cells. After an injury, repair of muscular tissue can occur by recruiting satellite cells as the source of nuclei for new muscle cells.[35]

Maturation Phase

The maturation phase marks the conclusion of the proliferation phase of injury response and is characterized by "cleaning up" the area and increased strength of the repaired or replaced tissues. This is the final phase of the injury response process and may last a year or more.

At the conclusion of the wound contraction, the number of fibroblasts, myofibroblasts, and macrophages is reduced to the preinjury state. Because these repair agents no longer need to be delivered to the area, the number of capillaries, the overall vascularity of the area, and the water content are reduced. In the case of superficial wounds, these events are indicated by the fading redness of the scar and the eventual return to near-normal skin color and texture.

The proportion of type I collagen continues to increase, replacing the existing type III collagen and other parts of the collagen lattice. As the amount of type I collagen continues to grow, the tissue's tensile strength increases. Because most musculoskeletal injuries are repaired by the replacement of tissues, increasing stresses must be applied to the collagen to encourage its proper organization and to allow maximum tensile strength.

CHRONIC INFLAMMATION

Inflammation that persists for longer than 1 month beyond its normal healing time is considered chronic. In this case, the inflammatory response is marked only by loss of function. The remaining cardinal signs need not be present. During this phase of the inflammatory process, the body is still reacting to the presence of foreign material and/or infection.

Fibroblastic activity continues to the point at which large quantities of collagen envelop the affected area, forming a *granuloma*. This granuloma affects the function of the involved part, leading to a loss of full function and to development of secondary reactions in associated structures. A baseball pitcher with chronic rotator cuff inflammation may demonstrate this. The presence of a granuloma in the supraspinatus may decrease the range of motion and strength of the joint. By continuing to pitch, the athlete is further irritating the tendon.

THE ROLE OF THERAPEUTIC MODALITIES

We began this chapter by noting that the use of therapeutic modalities does not actually hasten the healing process; rather, they attempt to provide the optimal environment for healing to take place. But what is considered a modality? Quite simply stated, it is the application of some form of stress to the body for the purpose of eliciting an adaptive response.

The term "therapeutic" is essential to fully describe the principles behind the application of thermal, mechanical, electrical, or chemical energy to the body. To be deemed therapeutic, the stress applied to the body must be conducive to the healing process of the injury in its current state. The optimum conditions for healing require a balance between protecting the area from further distresses and returning the body segment to normal function at the earliest possible time.[8] Hence, the application of a modality at an improper point in its recovery phase may hinder, if not actually set back, the healing process.

SUMMARY

Life is a series of positive and negative stressors. When the negative stresses outweigh the positive ones, or the intensity of the negative stress is too great, injury

---

Granuloma: A hard mass of fibrous tissue.

occurs. The resultant damage, the primary injury, leads to a sequence of events creating a self-perpetuating cycle that causes further cell death in the form of secondary hypoxic injury.

The body reacts to this through a defensive mechanism, inflammation. Although inflammation is needed for healing, its effects must be controlled because prolonged inflammation is detrimental to the healing process. The process of healing is characterized by revascularization, wound contracture, and remodeling.

Therapeutic modalities are used to control and limit the negative effects of inflammation by providing the optimum environment for healing to occur. Each modality used in the treatment of an injury should be judged for the effect it will have on the injury response process in the current stage of healing. Applying the wrong modality at the wrong stage is not therapeutic and causes a delay in the healing process.

The missing element in the injury response process, pain, is a complex and diffuse entity. The body's physiological and psychological responses to pain are discussed in Chapter 2.

Chapter Quiz

1. Which of the following physiological events occurs during the alarm stage of the general adaptation syndrome?
   A. Cell death occurs.
   B. Proteins are broken down into amino acids.
   C. The cardiac stroke volume is decreased.
   D. Vasodilation occurs in nonessential muscle groups.

2. An example of an injury caused by macrotrauma is:
   A. Stress fracture
   B. Sprain
   C. Tendinitis
   D. Pes planus

3. Stress fractures result when:
   A. Osteoclastic activity is greater than osteoblastic activity
   B. Osteoblastic activity is greater than osteoclastic activity
   C. Osteoclastic activity and osteoblastic activity are equal
   D. The body reaches the stage of resistance

4. Which of the following tissue types has the best potential to reproduce itself after an injury?
   A. Epithelial tissue
   B. Muscular tissue
   C. Nervous tissue
   D. Connective tissue

5. Water leaves the cell and enters the interstitial space by following:
   A. Histamine
   B. Debris
   C. Cortisol
   D. Proteins

6. Which of the following cell types is anaerobic and therefore is able to withstand a low-oxygen environment?
   A. Fibrocyte
   B. Granuloma
   C. Macrophage
   D. Anerocyte

7. After depolarization of the nerve, the period during which a stronger-than-normal stimulus is required to initiate another action potential is the:
   A. Absolute refractory period
   B. Relative refractory period
   C. Silent refractory period
   D. Latent refractory period

8. Which of the following inflammatory mediators inhibits coagulation of blood?
   A. Histamine
   B. Heparin
   C. Kinins
   D. Leukotrienes

9. Which of the following structures has the poorest blood supply?
   A. Muscle
   B. Fascia
   C. Meniscal cartilage
   D. Bone

10. The rate of atrophy is accelerated through the stimulation of:
    A. Golgi tendon organs
    B. Phasic stretch receptors
    C. Actin and myosin filaments
    D. Blood flow

11. The healing process begins with:
    A. Inflammation
    B. Coagulation
    C. Phagocytosis
    D. Repair phase

12. All of the following aid in venous return **except:**
    A. Gravity
    B. Muscular contractions
    C. The sodium-potassium pump
    D. One-way valves

13. If vascular hydrostatic pressure exceeds the plasma colloid osmotic pressure:
    A. Edema forms
    B. Edema reduces
    C. Edema remains constant

14. List the five cardinal signs of inflammation and indicate the events that cause them:

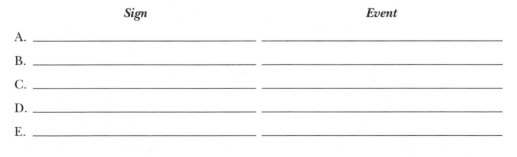

Sign	*Event*
A. _____	_____
B. _____	_____
C. _____	_____
D. _____	_____
E. _____	_____

15. The attraction of one chemical to an area because of the presence of another is called _____ .

16. Decribe the mechanisms for removing blood and exudate from the injured area. How can the care provider facilitate this process? What is the only mechanism available to remove proteins?

REFERENCES

1. Allen, RJ: Human Stress: Its Nature and Control. Burgess Publishing, Minneapolis, 1983.
2. Fahey, TD: Athletic Training: Principles and Practice. Mayfield Publishing, Minneapolis, 1986.
3. Reed, B: Wound healing and the repair in the use of thermal agents. In Michlovitz, S (ed): Thermal Agents in Rehabilitation, ed 3. FA Davis, Philadelphia, 1996, pp 3–27.
4. Enwemeka, CS: Inflammation, cellularity, and fibrillogenesis in regenerating tendon: Implications for tendon rehabilitation. Phys Ther 69:816, 1989.
5. Gross, MT: Chronic tendinitis: Pathomechanics of injury, factors affecting the healing response, and treatment. J Orthop Sports Phys Ther 16:248, 1992.
6. Wilkerson, GB: Inflammation in connective tissue: Etiology and management. Athletic Training 20:298, 1985.
7. Kloth, LC and Miller, KH: The inflammatory response to wounding. In Kloth, LC, McCulloch, JM, and Feedar, JA (eds): Wound Healing: Alternatives in Management. FA Davis, Philadelphia, 1990, pp 1–13.
8. Knight, KL: Cryotherapy in Sport Injury Management. Human Kinetics, Champaign, IL, 1995.
9. Salter, RB, et al: The biological effect of continuous passive motion on the healing of full thickness defects in articular cartilage. J Bone Joint Surg 62:A1232, 1980.
10. Denegar, CR, et al: Influence of transcutaneous electrical nerve stimulation on pain, range of motion, and serum cortisol concentration in females experiencing delayed onset muscle soreness. J Orthop Sports Phys Ther 11:100, 1989.
11. Beetham, WP Jr, et al: Physical Examination of the Joints. Philadelphia, WB Saunders, 1965.
12. Voight, ML: Reduction of post traumatic ankle edema with high-voltage pulsed galvanic stimulation. Athletic Training 19:278, 1984.
13. Vander, AJ, Sherman, JH, and Luciano, DS: Human Physiology: The Mechanisms of Body Function, ed 3. McGraw-Hill, New York, 1980.
14. Vanudevan, SV and Melvin, JL: Upper extremity edema control: Rationale of the techniques. Am J Occup Ther 33:520, 1980.
15. Rucinski, TJ, et al: The effects of intermittent compression on edema in postacute ankle sprains. J Orthop Sports Phys Ther 14:65, 1991.
16. Gilbart, MK, et al: Anterior tibial compartment pressures during intermittent sequential pneumatic compression therapy. Am J Sports Med 23:769, 1995.
17. Halvorson, GA: Therapeutic heat and cold for athletic injuries. Physician and Sportsmedicine 18:87, 1990.
18. Kolb, P and Denegar, C: Traumatic edema and the lymphatic system. Athletic Training 18:339, 1983.
19. McCulloch, J and Boyd, VB: The effects of whirlpool and the dependent position on lower extremity volume. J Orthop Sports Phys Ther 16:169, 1992.
20. Von Schroeder, et al: The changes in intramuscular pressure and femoral vein flow with continuous passive motion, pneumatic compressive stockings, and leg manipulations. Clin Orthop 218, May, 1991.
21. Kisner, C and Colby, LA: Therapeutic Exercise: Foundations and Techniques. FA Davis, Philadelphia, 1990.
22. Cailliet, R: Soft Tissue Pain and Disability. FA Davis, Philadelphia, 1977.
23. Urbancova, H, Hnik, P, and Vejsada, R: Bone fracture influences reflex muscle atrophy which is sex-dependent. Physiol Res 42:35, 1993.
24. DeVahl, J: Neuromuscular electrical stimulation (NMES) in rehabilitation. In Gersh, MR (ed): Electrotherapy in Rehabilitation. FA Davis, Philadelphia, 1992, pp 218–268.
25. Spence, AP and Mason, EB: Human Anatomy and Physiology, ed 3. Benjamin/Cummings, Menlo Park, CA, 1987.
26. Hunter-Griffin, L: Athletic Training and Sports Medicine. American Academy of Orthopaedic Surgeons, Park Ridge, IL, 1991.
27. Lieher, RL and Kelly, MJ: Factors influencing quadriceps femoris muscle torque using transcutaneous neuromuscular stimulation. Phys Ther 71:715, 1991.

28. Houglum, PA: Soft tissue healing and its impact on rehabilitation. Journal of Sports Rehabilitation 1:19, 1992.

29. Hebda, PA, Collins, MA, and Tharp, MD: Mast cell and myofibroblast in wound healing. Dermatol Clin 11:685, 1993.

30. Tranquillo, RT and Murray, JD: Mechanistic model of wound contraction. J Surg Res 55:233, 1993.

31. Daly, TJ: The repair phase of wound healing: Re-epithelialization and contraction. In Kloth, LC, McCulloch, JM, and Feedar, JA (eds): Wound Healing: Alternatives in Management. FA Davis, Philadelphia, 1990, pp 14–30.

32. Dickinson, A and Bennett, KM: Therapeutic exercise. Clin Sports Med 4:417, 1985.

33. Garrett, WE: Muscle strain injuries: Clinical and basic aspects. Med Sci Sports Exerc 22:436, 1990.

34. Lechner, CT and Dahners, LE: Healing of the medial collateral ligament in unstable rat knees. Am J Sports Med 19:508, 1991.

35. Russell, B, et al: Repair of injured skeletal muscle: A molecular approach. Med Sci Sports Exerc 24:189, 1992.

CHAPTER 2

The Physiology and Psychology of Pain

Barton P. Buxton, EdD, ATC

Of all the components of the injury response, none is less consistent or less understood than an individual's response to pain. The sensation of pain is a diffuse entity inherent to the nervous system and basic to all people. It is a personal experience that all humans endure. Acute pain is the primary reason why people seek medical attention and the major complaint that they describe on initial evaluation. Chronic pain may be more debilitating than the trauma itself and, in many instances, is so emotionally and physically debilitating that it is a leading cause of suicide.[1–3]

Pain serves as one of the body's defense mechanisms by warning the brain that its tissues may be in jeopardy, yet pain may be triggered without any physical damage to tissues.[4] The pain response itself is a complex phenomenon involving sensory, behavioral (motor), emotional, and cultural components. Once the painful impulse has been initiated and received by the brain, the interpretation of pain itself is based on interrelated biological, psychological, and social factors.[5]

When certain nerve fibers, **nociceptors,** are stimulated, "pain" impulses are sent to the brain as a warning that the body's integrity is at risk. The evaluative portion of the brain interprets these signals as pain. The emotional response may be expressed by screaming, crying, fainting, or just thinking, "%@!#, that hurts!" When the pain is intense or unexpected, an immediate reflex loop activates the behavioral response by sending instructions to motor nerves to remove the body part from the stimulus. An example of this is accidentally sticking your finger with a pin. In this case, the pin activates specialized nerve fibers to send signals through

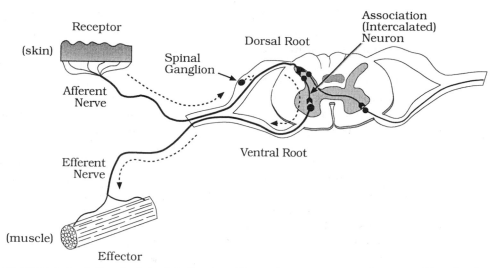

FIGURE 2–1 **A Simple Spinal Reflex Arc.** Figure demonstrates a reflex caused by stimulation of pain receptors in the skin. On reaching the spinal cord, the afferent pain impulses excite an association neuron, which routes efferent impulses to the appropriate muscle group, causing them to contract and withdraw from the painful stimulus. The afferent impulses are also routed up the spinal cord and into the brain, where the stimulus is interpreted as pain.

a peripheral nerve network, routing the impulses up the spinal cord to the brain. When the afferent impulses reach the spinal cord, a reflex loop is formed within one to two levels of the spinal input. One portion of the loop is sent back down the tract to activate the muscles necessary to remove your finger from the stimulus (Fig. 2–1). The remaining impulses of the reflex continue on to the brain, where they are translated as pain, and you respond by saying, "Ouch!"

If an individual has knowledge about a potentially painful stimulus, such as receiving an injection, cognitive mechanisms can inhibit the reflex loop and block portions of the behavioral response. As the painful stimulus increases, so does the conscious effort required to keep from trying to escape from the stimulus. The emotional component may still be in place as you grimace, make a fist, or think, "What's this jerk doing to me!"

The cultural components of pain are almost too complex to define. However, pain perception has been linked to ethnicity and socioeconomic status.[6–8] For example, Italian patients are less inhibited in the expression of pain than are Irish or Anglo-Saxon patients.[7,8] Ultimately, cultural components can be viewed as any variable that relates to the environment in which a person was raised and how that environment deals with pain and responses to pain.

THE PAIN PROCESS

Noxious input or *nociceptive stimulus* causes the activation of pain fibers. **Chemical irritation** or **mechanical deformation** of nerve endings results in the depolariza-

---

Noxious: Harmful, injurious.
Nociceptive stimulus: Impulse giving rise to the sensation of pain.

tion of pain fibers. The painful impulse is triggered by the initial mechanical force of the injury (whether sudden or gradual in onset) and is continued by chemical irritation resulting from the inflammatory process. In subacute and chronic conditions, pain may be continued by reflex muscle spasm in a positive feedback loop or through the continued presence of chemical irritation.[9]

The pain response is initiated by stimulation of nociceptors, specialized nerve endings that respond to painful stimuli. Mechanical stress or damage to the tissues excites **mechanosensitive** nociceptors. Various chemical substances released during the inflammatory response, such as bradykinin, serotonin, histamine, and prostaglandins, excite **chemosensitive** nociceptors (see Table 1–4). Chemical irritation of nerve endings may produce a severe pain response without true tissue destruction.[10] Unlike other types of nerve receptors, nociceptors display *sensitization* to repeated or prolonged stimulation. During the inflammatory process, the threshold required to initiate an action potential is lowered, and the continued stimulation of the chemosensitive receptors perpetuates the cycle.[11]

To begin to understand the complexity of pain, comprehension of the various neurophysiological pathways involved in the transmission, perception, and inhibition of pain is critical. The nervous system (the peripheral sensory and motor nerves, spinal cord, brain stem, and brain) forms a complex network of **afferent** and **efferent** pathways for transmitting and reacting to impulses that the brain "perceives" as being painful. All noxious impulses are transmitted via the afferent pathways to the thalamus, where the "painful" stimulus triggers the physiological and psychological processes described in the introduction to this chapter. The neurophysiological foundations of pain are appropriately explained by the discussion of the pathways leading to the pain response.

Modulation of Pain

The acute pain response begins with a noxious stimulus. External sources, such as a burn or a cut, or internal sources, such as a muscle strain or a ligament sprain, can generate this stimulus. After trauma, substances such as bradykinin, prostaglandins, substance P (SP), and other chemicals are released in and around the surrounding tissues (Table 2–1).[12] Immediately after the trauma, **primary hyperalgesia** occurs, lowering the nerve's threshold to noxious stimuli and magnifying the pain response. Within hours, **secondary hyperalgesia** increases the size of the painful area as the chemicals diffuse into the surrounding tissues, causing them to become *hypersensitive.*

The initiation of the pain process always begins with a chemical stimulus. A review of the chemical *precursors* to nociception may help in the understanding of the overall process. During acute trauma, the cell walls become damaged. This event causes dopamine and norepinephrine (NE) to be released from precursors in the cell membrane, which in turn causes the activation of phospholipase, allowing the cell membrane to release arachidonic acid. When arachidonic acid is re-

---

Sensitization: The process of being made sensitive to a specific substance.
Hypersensitivity: Abnormally increased sensitivity, a condition in which there is an exaggerated response by the body to a stimulus.
Precursor: A substance that is formed before changing into its final state or substance.

TABLE 2–1   **Inflammatory Integration of Pain Response**

Mediator	Action
Bradykinins	Direct stimulation of nerve fiber carrying the noxious stimuli
Prostaglandin	Sensitization of the nerve fibers so that other mediators can initiate nociception
Substance P	Extravasation of substances that can cause nociception

leased in the presence of cyclooxygenase, it is converted to prostaglandin (Fig. 2–2).[13] Prostaglandins have many roles in inflammation, but they also sensitize the nerve endings to other chemicals, such as bradykinin, which in turn initiate nociception. Found in plasma and released during coagulation that follows the injury, bradykinins are direct activators of nociception. The bradykinins also act as powerful vasodilators and increase vascular permeability during the inflammatory response. Nonsteroidal anti-inflammatory drugs (NSAIDS) play an important role in the treatment of acute pain in that they block the formation of cyclooxygenase

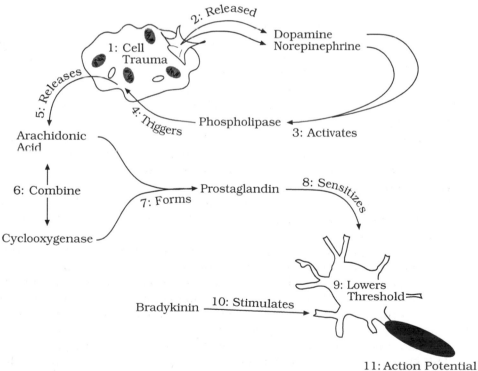

FIGURE 2–2   **Chemical Initiation of Nociception.** When a cell is damaged (1), it releases dopamine and norepinephrine (2). These two chemicals activate phospholipase (3), which triggers the cell membrane to release arachidonic acid (4 and 5). Arachidonic acid then combines with cyclooxygenase (6) to form prostaglandin (7), which sensitizes (8) and lowers the depolarization threshold of nociceptors (9). Other chemical agents such as bradykinin (10) stimulate the dendrite, resulting in the initiation of a noxious nerve impulse (11).

and prevent the synthesis of prostaglandin. Therefore, NSAIDs are an important early mediator for the interruption of the pain and inflammation cycle.

Substance P (SP) is a peptide that is manufactured in the spinal cord's dorsal root ganglia and is stored in the terminals of the peripheral afferent nerves. The release of SP influences pain transmission by triggering vasodilation and *extravasation* of bradykinin from the plasma, histamine from the mast cells, and serotonin from the platelets.[12] Once the substances are released and the nociception has been initiated, SP is also released by the axon terminals of **C fibers** in the dorsal horn, where it acts to transmit the impulse via the dorsal horn neurons.

The nociceptors activated by these substances and their cell bodies are located in the dorsal root ganglia and consist of a subgroup of nerve endings made up of small, unmyelinated C fibers and larger, thinly myelinated **A-delta fibers.**[14] Through a process termed transaction, the chemical substances cause a change in the nerve or the nerve environment and allow an action potential to occur. The action potential then sets up a condition that permits the impulse to be transmitted along the entire length of the nerve through the process of depolarization (see Box 1–2). The depolarization of myelinated and unmyelinated nerve fibers occurs because of an increase in the permeability of sodium and the loss of potassium from inside the nerve fiber. Depolarization occurs at the nodes of Ranvier in the myelinated nerve fibers and is responsible for the increase in nerve conduction velocity.

After an injury, A-delta and C fibers carry noxious stimuli from the periphery via afferent pathways to the dorsal horn of the spinal cord. The noxious stimuli activate 10 to 25 percent of the A-delta fibers and 50 to 80 percent of the C fibers.[14] Triggered by strong mechanical pressure or intense heat, A-delta fibers produce a fast, bright, localized pain sensation.[15] C fibers are *polymodal* nociceptors that are triggered by thermal, mechanical, and chemical stimuli and generate a more diffuse, nagging sensation.[14]

When an injury, such as a sprained ankle, occurs, the person experiences a sharp, well-localized, stinging or burning sensation arising from activation of the A-delta fibers. This initial reaction, **protopathic pain** (first pain), allows the individual to realize that trauma has occurred and to recognize the response as pain. Very quickly, the stinging or burning sensation becomes an aching or throbbing sensation, a response marking activation of C fibers termed **epicritic pain** (second pain).[16]

A third type of peripheral afferent nerve fiber that warrants mention is the A-beta fiber. A-beta fibers are large, myelinated, low-threshold mechanoreceptors that respond to light touch and low-intensity mechanical information. Stimulation of these A-beta fibers may interrupt nociception in the dorsal horn of the spinal cord.[17] This concept can be illustrated by the instinctive reaction to rub an injured area (e.g., when you bump your head). The process of rubbing the skin activates A-beta fibers that, in turn, inhibit transmission of the painful impulses. This same process can be initiated by using large-fiber (A-beta), sensory, electrical

---

Extravasation: To exude from or pass out of a vessel into the tissues, said of blood, lymph, or urine.
Polymodal: Capable of being depolarized by different types of stimuli.

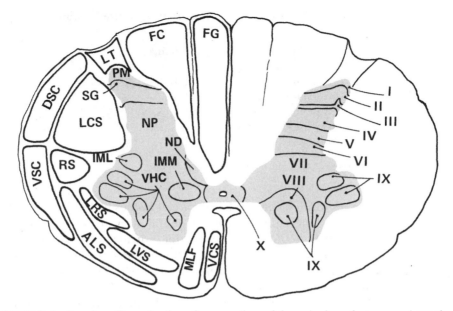

FIGURE 2–3 **Laminar Organization.** Cross section of the spinal cord at approximately the C8-T1 segmental level. The right side of this illustration indicates the location of the laminae, depicted by Roman numerals. The left side illustrates the tracts and nuclei of the spinal cord:

ALS = anterolateral system	MLF = medial longitudinal fasciculus
DSC = dorsal spinocerebellar tract	ND = nucleus dorsalis
FC = fasciculus cuneatus	NP = nucleus proprius
FG = fasciculus gracilis	PM = posteromarginal nucleus
IML = intermediolateral cell column	RS = rubrospinal tract
IMM = intermediomedial cell column	SG = substantia gelatinosa
LCS = lateral corticospinal tract	VCS = ventral corticospinal tract
LRS = lateral reticulospinal tract	VHC = ventral horn cell columns
LT = Lissauer's tract	VSC = ventral spinocerebellar tract
LVS = lateral vestibulospinal tract	

(From Gilman, S and Newman, SW: Manter and Gatz's Essentials of Chemical Neuroanatomy and Neurophysiology, ed 9. FA Davis, Philadelphia, 1996, p 13, with permission.)

stimulation. As we will see later, this is the basis of the gate control theory of pain reduction.

Ascending Pain Pathways

Because A-beta, A-delta, and C nerve fibers all originate in the periphery and terminate in different areas of the dorsal horn, they are termed *first-order neurons*. An understanding of the anatomy of the dorsal horn is needed to comprehend the neurological synapses that *modulate* pain outside of the brain. The gray matter of

---

First-order neuron: Sensory nerve that courses outside the central nervous system and has its body in a dorsal root ganglion.
Modulate: To regulate or adjust.

TABLE 2–2   Nerve Fibers Terminating in the Laminae

Nerve Type	Laminae
Cutaneous C fibers	I, II, V
Visceral C fibers	I, V
Cutaneous A-delta fibers	I, II, V, X
Visceral A-delta fibers	I, V
Larger A-delta fibers	III, IV, V

Source: Adapted from Bowsher,[15] pp 22–23.

the spinal cord is divided into 10 layers of cell bodies called **laminae** (Fig. 2–3). Before synapsing in the laminae, the peripheral afferent nerves course into the tract of Lissauer,[15] where the A-delta and C fibers divide and send impulses up and down one to two segments of the spinal column. Once in the dorsal horn of the spinal cord, the small A-delta and C fibers synapse with neurons and terminate in various laminae (Table 2–2).

Several types of neurons are found within lamina I. The two of interest to us are the wide–dynamic-range (WDR) neurons and the nociceptive-specific (NS) neurons.[18] The wide-dynamic-range neurons respond to both noxious and non-noxious stimuli, whereas the nociceptive-specific neurons respond only to noxious stimuli. These neurons in lamina I are part of the cells that make up the long spinothalamic tract (STT).

The substantia gelatinosa (SG), which is partially located within lamina II, contains small internuncial neurons that can excite (stalked cells) or inhibit (islet cells) the transmission of noxious stimuli (Fig. 2–4). The small internuncial neurons in the SG send axons to lamina I and release *enkephalin* and gamma-aminobutyric acid, both of which inhibit the transmission of noxious stimuli.[18]

Laminae III and IV are composed of wide-dynamic-range neuron cells and low-threshold mechanoreceptors that play a limited role in the modulation and transmission of pain. Lamina V is a major synapse of A-delta and C fibers in the dorsal horn. Lamina V has a large number of wide-dynamic-range cells that respond to a spectrum of stimuli from light touch to mechanical pressure and heat. The wide-dynamic-range cells from laminae I and V make up the majority of fibers in the spinothalamic tract, where first-order neurons terminate and *second-order neurons* originate.

All first-order neurons course from the periphery to synapse in the dorsal root ganglion and the laminae before crossing the spinal cord to the spinothalamic tract. Once in the spinothalamic tract, the noxious stimulus is then transmitted to the brain via two different portions of the spinothalamic tract, the

---

Enkephalin: A substance released by the body that reduces the perception of pain by bonding to pain receptor sites.

Second-order neuron: A nerve having its body located in the spinal cord. It connects second- and third-order neurons (a nerve having its body in the thalamus and extending into the cerebral cortex).

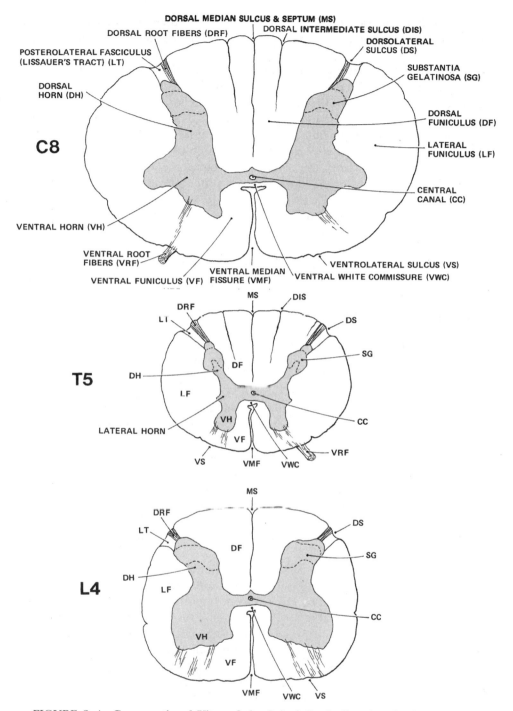

FIGURE 2–4 **Cross-sectional View of the Spinal Cord.** Showing the location of various tracts in the eighth cervical (C8), fifth thoracic (T5), and fourth lumbar (L4) spinal regions. (From Gilman, S and Newman, SW: Manter and Gatz's Essentials of Clinical Neuroanatomy and Neurophysiology, ed 9. FA Davis, Philadelphia, 1996, p 12, with permission.)

neospinothalamic tract (NSTT) and the **paleospinothalamic tract** (PSTT). These tracts are also referred to as the lateral and ventral spinothalamic tracts, respectively.

This dual-tract system of afferent pain pathways enables the body to have immediate warning of the presence, location, and intensity of an injury as well as the slow, aching reminder that tissue damage has occurred. The neospinothalamic tract receives input from A-delta fibers that synapse with the nociceptive-specific neurons and the wide-dynamic-range neurons in laminae I and V. These nociceptive-specific neurons and the wide-dynamic-range neurons of the neospinothalamic tract immediately cross the ventral white column of the spinal cord to the opposite anterolateral white column.[19] Once in the anterior horn, the fibers of the neospinothalamic tract and a portion of the spinothalamic tract synapse with motor units or stimulate preganglionic neurons of the sympathetic or parasympathetic system and then communicate with the thalamus.[14] This transmission is responsible for the motor and autonomic responses associated with tissue damage and information pertinent to the site, intensity, and duration of the painful stimulus.[20] Melzack and Wall[21] describe the neospinothalamic tract as the **sensory-discriminative pathway of pain** (Fig. 2–5).

The second portion of the STT, the PSTT, is located more medially, but still in the anterolateral portion of the white matter of the spinal cord. The PSTT receives its input predominantly from C fibers that synapse with the nociceptive-specific neurons and the wide-dynamic-range neurons in laminae I and V. The second-order neurons of laminae I and V then cross over the spinal cord and project to the *reticular formation* (RF), located in the central portion of the brain stem. The neurons then course through a complicated network of synapses to the medulla oblongata, midbrain, hypothalamus, thalamus, limbic system, and periaqueductal gray (PAG), hence the name paleospinothalamic tract (Table 2–3).[22]

The **reticular formation** is responsible for evoking motor, sensory, and autonomic responses to noxious stimuli, allowing the injured person to respond rapidly to the stimuli.[14,19] The paleospinothalamic tract has multiple synapses with other areas of the central brain (the medulla, the midbrain, the PAG, the hypothalamus, and the medial portions of the thalamus) responsible for poorly localized, dull, aching pain as well as for the behavioral, emotional, and affective aspects of pain.[19,20,23]

The brain's limbic system aids in integrating higher brain function with motivational and emotional reactions. It contains afferent nerves from the hypothalamus and the brain stem and receives descending influence from the cortex.[24] This communication is responsible for the emotional response to painful experiences. When an injury occurs, the neural communication between the limbic system, thalamus, RF, and cortex produces reactions such as fear, anxiety, or crying. In short, the limbic system is responsible for the body's affective qualities of reward, punishment, aversive drives, and fear reactions to pain.[19] Melzack and Wall[21] have referred to this as the **motivational-affective system.**

The integration of the cortex is an important component in both the ascending and descending aspects of pain modulation.[24] Via axons, ascending pain stim-

---

Reticular formation: A diffuse network of cells and fibers located in the brain stem. The reticular formation influences alertness, waking, sleeping, and certain reflexes.

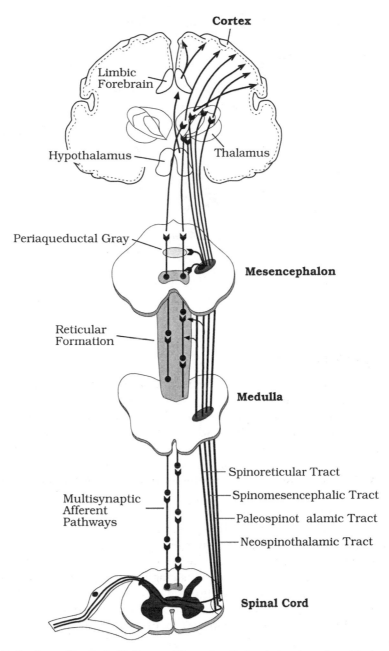

FIGURE 2–5 Ascending Pain Pathways. The spinothalamic tracts and multisynaptic afferent systems. (Adapted from Bonica, JJ: The Management of Pain [V 1]. Lea & Febiger, Philadelphia, 1990, p 89.)

uli are transmitted from the thalamus to the central sulcus in the parietal lobe (somatosensory cortex), where the pain is discriminated and localized. Because of the proliferation of nerve cells and the cortex's functions (consciousness, speech, hearing, memory, and thought), it is unlikely that the afferent synapses that occur during noxious stimulation affect only one efferent neuron. Thus, many areas of the cortex can be stimulated during a painful experience.

TABLE 2–3   **The Areas of the Paleospinothalamic Tract**

Area	Function
Medulla oblongata	Controls autonomic functions such as heart rate, respiration, and vomiting.
	Connects the spinal cord to the brain.
Midbrain	Serves as center for many reflexes and assists in coordinating movement and visual tracking.
Hypothalamus	Controls the endocrine system's release of hormones. Through this mechanism, the hypothalamus regulates metabolism and stress response.
Thalamus	Influences mood and body movements that are associated with fear, anxiety, pain, and rage.
Limbic system	Linked to emotions and, through the cingulate gyrus, controls the visceral response to emotions and the sensation of pain and pleasure.
Periaqueductal gray	Hormonally controls the release of β-endorphin and other pain-reducing chemicals.

Descending Pain Pathways

The descending pain modulation mechanisms could influence both the input and the mediation of the noxious stimuli.[25] One of these descending mechanisms originates in the cortex's corticospinal tract. The corticospinal tract descends from the cortex to the medulla, where its fibers cross over to the opposite side of the medulla and to lower levels of the spinal cord, where it terminates in laminae I through VII and transcends through the dorsolateral funiculus (large fiber tract). The corticospinal tract could act to exert postsynaptic (descending) control over the afferent transmission of thermal, mechanical, and C-fiber input at laminae I and II.[25]

A second structure exerting descending control of noxious stimuli is the PAG. The PAG receives input from the cortex, limbic system, hypothalamus, and PSTT (Fig. 2–6). The hypothalamus sends *β-endorphins* via neurons to the PAG, where they are routed to the nucleus magnocellularis of the rostral medulla that descends laterally to the dorsal horn. The neurons from this descending system terminate in laminae I, II, IV, V, VI, and X, where they release NE, a chemical neurotransmitter exerting postsynaptic control over the noxious input at laminae I, II and V.[12]

Another descending control system arises from the nucleus raphae magnus in the upper medulla. Descending axons from this region of the brain track down to the lower medulla and the spinal cord, where they release serotonin (5-HT) at their terminal end, producing analgesia at laminae I, II, and V.[12]

β-endorphin: A morphinelike neurohormone produced from β-lipotropin in the pituitary. Endorphins are thought to increase the pain threshold by binding to receptor sites.

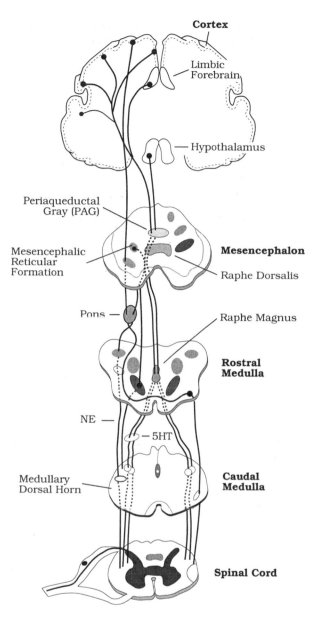

FIGURE 2–6 **Descending Pain Pathways.** The distal terminals of these axons release norepinephrine and 5-HT that produce analgesia by blocking noxious stimuli. (Adapted from Bonica, JJ: The Management of Pain (V 1). Lea & Febiger, Philadelphia, 1990, p 106.)

The notion of central control and descending inhibition of pain is based on the body's ability to use and produce various forms of *endogenous opiates,* each having a distinct function and a specific receptor affinity (Table 2–4). Enkephalins are found throughout the central nervous system, but particularly in the dorsal horn. Descending input from the PAG activates enkephalin release in laminae I, II, III, and V.[18] Thus, the aggregation of noxious stimuli may cause both presynaptic and postsynaptic control of nociception in the dorsal horn via enkephalin release.

Endogenous opiates: Pain-inhibiting substances produced in the brain. These include endorphins and enkephalins.

TABLE 2–4   **Classification of Human Endogenous Opiates and Their Precursors**

Endogenous Opiate	Precursor
Enkephalin	Proenkephalin A
Dynorphins	Proenkephalin B
ACTH	Propiomelanocortin (POMC)
Endorphins	POMC, β-Lipotropin

Source: Adapted from Bonica,[12] pp 95–121.

Dynorphins are primarily located in laminae I and V, making it feasible for them to inhibit pain. Levels of dynorphin increase in laminae I and V during periods of hyperstimulation.[18] However, their rapid degradation limits their role in long-term pain reduction.

As previously mentioned, β-endorphin cell bodies are strongly influenced by β-endorphin and project from the thalamus to the PAG.[15] During periods of intense noxious input, β-endorphins are released and provide temporary inhibition to noxious stimulation. This concept is based on their location in the PAG and the idea that their release would block *interneuron* interaction.[15]

Review of the Process of Pain Transmission

Much decision making in the treatment of pain can be based on the understanding of the physiological and chemical interaction that occurs after trauma. In simple terms, pain transmission appears to be fairly straightforward. The acute pain response is initiated when substances are released from injured tissues, causing a noxious stimulus to be transmitted via A-delta and C fibers to the dorsal horn. Once in the dorsal horn, the stimulus is transmitted to the higher brain centers via the STT, which bifurcates into two tracts. The impulse is propagated via the NSTT to the thalamus and then to the cortex, where discrimination and location of the stimulus are assessed. At the same time, noxious stimulation is projected upward toward the RF, the PAG matter, the hypothalamus, and the thalamus via the PSTT. Neurons in the thalamus send axon projections to the limbic system and the cortex. Once the noxious stimuli have reached the higher centers of the brain, the descending control mechanisms are activated, the incoming noxious stimuli can be inhibited at various levels (laminae I, II, and V and PAG), and endogenous opiates can be released.

PAIN THEORY: HISTORICAL PERSPECTIVES

Theories regarding the cause, nature, and purpose of pain have been debated since the dawn of humankind.[26] Most early theories were based on the assumption that pain was related to a form of punishment. Indeed, the word "pain" is derived

---

Interneuron: A neuron connecting two nerves.

from the Latin word "poena," meaning a fine, penalty, or punishment. The ancient Greeks believed that pain was associated with pleasure because the relief of pain was both pleasurable and emotional.[26] Aristotle reassessed the theory of pain and declared that the soul was the center of the sensory processes and that the pain system was located in the heart.[26]

The Romans, coming closer to contemporary thought, viewed pain as something that accompanied inflammation. In the second century, Galen offered the Romans his works on the concepts of the nervous system. However, the views of Aristotle weathered the winds of time. In the fourth century, successors of Aristotle discovered anatomic proof that the brain was connected to the nervous system. Despite this, Aristotle's belief prevailed until the 19th century, when German scientists provided irrefutable evidence that the brain is involved with sensory and motor function.[26]

Specificity Theory of Pain Modulation

Modern concepts of pain theory continue to advance from the ideas of Aristotle. However, controversy still exists as to which theories are correct. The theories accepted at the turn of the century were the specificity theory and the pattern theory, two completely different and seemingly contradictory views. The specificity theory suggests that there is a direct pathway from peripheral pain receptors to the brain (Fig. 2–7). The pain receptors are located in the skin and are purported to carry pain impulses via a continuous fiber directly to the brain's pain center. This pathway includes the peripheral nerves, the lateral STT in the spinal cord, and the hypothalamus (the brain's pain center). This theory was examined and refuted using clinical, psychological, and physiological evidence by Melzack and Wall in 1965.[27]

Melzack and Wall[27] discussed clinical evidence describing pain sensations in severe burn patients (with lesions to a peripheral nerve), amputee patients (phantom limb pain), and patients with degenerative nerve disease (peripheral neural-

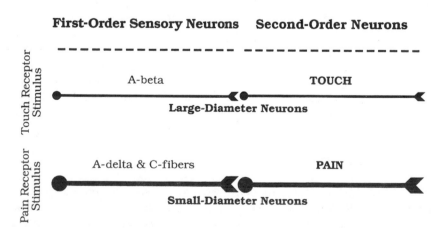

FIGURE 2–7 **The Specificity Theory of Pain Modulation.** This theory proposed that the body contained only four types of sensory nerve endings. A single nerve would respond only to a specific stimulus such as temperature, pain, or touch.

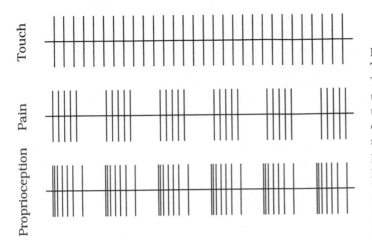

FIGURE 2–8 **The Pattern Theory of Pain Transmission.** This theory proposed that the body contained only one type of nerve ending that, depending on the type of stimulus, would code the impulse accordingly. This figure provides an example of how the impulses arising from touch, pain, and proprioception would be encoded along the same nerve.

gia). These pain syndromes do not occur in a fixed, direct linear system. Rather, the quality and quantity of the perceived pain are directly related to psychological variables and sensory input. This theory had been previously addressed by Pavlov, who inflicted dogs with a painful stimulus, then immediately gave them food.[28] The dogs eventually responded to the stimulus as a signal for food and showed no responses to the pain.

The psychological aspect of pain perception was later addressed by Beecher,[29] who studied 215 soldiers seriously wounded in the Battle of Anzio, finding that only 27 percent requested pain-relieving medication (morphine). When the soldiers were asked if they were experiencing pain, almost 60 percent indicated that they suffered no pain or only slight pain, and only 24 percent rated the pain as bad. This was most surprising because 48 percent of the soldiers had received penetrating abdominal wounds. Beecher also noted that none of the men were suffering from shock or were insensitive to pain because inept intravenous insertions resulted in complaints of acute pain.

The conclusion was drawn that the pain experienced by these men was blocked by emotional factors. The physical injuries that these men had received represented an escape from the life-threatening environment of battle to the safety of a hospital, or even release from the war. This relationship suggests that it is possible for the central nervous system to intervene between the stimulus and the sensation in the presence of certain psychological variables. The idea of this relationship further refutes a fixed-gain transmission nervous system. No physiological evidence has been found to suggest that certain nerve cells are more important for pain perception and response than others; therefore, the specificity theory can be discounted.

Pattern Theory of Pain Modulation

According to the pattern theory, there are no specialized receptors in the skin. Rather, a single "generic" nerve responds differently to each type of sensation by creating a uniquely coded impulse formed by a spatiotemporal pattern involving the frequency and pattern of nerve transmission. An analysis of the word's elements, "spatio" and "temporal," further defines this theory. The distance between the nerve's impulses (space) comprises the spatial coding, whereas the frequency of the transmission accounts for the temporal component (Fig. 2–8). An example of this type of coding can be found with most institutional phone systems. A call from inside a university has a different ring from an outside call.

Although the pattern theory was closer to being neurologically correct than the specificity theory, it still had shortcomings. Melzack and Wall[27] refuted this theory as well, based on the physical evidence of physiological specialization of receptor-fiber units. In addition, this theory failed to account for the role played by the brain in pain perception as described in the specificity theory.

CONTEMPORARY PAIN CONTROL THEORIES

Although both the specificity and pattern theories of pain transmission were eventually refuted, they did provide some lasting principles that are still present in contemporary pain modulation theories. The strengths of these two theories, plus findings obtained through additional research, were factored together to form the basis of the current perspective regarding pain transmission and pain modulation. Still, there is much to be learned and studied before the exact mechanisms of pain transmission and perception are understood.

Gate Control Theory of Pain Modulation

In examining the available theories of pain transmission, Melzack and Wall[27] incorporated features of physiological receptor specialization from specificity theory and spatiotemporal coding of action potentials from the pattern theory, while also including the physiological evidence of the spinal mechanism and of the central control over afferent input. This offered a new theory of pain consistent with the concept of central summation and input control.[27,30] The theory of gate control for the modulation of pain was developed and simply implies that **a nonpainful stimulus can block the transmission of a noxious stimulus.**

The gate control theory is based on the premise that the **SG,** located in the dorsal horn of the spinal cord, modulates the afferent nerve impulses. This then influences the first central transmission (**T**) cells, which correspond to either the neospinothalamic or paleospinothalamic tract and activate a central control triggering the mechanisms responsible for the response and perception of pain. Incorporated in Lissauer's tract, the SG acts as a modulating gate or a control system between the peripheral nerve fibers and central cells that permits only one type of nerve impulse (pain or no pain) to pass through. Serving in a capacity similar to that of a "switch operator" in a railroad yard, the SG monitors the amount of activity occurring on both incoming tracts in a *convergent* system, opening and closing the gate to allow the appropriate information to be passed along to the *T cell.* Impulses traveling on the fast, nonpain fibers increase activity in the SG. Impulses on the

---

Convergent: Two or more input routes are reduced to a single route.
T cell: A transmission cell that connects sensory nerves to the central nervous system. Not to be confused with T cells found in the immune system.

slower pain fibers exert an inhibitory influence. When the SG is active, the gate is in its "closed" position and a nonpainful stimulus is allowed to pass on to the T cell.

If we look back to our previous example of bumping the head, the initial trauma activates A-delta and, eventually, C fibers. Rubbing the traumatized area stimulates A-beta fibers, which activate the SG to close the spinal gate, thus inhibiting transmission of the painful impulses. However, rubbing the injured area does not completely remove all the pain because the transmission of pain involves hundreds and thousands of gates. For complete pain removal, each of the gates must be activated. If they are not all activated, a decrease, rather than a complete inhibition, of pain results.

The gate control theory is predominated by three features of afferent input: (1) ongoing activity before the stimulus, (2) stimulus response, and (3) relationship between small- and large-diameter fibers. The spinal cord constantly receives nerve impulses from the periphery. Small myelinated and unmyelinated fibers transmit nerve impulse activity. These small fibers tend to be tonically active and slow to adapt, holding the gate in an open position.[27] They are characteristically "pain" fibers. Benign sensory stimulation causes an increase in large-fiber activity. Large-fiber impulses activate the T cell and partially close the presynaptic gate. Figure 2–9 represents the gate theory of Melzack and Wall through a schematic diagram. Somatic input is subjected to the modulating control of the gate.[25]

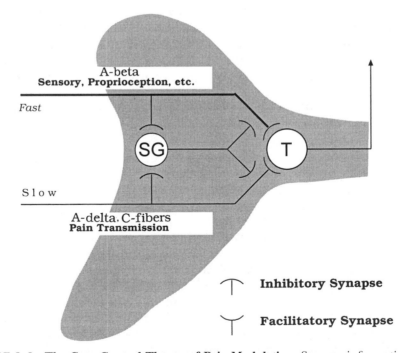

FIGURE 2–9 **The Gate Control Theory of Pain Modulation.** Sensory information enters the spinal gate located in the dorsal horn of the spinal cord (located by the gray area) along large, fast, myelinated, A-beta fibers. Painful impulses enter the gate along slower, small-diameter A-delta and C-fibers. Interneurons from each of these tracts project into the substantia gelatinosa (SG) (located in laminae I and II) and then from the SG affect the T cell. Activity along the fast A-beta fibers excites the SG to exert an inhibitory influence on the painful impulses traveling along the pain tract.

Descending efferent fibers after stimulation of the brain activate the central control mechanism. This trigger mechanism has a profound influence on the gate and affects afferent activity at early synaptic levels in the somatic system.[25] Despite controversy and minor evolution, Melzack and Wall's concept of "gating" or "input modulation" is presently recognized as the major basis of pain theory.

Levels Theory of Pain Control

The gate control theory has spawned a new generation of pain control research. One area of study centers on the levels of the central nervous system in which pain control occurs. The three levels of this model are shown in Table 2–5.[31]

Pain perception can be broken down into two distinct categories: (1) pain threshold and (2) pain tolerance. **Pain threshold** is the level of noxious stimulus required to alert the individual to a potential threat to tissue. The pain threshold can be measured experimentally by introducing a painful stimulus (e.g., cold water, pressure, or heat) to tissue to a point at which the individual reports "pain." In experimental pain models, researchers use water maintained at 1° to 3°C (cold pressor test), radiant heat, or mechanical pressure created by placing dull metal spikes

TABLE 2–5 Spinal Levels of Pain Control

Spinal Level	Theory	Activating Stimuli	Physiological Events
I	Presynaptic inhibition	Sensory stimulation of A-beta fibers	Enkephalin interneurons block the transmission of impulses traveling along small C fibers within the dorsal horn T cell.
		Pulse width/phase duration 75 μsec	
II	Descending inhibition	Intense (high-frequency) stimulation of C fibers	Central biasing mechanisms in the periaqueductal gray matter and the raphe nucleus activate descending influences along the dorsolateral tract of the spinal cord.
		Pulse width/phase duration 1000 μsec	
III	β-Endorphin modulation	Noxious, low-frequency, motor stimulation (A-delta)	Activates the tract cell and reticular formation, resulting in the release of β-endorphin from the anterior pituitary gland, causing the degeneration of prostaglandin and dorsal horn inhibition.
		Pulse width/phase duration 250–300 μsec	

Source: Adapted from Castel.[31]

inside a blood pressure cuff to measure pain threshold and tolerance. You can per-form a simple experiment on yourself by squeezing your fingernail. The point at which you subjectively first experience pain could be quantitatively measured as your pain threshold by recording the amount of foot-pounds of pressure used.

Clinically, the pain threshold is represented by the complaint of pain after an injury. This response, first pain, represents an individual's pain threshold. Pain threshold is a product of the noxious stimuli being transmitted via the A-delta fibers (first pain fibers) to the synapse with the NS neurons and the WDR neurons in lamina I, where they are transmitted to the thalamus. Therefore we can assess pain threshold as a very physiological mechanism.

Pain tolerance, on the other hand, is a measure of how much pain a person can or will withstand. In an experimental model, pain tolerance is measured by the amount of pain or "quantity" of exposure (cold water, pressure, heat) that an indi-vidual can or will endure. Clinically, pain tolerance can be related to a person losing consciousness because of pain or declaring in a half-lucid state, "I can't take this any more." In assessing the physiological model of pain transmission, pain tolerance is associated with the PSTT communication with the limbic system and the cortex. Within these structures, many synaptic interactions occur, and various levels of cog-nition can help the individual to determine the maximum level of noxious stimula-tion that can be tolerated. Examination of the physiology of noxious transmission and experimental research indicate that pain threshold and pain tolerance are not correlated.[32] Therefore, an athlete who reports feeling excessive pain immediately after an injury may be able to endure the pain and continue to participate because of a high level of pain tolerance. An athlete having a low pain tolerance may declare that an otherwise minor injury is prohibiting normal activity.

Several intrinsic factors influence an individual's perception of pain. For ex-ample, extroverts express pain more freely than introverts, but introverts are more sensitive to pain.[33] Cognitive-evaluative influences include the activities in which the person is involved, the perceived impact that the injury may have, and past experiences.

Perhaps the largest social and cultural influence on pain perception in the United States is that of gender role stereotypes. As young children, we often heard, "Big boys don't cry." Children often have engraved into their minds that boys are not supposed to cry, but it is appropriate for girls to cry. Although social consciousness has helped decrease this and other types of stereotyping, its influ-ences are still with us.

When comparing pain response between genders, the literature indicates that women have lower pain thresholds and pain tolerances than men as reported in epidemiological, experimental, and clinical studies. Further research indicates that women are more likely than men to experience a variety of types of recurrent pain and have more severe levels of pain, more frequent pain, and pain of longer duration than men.[34] In some clinical studies, female subjects reported greater pain than male subjects at high levels of stimulation, greater pupil dilation with noxious stimuli,[35] shorter time to ischemic pain tolerance,[36] and lower threshold to esophageal pain.[37] Male college students have a statistically significant higher pain tolerance than their female counterparts, and the female subjects had signif-icantly higher scores of fearful thoughts related to the experience of pain.[38]

Gender differences have also been noted in pain response in their relation-ship to expenditures for healthcare services. Women use more specific healthcare services based on psychological need and screening than men.[39] Female patients described significantly more pain than male patients and were perceived by their caregivers to experience more pain, resulting in more and stronger pain medications being prescribed for women than for men. Likewise, female patients were less likely than male patients to receive no medication for their pain.

Although these studies seemingly indicate significant gender differences in pain tolerance and pain threshold, it is unclear whether these differences are biologically, psychologically, or socially generated. It is unclear whether women are simply more willing to report and express pain than men.[40] Although the root of these differences is unclear, clinicians should consider that possible differences in pain threshold and pain tolerance may exist between men and women.

In young athletes, pain perception may be influenced by the presence of peers. Children have been found to "tolerate" pain to a higher level when observed by their peers than when alone.[41] The perception of pain is also negatively correlated with anxiety levels about pain.[42] This would indicate that patients who are anxious or fearful about pain may have a lower tolerance to pain than their less anxious counterparts.

As previously mentioned, differences in the definition and expression of pain based on culture and ethnicity have been documented.[33,43] A person's past experience influences the pain perception of a current injury. The experience may be recalling a previous injury that required surgery, or even the image of a similar injury on television. A fear of doctors or hospitals may cause increased anxiety because the person is afraid of being exposed to these stressors when an injury occurs. Likewise, if an injury is potentially career-threatening, the reaction may be increased.

Athletic participation and the type of sport played also appear to influence an individual's response to pain.[44–48] Athletes who participate in contact sports are able to tolerate significantly higher levels of pain than athletes who participate in noncontact sports or nonathletes, although no significant differences in the pain threshold between athletes and nonathletes were found.[49] Professional ballet dancers were found to have significantly higher pain thresholds and pain tolerances than a group of nonathletes of the same age.[50] Likewise, competitive swimmers had significantly higher tolerances of ischemic pain than did a comparable group of club swimmers.[51]

Sometimes other events override the processing of pain because the brain is preoccupied with more urgent matters. Immediate processing of information not related to pain may push the processing of the pain response to the background. A good example of this is the typical movie portrayal of British soldiers just after a fierce battle:

"I say, old chap, that was a nasty one, wasn't it? Too bad about your leg."

"My leg?"

"Your leg. You've been hit."

"Oh, bloody 'ell. Cup of tea, then?"

In this case, the soldier was so happy to make it out of combat alive, and his brain was so focused on analyzing the situation that he did not realize an injury had occurred. This same type of processing occurs in athletics. An athlete may be so focused on the competition that, when an injury occurs, its magnitude may not be immediately recognized.

Based on this integrative process, the perception of pain is subjective and variable in nature. Notwithstanding, it does consist of several measurable objective parameters. When you ask a patient how he or she feels today, the response is usually "better," "worse," or "the same." By asking, you are requiring the person to measure the pain and compare it to the way it felt yesterday. Several standardized methods are available to measure the amount of pain in relatively objective terms. Through the use of these tools, the location, intensity, and duration of the pain may be ascertained. Other methods exist that assess activities, emotions, and/or personality traits that influence the perception of pain.

ASSESSMENT OF PAIN

Pain is a personal expression of what one person feels. The feeling is based on a discriminative, effectual, and evaluative process. Therefore, the assessment of pain becomes very challenging to the clinician. The assessment process should encompass both the subjective and objective evaluations to properly document the level and amount of pain that the patient is experiencing.

A subjective assessment of pain is commonplace in all evaluations. The patient is queried about the location, duration, and type of pain being experienced (Table 2–6). The responses to these questions allow the clinician to chart a subjective baseline of the patient's present pain status. In turn, these responses can also help in further evaluation of the underlying pathology.

Visual Analogue Scale

Once the subjective evaluation is made, the clinician should also gain a baseline of the patient's objective response to pain. This allows the clinician to measure the decreases or increases in the levels or types of pain felt by the patient. There are several types of objective pain scales that can be used. The most common and most reliable is the Visual Analogue Scale (VAS) (Fig. 2–10).[52] The patient marks on the line where he or she feels that the pain is best represented. The clinician then measures the distance from the right side of the line to the "mark" of pain. A new VAS should be used for every assessment, and the patient should not see or be allowed to use prior responses for reference. The VAS is consistent, reliable, and easy to use. It can be used before and after treatments to measure the effectiveness of treatment or day to day to measure a patient's progress.

TABLE 2–6 **Subjective Assessment of Pain**

Where is your pain?
When did your pain begin?
What is the duration of your pain?
Have you ever experienced this pain before?
Can you describe how the pain feels?
Is the pain getting better or worse?
Does your pain increase with activity?
Do you have more pain after activity?
Do you have pain at night?

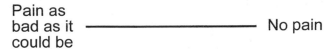

FIGURE 2–10 **Visual Analogue Scale.** The patient is asked to indicate the amount (intensity) of pain being experienced by placing a mark along the above line. This rating is quantitatively assessed by measuring (in centimeters) the distance from the left edge of the line to the patient's mark. For example a mark along the center of the line would be given a rating of 5.0.

McGill Pain Questionnaire

Another tool that has been used to assess pain is the McGill Pain Questionnaire (MPQ) (Fig. 2–11).[53] This instrument usually consists of three parts: Part 1 is used to localize the area of pain and identify whether the perceived source of the pain is superficial (external), internal, or both. Part 2 incorporates the VAS that was described in the previous section. Part 3 is the Pain Rating Index, a collection of 76 words grouped into 20 categories. A patient is instructed to circle or underline the words in each group that best describe the sensation of pain being experienced. The patient may pick only one word in each category, but each category need not be used. The words in groups 1 to 10 are somatic in nature and relate to the physiology of the pain. The words in groups 11 to 15 are affective and group 16 is evaluative. The words in groups 17 to 20 are miscellaneous words that are used only in the scoring process.

To score the MPQ, the clinician simply adds up the total number of words chosen, up to the maximum of 20 words (one for each category). The level of the pain intensity is determined by assigning a value to each word by its order (first word equals 1, second word equals 2, and so on). Therefore, a patient could have a high MPQ score of 20 (selecting a word in each group), but have a low-intensity score by selecting the first word in every group.

The MPQ takes longer (approximately 10 minutes) to complete and score than the VAS, but it can be a useful tool in the objective assessment of pain. It is primarily used during the first visit to a clinic, as there is some debate concerning its usefulness during subsequent visits.[54]

Submaximal Effort Tourniquet Test

In 1966, Smith et al.[55] described a method of "matching" a patient's pain using a Submaximal Effort Tourniquet Test (SETT). The SETT is performed by inflating a sphygmomanometer cuff to above systolic blood pressure on the patient's elevated arm. Once the cuff is inflated, the patient is instructed to open and close the hand or fist rhythmically. A handgrip dynamometer and a metronome can be used for standardization. The patient should continue opening and closing the hand or fist until the cramping sensation that he or she feels "matches" the pain from the "original" pathology. The amount of time that elapses from onset to fruition of matched pain is the recorded objective measure. The SETT can be repeated at every treatment session to gauge treatment progress and is effective in "matching" all types of pain.[54]

A. Where is your pain?

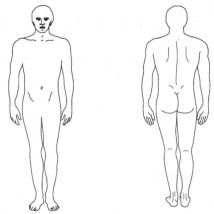

Using the above drawing, please mark the area(s) where you feel pain. Mark an "E" if the source of the pain is external or "I" if it is internal. If the source of the pain is both internal and external, please mark "B".

B. Pain rating index

Many different words can be used to describe pain. From the list below, please circle those words that best describe the pain you are currently experiencing. Use only one word from each category. You do not need to mark a word in every category -- **Only mark those words that most accurately describe your pain.**

1.	2.	3.	4.
Flickering	Jumping	Pricking	Sharp
Quivering	Flashing	Boring	Cutting
Pulsing	Shooting	Drilling	Lacerating
Throbbing		Stabbing	
Beating			
Pounding			

5.	6.	7.	8.
Pinching	Tugging	Hot	Tingling
Pressing	Pulling	Burning	Itchy
Gnawing	Wrenching	Scalding	Smarting
Cramping		Searing	Stinging
Crushing			

9.	10.	11.	12.
Dull	Tender	Tiring	Sickening
Sore	Taut	Exhausting	Suffocating
Hurting	Rasping		
Aching			
Heavy			

13.	14.	15.	16.
Fearful	Punishing	Wretched	Annoying
Frightful	Grueling	Blinding	Troublesome
Terrifying	Cruel		Miserable
	Vicious		Intense
	Killing		Unbearable

17.	18.	19.	20.
Spreading	Tight	Cool	Nagging
Radiating	Numb	Cold	Nauseating
Penetrating	Drawing	Freezing	Agonizing
Piercing	Squeezing		Dreadful
	Tearing		Torturing

FIGURE 2–11   **Adaptation of the McGill Pain Questionnaire.** This multipart instrument is often used during the patient's first visit. In part A the patient is asked to localize the area(s) of pain and indicate if the source of the discomfort is superficial (external) or deep (internal). The pain rating index, Part B, is used to assess the level and nature of the patient's pain. These words are categorized as somatic (groups 1 to 10), affective (11 to 15), evaluative (16), and miscellaneous (17 to 20). Please refer to the text for instructions on scoring this portion of the questionnaire. Many McGill Pain Questionnaires also contain a visual analogue scale similar to that presented in Figure 2–9.

PLACEBO EFFECT

Placebo, stemming from the Latin word for "I shall please," is the term used to describe pain reduction obtained through mechanisms other than those related to the physiological effects of the treatment. The placebo effect is linked to a psychological mechanism whereby, if the patient thinks that the treatment is beneficial, a degree of pain reduction occurs.

All therapeutic modalities have some degree of placebo effect. This effect may be increased when the modality is applied with a sense of enthusiasm and faith. Indeed, most studies involving the use of a sham therapeutic modality (e.g., an ultrasound unit with the intensity set to zero) and an actual treatment have shown decreased levels of pain in each group. The placebo effect is so powerful that, in one instance, patients who received sugar pills but who were told that they were taking a specific medication, actually displayed the side effects of the medication.[33]

The placebo effect can be exploited in the application of therapeutic modalities. Changing modalities and new approaches in the treatment of an injury can positively influence the patient's perception and result in decreased pain.

REFERRED PAIN

Many times clinicians are faced with a patient who is complaining about pain in an area where no clinical signs of injury are exhibited. This phenomenon, known as referred pain, may be described as the brain's error in localizing the source of the noxious input[30] or as "displaced" pain.[56]

Mechanisms involved in referred pain may occur because the pain fibers emerging from the injured site split into several branches within the spinal cord. Some of these branches make contact with other branches that carry only painful impulses. The rest connect with sensory nerve pathways arising from the skin. During this cross-branching, the signals become mixed up, causing the brain to misinterpret the true source of the noxious stimulus.[57]

An example of referred pain is seen when a nerve root is pinched. Pinching of the nerve produces a burning and aching sensation that radiates away from the vertebral column. Although the actual damage has occurred close to the spinal cord, the pain is perceived in the person's arm, leg, or trunk (depending on the location of the nerve root impinged on).

Trigger points are hypersensitive areas that form within muscle or connective tissue. The term "trigger point" was coined because pressure on these spots resulted in the "triggering" of referred pain.[56] These areas result from macrotrauma or microtrauma, postural abnormalities, or psychological stress, and send noxious impulses to the brain, which misinterprets the location and intensity of the stimulus. This type of pain does not follow normal sensory distribution patterns, such as those of the *dermatomes* (Fig. 2–12), so the sensation is felt in an area other than the actual location of the trigger point (see Appendix A).

Dermatome: A segmental skin area supplied by a single nerve root.

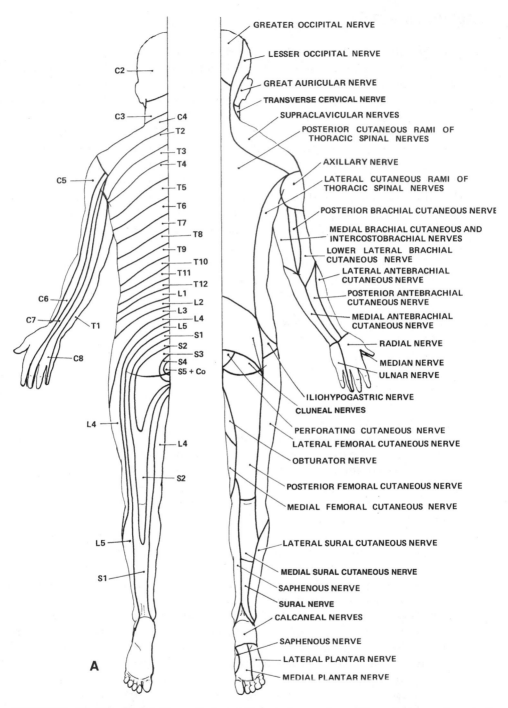

GREATER OCCIPITAL NERVE

LESSER OCCIPITAL NERVE

GREAT AURICULAR NERVE

TRANSVERSE CERVICAL NERVE

SUPRACLAVICULAR NERVES

POSTERIOR CUTANEOUS RAMI OF
THORACIC SPINAL NERVES

AXILLARY NERVE

LATERAL CUTANEOUS RAMI OF
THORACIC SPINAL NERVES

POSTERIOR BRACHIAL CUTANEOUS NERVE

MEDIAL BRACHIAL CUTANEOUS AND
INTERCOSTOBRACHIAL NERVES

LOWER LATERAL BRACHIAL
CUTANEOUS NERVE

LATERAL ANTEBRACHIAL
CUTANEOUS NERVE

POSTERIOR ANTEBRACHIAL
CUTANEOUS NERVE

MEDIAL ANTEBRACHIAL
CUTANEOUS NERVE

RADIAL NERVE

MEDIAN NERVE

ULNAR NERVE

ILIOHYPOGASTRIC NERVE

CLUNEAL NERVES

PERFORATING CUTANEOUS NERVE

LATERAL FEMORAL CUTANEOUS NERVE

OBTURATOR NERVE

POSTERIOR FEMORAL CUTANEOUS NERVE

MEDIAL FEMORAL CUTANEOUS NERVE

LATERAL SURAL CUTANEOUS NERVE

MEDIAL SURAL CUTANEOUS NERVE

SAPHENOUS NERVE

SURAL NERVE

CALCANEAL NERVES

SAPHENOUS NERVE

LATERAL PLANTAR NERVE

MEDIAL PLANTAR NERVE

FIGURE 2–12   **The Body's Dermatomes.** (*A*) Anterior surface, (*B*) posterior surface. Individual areas of the skin are innervated by a single spinal nerve root and may be further divided by individual nerves supplying the area. (From Gilman, S and Newman, SW: Manter and Gatz's Essentials of Clinical Neuroanatomy and Neurophysiology, ed 9. FA Davis, Philadelphia, 1996, pp 49, 50, with permission.)

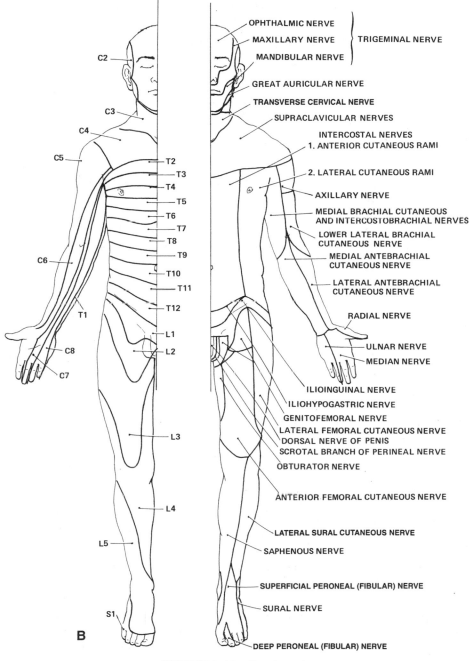

FIGURE 2–12 Continued.

Although referred pain may appear to be haphazard and random, it does have some logical, orderly constructs. Pain from within the abdomen and/or thorax is generally projected outward to the corresponding cutaneous dermatomes. Examples of this are demonstrated in the symptoms of heart attacks or a ruptured spleen or kidney. When the trigger point lies in the extremity, pain tends to be referred distally, rather than proximally, to the true source of the pain.

Table 2–7 **Characteristics of Chronic Pain**

Symptoms last longer than 6 months
Few objective medical findings
Medication abuse
Difficulty in sleeping
Depression
Manipulative behavior
Somatic preoccupation

Clinicians must perform a careful, thorough history and evaluation of patients who are suffering from symptoms of referred pain. Ultimately, the underlying pathology of the pain should be clear before treatment is prescribed. In cases in which the true cause of the pain is suspect, or if there is uncertainty of the nature of the pain, the patient should be referred to a physician for further evaluation. Ultimately, you don't want to be treating a painful hip when the pathology is in the low back.

CHRONIC PAIN

Pain extending beyond the normal course of an injury or illness is considered chronic. A benchmark time frame for determining chronic pain is 6 months after the injury.[58,59] Individuals suffering from chronic pain live in a world where the pain dictates their lives, and they develop a pattern of pain behavior (Table 2–7). In these cases, pain can no longer be considered merely a symptom. It is a disease in itself.[60] Chronic pain may be considered a learned response in which a positive feedback loop is formed in the spinal cord.[61]

This produces a mechanism in which the spinal gate remains open because of an imbalance between the stimuli allowed to enter the gate. The input accepted from the large-diameter (nonpain) fibers is less than the input accepted from the small-diameter (pain) fibers.

Treatment regimens for acute pain problems are ineffective and often *contraindicated* when applied to patients suffering from chronic pain.[62] The goal in the treatment of chronic pain is to break the positive feedback loop and essentially "unlearn" the pain. Exercise may increase an individual's endorphin level, assisting in the reduction of chronic pain. Also, exercise may affect the patient's perception of pain simply by distracting the attention from the pain to the exercise.[63] The importance of guidance by a licensed physician in the treatment of chronic pain to ensure the absence of an advanced underlying disease state cannot be understated.

PAIN MANAGEMENT TECHNIQUES

Pain management techniques may be classified as physical, behavioral, or cognitive. Healthcare practitioners tend to focus their pain control programs on physi-

---

Contraindicate: To make inadvisable.

cal means using therapeutic modalities.[64] A comprehensive pain management plan should encompass all three techniques.

The physical measures used to control pain include thermal, electrical, and mechanical modalities; medication; and surgery. This text focuses on the use of therapeutic modalities to control the effects of both injury and pain.

Behavioral and cognitive approaches to pain management may be implemented by decreasing the individual's anxiety about the injury. Explaining the effects and sensations of the treatment and using soothing or distracting stimuli move attention away from the pain. These first elements require that the clinician communicate with the patient and attempt to remove the fear of the unknown. The use of stereo headphones, television, books, conversation, or any other similar device may distract the patient's attention from the pain of the injury or discomfort caused by the treatment.

A full understanding of the differences between symptomatic and curative treatments is also required. Techniques that address only the pain associated with the injury (electrical stimulation, medication, and so on) have little influence on the injury itself. Most treatment regimens are designed to reduce the physical damage resulting from the injury and thus truly relieve the cause of the pain.

SUMMARY

Pain is a multitentacled beast that is ingrained throughout our bodies. Rather than being a "simple" physiological stimulus-response entity, pain, pain perception, and the reaction to pain involve physiological, psychological, cognitive, and affective components. Likewise, cultural, social, and other factors influence the behavioral reaction to pain.

Injured tissues transmit painful impulses along A-delta and C fibers. Once in the dorsal horn of the spinal cord, these impulses are transmitted to higher processing centers along the STT. One portion of this tract, the NSTT, is responsible for the discrimination of the type and intensity of the pain and the pain's location in the body. The second part of the STT, the PSTT, is responsible for the physiological and psychological reaction to the stimulus.

Although pain is an individual event that is inherently subjective in nature, it can be quantitatively and qualitatively measured with a reasonable degree of accuracy. The Visual Analogue Scale, McGill Pain Questionnaire, and other tests provide a unique view of an individual's perception of pain, although caution should be used when attempting to correlate one person's pain with another's.

With therapeutic modalities, pain can be controlled through one of two mechanisms. The better of these is to restore the body's homeostasis and provide the optimal environment for healing to occur. Once the inflammatory process subsides and the mechanical and chemical stimulation of the nociceptors has ceased, pain should be eliminated. Modalities may also be used to effect the transmission of the painful impulses. As we will see throughout this text, heat, cold, electrical stimulation, and other therapeutic techniques can be used to disrupt the pain process.

In certain cases, the pain experienced by the patient is not related to underlying tissue trauma, or the location of the pain is not associated with the area of tissue trauma. These cases require keen evaluative skills and atypical treatment protocols.

Chapter Quiz

1. Which of the following chemicals is the primary activator of nociception?
   A. Histamine
   B. Arachidonic acid
   C. Potassium
   D. Bradykinins

2. Which of the following chemicals is the precursor of prostaglandin?
   A. Cyclooxygenase
   B. Arachidonic acid
   C. Phospholipase
   D. Dopamine

3. Where in the body is substance P produced?
   A. Substantia gelatinosa
   B. Anterior commissure
   C. Peripheral afferent nerves
   D. Dorsal root ganglia

4. The change of a chemical stimulus to an electrical action potential is termed:
   A. Nociception
   B. Myelination
   C. Saltatory conduction
   D. Transaction

5. A typical noxious stimulus activates _____ percent of the A-delta fibers and _____ percent of the C fibers.
   A. 10 to 25 percent/50 to 80 percent
   B. 5 to 8 percent/10 to 30 percent
   C. 60 to 80 percent/15 to 30 percent
   D. 100 percent/100 percent

6. Which of the following types of nerves is polymodal?
   A. A-alpha
   B. A-beta
   C. A-delta
   D. C fibers

7. Which of the following types of nerves creates epicritic pain?
   A. A-alpha
   B. A-beta
   C. A-delta
   D. C fibers

8. Which of the following nerve fibers is responsible for producing protopathic pain?
   A. A-alpha
   B. A-beta

C. A-delta

D. C fibers

9. Which of the following laminae is also referred to as the substantia gelatinosa?
   A. I
   B. II
   C. V
   D. X

10. In which of the following laminae do the primary first-order nociceptive fibers terminate?
    A. II
    B. I and II
    C. I and V
    D. VII and X

11. According to the gate control theory of pain modulation, what structure monitors the activity of the incoming nerves and subsequently opens or closes the gate?
    A. T cell
    B. Dorsal horn
    C. Paleospinothalamic tract
    D. Substantia gelatinosa

12. The forces that initiate the transmission of noxious impulses are:

    A. _____

    B. _____

13. Describe the techniques that can be used to decrease a patient's perception of pain.

REFERENCES

1. Lester, D and Yang, B: An approach for examining the rationality of suicide. Psychol Rep 79:405, 1996.
2. Orbach, I: Dissociation, physical pain, and suicide: A hypothesis. Suicide Life Threat Behav 24:68, 1994.
3. Fishbain, DA: Completed suicide in chronic pain. Clin J Pain 7:29, 1991.
4. Roeser, WM, et al: The use of transcutaneous nerve stimulation for pain control in athletic medicine. A preliminary report. Am J Sports Med 4:210, 1976.
5. Monks, R and Taenzer, P: A comprehensive pain questionnaire. In Melzack, R (ed): Pain Measurement and Assessment. Raven Press, New York, 1983, pp 233–237.
6. Garron, D and Leavitt, F: Demographic and affective covariates of pain. Psychosom Med 41:525, 1979.
7. Zombroski, M: Cultural components in response to pain. Journal of Social Issues 8:15–35, 1952.
8. Zola, I: Culture and Symptoms: An analysis of patients presenting complaints. American Social Review 31:615, 1966.
9. Halvorson, GA: Therapeutic heat and cold for athletic injuries. Physician and Sportsmedicine 18:88, 1990.
10. Wilkerson, GB: Inflammation in connective tissue: Etiology and management. Athletic Training 20:298, 1985.
11. Walsh, DL: Nociceptive pathways: Relevance to the physiotherapist. Physiothcrapy 77:317, 1991.
12. Bonica, JJ, et al: Biochemistry and the modulation of nociception and pain. In Bonica, JJ (ed): The Management of Pain, ed 2. Lea & Febiger, Philadelphia, 1990, pp 95–121.

13. Insel, PA: Analgesics, antipyretics and antiinflammatory agents: Drugs employed in the treatment of rheumatoid arthritis and gout. In Gilman, AG, et al (eds): The Pharmacological Basis of Therapeutics, ed 8. Pergamon Press, New York, 1990, pp 638–681.

14. Chapman, CR: Pain, perception and illusion. In Sternbach, RA (ed): The Psychology of Pain. Raven Press, New York, 1986, pp 153–180.

15. Bowsher, D: Central pain mechanisms. In Wells, PE, Frampton, V, and Bowsher, D (eds): Pain Management in Physical Therapy. Appleton & Lange, Norwalk, CT, 1988, p 22–29.

16. Price, DD: Psychological and Neural Mechanisms of Pain. Raven Press, New York, 1988.

17. Melzack, R: The Puzzle of Pain. Basic Books, New York, 1973.

18. Bonica, JJ: Anatomic and physiologic basis of nociception and pain. In Bonica JJ (ed): The Management of Pain (ed 2). Lea & Febiger, Philadelphia, 1990, pp 28–94.

19. Guyton, AC: Textbook of Medical Physiology, ed 6. WB Saunders, Philadelphia, 1980.

20. Willis, WD: The pain system: The neural basis of nociceptive transmission in the mammalian nervous system. In Gildenberg, PL (ed): Pain and Headache. Karger, New York, 1985, pp 77–92.

21. Melzack, R and Wall, PD: The gate control theory of pain. In Soulairac, A, Cahn, J, and Carpentier, J (eds): Pain: Proceedings of the International Symposium on Pain. Academic Press, London, 1968.

22. Wallace, KG: The physiology of pain. Critical Care Nursing Quarterly 15(2):1–13, 1992.

23. Clark, RG: Essentials of Clinical Neuroanatomy and Neurophysiology. FA Davis, Philadelphia, 1975.

24. Mitchell, GAG and Mayor, D: The Essentials of Neuroanatomy, ed 4. Churchill Livingstone, London, 1989.

25. Melzack, R: Neurophysiology foundations of pain. In Sternbach, RA (ed): The Psychology of Pain. Raven Press, New York, 1986, pp 1–24.

26. Procacci, P and Maresca, M: Advances in Pain Research and Therapy. Raven Press, New York, 1984, pp 1–12.

27. Melzack, R and Wall, PD: Pain mechanisms: A new theory. Science 150:971–979, 1965.

28. Pavlov, IP: Conditioned Reflexes. Milford, Oxford, 1927.

29. Beecher, HK: Pain in men wounded in battle. Ann Surg 123:96, 1946.

30. Newton, RA: Contemporary views on pain and the role played by thermal agents in managing pain systems. In Michlovitz, S (ed): Thermal Agents in Rehabilitation, ed 2. FA Davis, Philadelphia, 1990, p. 20.

31. Castel, JC: Pain Management with Acupuncture and Transcutaneous Electrical Nerve Stimulation Techniques. Pain Control Services, Lake Bluff, IL, 1979.

32. Buxton, BP and Perrin, DP: The relationship between personality characteristics and pain response. Journal of Sport Rehabilitation 1:111, 1992.

33. French, S: Pain: Some physiological and sociological aspects. Physiotherapy 75:255, 1989.

34. Unruh, AM: Gender variations in clinical pain experience. Pain 65:2, 1996.

35. Ellermeier, W and Westphal, W: Gender differences in pain ratings and pupil reactions to painful pressure stimuli. Pain 61:435, 1995.

36. Fillingim, RB and Maixner, W: The influence of resting blood pressure and gender on pain response. Psychosom Med 58:326, 1996.

37. Nguyen, P, Lee, SD, and Castell, DO: Evidence of gender differences in esophageal pain threshold. Am J Gastroenterol 90:901, 1995.

38. Karchnick, KL, et al: Gender differences in pain threshold, tolerance and anxiety. Journal of Athletic Training 32:S44, 1997.

39. Weir, R, et al: Gender differences in psychosocial adjustment to chronic pain and expenditures for health care services used. Clin J Pain 12:277, 1996.

40. Vallerand, AH: Gender differences in pain. Image J Nurs Sch 27:235, 1995.

41. Lord, RH and Kozar, B: Pain tolerance in the presence of others: Implications for youth sports. Physician and Sportsmedicine 17:71, 1989.

42. Solsona, AM, et al: Relationship between acute pain and pain anxiety. Journal of Athletic Training 32:S43, 1997.

43. Buxton, BP, et al: Pain and ethnicity in athletes. Journal of Sport Rehabilitation 2:13, 1993.

44. Hall, EG and Davies, S: Gender differences in perceived intensity and affect of pain between athletes and non-athletes. Percept Mot Skills 73:779, 1991.

45. Jarmenko, ME, Silbert, I, and Mann, I: The differential ability of athletes and non-athletes to cope with two types of pain: A radical behavioral model. Psychological Record 31:265, 1981.

46. Newman, S: Dealing with pain. Coaching Review 6:25, 1983.

47. Walker, J: Pain distraction in athletes and non-athletes. Percept Mot Skills 33:1187, 1971.
48. Yamaguchi, AY, et al: Difference in pain response and anxiety between athletes and non-athletes. Journal of Athletic Training 32:S45, 1997.
49. Ryan, ED and Kovacic, CR: Pain tolerance and athletic participation. Percept Mot Skills 22:383, 1966.
50. Tajet-Foxell, B and Rose, FD: Pain and pain tolerance in professional ballet dancers. Br J Sports Med 29:31, 1995.
51. Scott, V and Gijsbers, K: Pain perception in competitive swimmers. BMJ 282:91, 1981.
52. Hussisson, EC: Visual analogue scales. In Melzack, R (ed): Pain Management and Assessment. Raven Press, New York, 1983.
53. Melzack, R: The McGill Pain Questionnaire: Major properties and scoring methods. Pain 1:277, 1975.
54. Bowsher, D: Acute and chronic pain and assessment. In Wells, PE, Frampton, V, and Bowsher, D (eds): Pain Management in Physical Therapy. Appleton & Lange, Norwalk, CT, 1988, pp 39–44.
55. Smith, GM, et al: An experimental pain method sensitive to morphine in man: The submaximal tourniquet technique. J Pharmacol Exp Therap 154:324, 1966.
56. Travell, JG and Simons, DG: Myofascial Pain and Dysfunction: The Trigger Point Manual. Williams & Wilkins, Baltimore, 1983.
57. Ottoson, D and Lundeberg, T: Pain Treatment by Transcutaneous Electrical Nerve Stimulation: A Practical Manual. Springer-Verlag, New York, 1988.
58. DeVahl, J: Neuromuscular electrical stimulation (NMES) in rehabilitation. In Gersh, MR (ed): Electrotherapy in Rehabilitation. FA Davis, Philadelphia, 1992, pp 218–268.
59. Spengler, DM, Loeser, JD, and Murphy, TM. Orthopaedic aspects of the chronic pain syndrome. In The American Academy of Orthopaedic Surgeons Instructional Course Lectures, Vol 29. CV Mosby, St. Louis, 1980, p 101.
60. Cailliet, R: Soft Tissue Pain and Disability. FA Davis, Philadelphia, 1977.
61. Smoller, BM and Schulman, BM: Chronic pain: Prevention through early intervention. Occup Health Saf 50:14, 1981.
62. Russell, B, et al: Repair of injured skeletal muscle: A molecular approach. Med Sci Sports Exerc 24:189, 1992.
63. Raithel, KS: Chronic pain and exercise therapy. Physician and Sportsmedicine 17:204, 1989.
64. Singer, RN and Johnson, PJ: Strategies to cope with pain associated with sports-related injuries. Athletic Training 22:100, 1987.

CHAPTER 3

Development and Delivery of Treatment Protocol

Jeff Ryan, PT, ATC

This chapter presents an overview of the decision-making process used in developing treatment plans and modality selection. Using the problem-solving approach, it presents the student with a series of case studies that reinforce the decision-making process. Administrative concerns as they relate to the delivery to treatment and rehabilitation programs are also discussed.

This text began by explaining that therapeutic modalities are used to create the proper environment for healing. Recall that many components of the injury response process are intertwined. Edema causes pain, pain causes spasm, and spasm causes pain. Although pain may be the patient's primary complaint, simply focusing your treatments on pain relief does little to resolve the underlying cause of the discomfort and the associated dysfunction. Approaching the patient's problems on a purely symptomatic basis often produces unsatisfactory results.

The ability to plan a treatment and rehabilitation program is perhaps the most complex skill that rehabilitation clinicians must master. This process integrates physical evaluation skills and knowledge of pathology with knowledge of applicable therapeutic techniques and principles, goal setting, and patient motivation and education. No one source is sufficient to gain proficiency in this skill. It is as much an art as it is a science, and your ability in this area will grow and be perfected with experience.

The problem-solving approach (PSA) is a logic-based technique used in developing the patient's treatment plan to achieve a long-term goal. Although "logical thinking" is something that we usually do not do consciously, we practice it as a part of our daily routine. It may involve such basic skills as getting dressed in the morning or more complicated tasks such as finding one's way around an unfamiliar city for a job interview. Either way, logical thinking is involved. The PSA extends this logical thinking into the treatment of the patient.

THE PROBLEM-SOLVING APPROACH

As described in Chapter 1, each individual responds to trauma differently. This fact alone should illustrate the need to treat each patient differently, based on his or her own needs. When based on *normative data,* generalized treatment protocols provide a reference point for determining where the patient "should be" and what treatment approaches can be used. Pre-established treatment protocols should not be viewed as, or used as, unyielding individual treatment plans. Individual treatment plans differentiate the specifics of each patient's case and lead to a more efficient and successful outcome.

The PSA describes an ongoing process of evaluation, analysis, and planning and is comprised of four steps: (1) recognition of the patient's problems, (2) prioritization of the problems, (3) goal setting, and (4) treatment planning (Table 3–1). To illustrate each of these components, an ongoing case study is presented throughout this chapter and continued in Chapters 4 through 7. Case studies also appear at the end of the chapter. Although the focus of this text is on therapeutic modalities, the role of these devices is to prepare the patient for therapeutic exer-

TABLE 3–1 **Components of the Problem-Solving Approach**

Component	Purpose
Recognition of the problems	Identify the type and depth of the involved tissues
	Identify the nature of the pathology
	Determine the stage of healing
	Recognize any contraindications to the use of modalities or exercises
Prioritization of the problems	Develop the logical treatment order based on a cause-and-effect relationship between the pathology and the signs and symptoms
Goal setting	Develop structure and sequence in the treatment plan
Treatment planning	Determine the modalities and exercises to be used and their sequence based on the patient's problems and treatment goals

---

Normative data: Information that can be used to describe a specific population.

cise and manual techniques. Modalities are also used after these techniques as a way of controlling exercise-induced inflammation.

Just as important as "knowing what you know" is "knowing what you don't know." Regardless of expertise and the number of years of experience, not every clinician is capable of managing every condition. Clinicians should not hesitate to seek the input and advice of others who possess more knowledge or have more experience managing a specific condition. The knowledge of when to refer a patient to a more appropriate rehabilitation setting or to another healthcare or medical professional should be considered a high ethical priority. This is also an important element in your learning process.

CASE STUDY 1

Scenario

A 22-year-old woman diagnosed as having patellofemoral pain syndrome after an anterior cruciate ligament (ACL) reconstruction of the right knee has been referred to you by an orthopedic surgeon for evaluation, treatment, and rehabilitation. The following information has been obtained from the patient and the patient's medical records:

Chief complaint: The patient reports intermittent pain "under her right kneecap" that increases when she goes up or down stairs and occasionally after long periods of sitting. The pain and the reported sensation that her knee "gives out" from time to time prohibit the patient from participating in a recreational soccer league or other strenuous activities.

History: While participating in a recreational soccer game, the patient twisted her knee while her foot remained planted on the ground, resulting in a complete tear of the ACL and a medial meniscus tear. She underwent ACL reconstruction with a bone-patellar tendon-bone autograft and had a partial medial menisectomy. She returned to play her senior season of intercollegiate soccer at $4\frac{1}{2}$ months after the surgery. Midway through the season she developed her present symptoms, and they have persisted intermittently for 9 months.

Diagnostic tests: Physician-ordered postsurgical x-rays and *magnetic resonance imaging* (MRI) scan of the knee joint were interpreted as normal.

Activity: The patient is now working for an accounting firm. She participates in adult league soccer, skates on roller blades, and works out lifting weights three times a week.

General medical conditions: No significant illnesses.

Medications: Nonsteroidal antiinflammatory drugs.

Contraindications to modality use: None.

Contraindications to therapeutic exercise: Painful arc of motion.

Patient goals: Pain-free *activities of daily living (ADLs)*. To return to recreational soccer competition.

Magnetic resonance image (MRI): A view of the body's internal structures obtained through the use of magnetic and radio fields.

Activities of daily living (ADLs): Fundamental skills that are required for a certain lifestyle, including mobility, self-care, and grooming.

Evaluation findings:

Function:	The patient cannot play soccer because of anterior knee pain.
	The patient cannot climb or descend stairs without pain.
	The patient cannot sit for more than 30 minutes without developing knee pain.
Observation:	One healed incision over the patellar tendon. *Keloid* formation is present.
Patellar mobility:	The patella is hypomobile superiorly. *Medial glide* is one quadrant, indicating tightness of the lateral *retinaculum* and *infrapatellar* scar formation. Inferior and lateral glides are within normal limits (WNL).
Patellar tracking:	The involved patella demonstrates increased lateral tracking relative to the opposite side.
	Moderate *crepitus* is felt.
Range of Motion:	Involved: $-2°$ of extension to $135°$ of flexion $(0° - 2° - 135°)$
	Uninvolved: $5°$ of hyperextension to $145°$ of flexion $(5° - 0° - 145°$.
Girth:	The girth of the involved knee is 1 cm greater than that of the uninvolved knee as measured over the joint line. Mild effusion is present.
Tone:	The patient displays poor control of the quadriceps muscle group. The vastus medius oblique (VMO) lacks tone and mass compared with that on the uninvolved side.
Strength:	Hip muscle groups are 5/5.
	Quadriceps are strong (5/5), but pain is elicited at the patellofemoral joint during maximum contraction.
	Hamstring groups are 5/5.
	Ankle groups are 5/5.
Flexibility:	All hip muscles are WNL.
	The quadriceps muscle is tight, demonstrating prone knee flexion to $125°$.
	Hamstrings are tight. The knee lacks $10°$ of extension with the hip at $90°$.
	Gastrocnemius and soleus muscles are tight. The ankle can be dorsiflexed only to $10°$ while the knee is extended.
Pain rating:	Patient describes pain as 5/10 when she is descending stairs, 1/10 while sitting.

Keloid: A nodular, firm, movable, and tender mass of dense, irregularly distributed collagen scar tissue in the dermis and subcutaneous tissue. Common in the African-American population, keloid scarring tends to occur after trauma or surgery.

Medial glide: The American Association of Orthopedic Surgeons (AAOS) evaluation technique of patellar mobility identifies two quadrants as normal.

Retinaculum: A fibrous membrane that holds an organ or body part in place.

Infrapatellar: The distal portion of the patella including the patellar tendon.

Crepitus: A grinding or crunching sound or sensation.

Special tests: Biomechanical	All demonstrate negative results.
analysis:	Feet excessively *pronate* (bilaterally) during walking gait. Shortened stance phase on the involved side.
Palpation:	The scar over the patellar tendon is adhered to the underlying tissues. Pain is produced during palpation along the medial retinaculum and at the inferior patellar pole.

Recognition of the Problems

Let's begin by stating the obvious: To provide proper care, you must know what condition(s) you are treating. However, again recalling the introduction to Chapter 1, you are treating more than a "sprained ankle." This stage of the PSA is designed to identify the type of tissues involved (e.g., anatomy, function, size, depth), the nature and effects of the pathology (e.g., pain, decreased range of motion (ROM), strength loss), and the stage of the healing process (e.g., acute inflammation, proliferation, maturation) (Table 3–2).

Each type of tissue responds differently to various modalities. The biological properties and functions of the traumatized tissues, their depth below the skin, and their stage in the inflammation and healing process dictate which modalities can effectively stimulate them. The use of a superficial modality to treat structures that are located deep within the tissues may produce little or no benefit. The application of a modality that accelerates the inflammatory response on tissues that are already actively inflamed can result in further cell destruction.

Begin the problem identification by reviewing any existing medical records describing the course of the patient's condition. Valuable information can be obtained from the records written by clinicians who have previously cared for the patient, including treatment notes, operative reports, diagnostic test reports, and the physician's prescription or referral notes. Other sources of information can include preparticipation medical examinations and notes pertaining to prior evaluation and treatment of unrelated conditions. All potential contraindications to treatment approaches, devices, and modalities should also be identified. Formal patient evaluations and re-evaluations should be conducted at timely intervals. Less detailed patient interviews should be performed before each treatment session to identify the patient's physical and mental status as well as to gain the patient's overall perspective on the treatment protocol.

TABLE 3–2 **Information Gained during the Patient Evaluation**

Subjective information (e.g., chief complaint, medical history, medications, mechanism of injury)
Nature of the trauma
Type of tissues involved
Stage of injury response
Patient goals
Contraindications to proposed modalities, exercises, and manual techniques

Pronation (Pronate): An inward flattening and tilting of the foot, resulting in the lowering of the medial longitudinal arch.

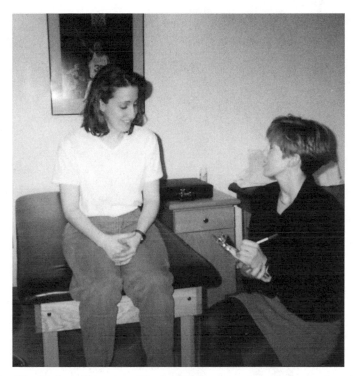

FIGURE 3–1   **The Patient Interview.** Much of the success in treatment planning lies in effective communication between the patient and the clinician.

A wealth of *subjective* information can be obtained during both the formal patient interview and during informal discussion (Fig. 3–1). Good clinical skills require keen listening skills and the ability to identify and solicit pertinent information offered by the patient. For instance, a patient comment such as "I am unable to tuck my shirt tail in" can identify restricted internal glenohumeral rotation.

FIGURE 3–2   **Return to Function after Injury.** The return to the preinjury level of activity follows a progressive sequence in which one level of function must be obtained before progressing to the next level.

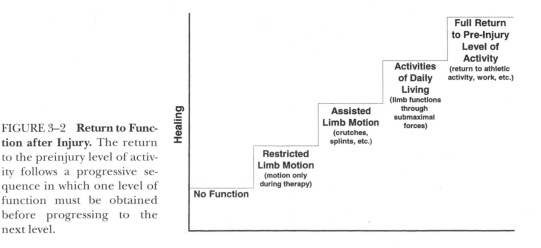

Subjective: Symptoms stated by the patient that are not externally apparent, such as pain. Personal beliefs and attitudes may alter subjective symptoms.

TABLE 3-3 Tools Used in the Evaluation of Orthopedic Injuries

Tool	How Measured	Information Gained
Subjective information	Active listening and note taking on the subjective information offered by the athlete, coach, teammates, and others.	(1) Injury mechanism, (2) inflammation based on reports of pain, swelling, warmth, etc., (3) functional limitations, and (4) treatment considerations based on previous successful or unsuccessful protocol.
Active range of motion	Goniometric measurement or a percentage of full movement in the case of the spine. This information can be used in terms of the raw values or relative to the opposite side.	Ability to move actively or passively with reference to specific motions.
Resisted range of motion (strength)	Measurement by manual muscle test using a grading scale, a hand-held *dynamometer*, or an isokinetic device. May also use descriptors describing the neuromuscular function and integrity of the involved tissues: strong and pain-free (normal), strong and painful (tendinitis), weak and painful (musculotendinous tear), or weak and pain-free (musculotendinous tear or neurological involvement).	Indication of the strength deficits of a muscle or group of muscles. Can also determine injury to a muscle or tendon by eliciting pain and/or weakness associated with contraction of the muscle or muscle group.
Edema/effusion	Circumferential measurement with a tape measure around specific landmarks or *volumetric measurement* in the case of a distal extremity.	Indication of the presence of swelling or edema relative to the opposite extremity.
Weight-bearing status	Measurement as full, partial, or non-weight bearing. Can also be described as a percentage of full weight bearing.	Ability of the patient to bear weight in the presence of pain, swelling, weakness, and/or decreased range of motion.
Atrophy or *hypertrophy*	Circumferential measurement with a tape measure and result compared with that for opposite extremity.	Determination of the decrease or increase of tissue mass. Note that there is little correlation between limb girth and strength.
Pain	Pain rating scale of 0 to 10, with 0 being no pain and 10 being the worst pain imaginable.	Presence of pain with a specific functional activity (squatting), movement (shoulder flexion), special test (valgus stress to the elbow), or at rest. Ratings can be used for a single patient but cannot be compared with those of other patients.
Deep tendon reflex	Grading system in an orthopedic population: 0 = absent, 1 = *hyporeflexia*, 2 = normal.	Determination of the functional level of the reflex arc.
Sensation	Light touch to bilateral areas of the body having the same dermatomal or specific nerve distributions.	Assessment of the function of the sensory nervous system. Note that dermatomal distributions may vary greatly from person to person.

Joint mobilization	Evaluation of the accessory motions found in joints. Graded as *hypomobile*, normal, and *hypermobile*.
	Determination of the presence of adequate accessory motion needed to produce normal physiological motion.
Balance and proprioception	Timed test of the ability to balance or successfully determine joint position compared to the contralateral limb or normative data. Can be a simple stance test, replication of joint position test, or use of a balance assessment system.
	Determination of the function of the proprioceptive receptors in a joint.
Flexibility	Assessment of muscle length by fixing one end of the muscle and moving the other end until maximum length is reached. Can sometimes be measured goniometrically or assessed as normal or tight compared to ranges of normative data.
	Determination of whether a muscle or muscle group is functioning at a normal length or if it is producing abnormal stresses because of tightness.
Posture	Inspection and observation of posture and comparison with normative information.
	Assessment of abnormal stresses put on tissues by poor postural control or habits. Such stresses can cause pain or paresthesia.
Special tests	Use of tests designed to (1) elicit pain in the presence of pathology, (2) laxity in ligaments, or (3) the integrity of structures, etc.
	Determination of clinical function and degree of pathology.
Biomechanical assessment	Observation and measurement of biomechanical problems that can alter function. It may be performed as a specific measurement (leg length) or observed as a part of a functional activity (gait analysis).
	Determination of the causes of abnormal stresses placed on the body by inherent biomechanical problems. Sometimes the effects of these problems can be decreased or eliminated with exercise or the use of *orthotics*.
Function	Measurement as the capability of a patient to perform activities of daily living at work or home as well as sport-specific function.
	Determination of the amount of function the patient has with regard to a specific injury.

Dynamometer: A device used for measuring muscular strength.
Volumetric measurement: Determination of the size of a body part by measuring the amount of water it displaces.
Hypertrophy: To develop an increase in bulk, for example, in the cross-sectional area of muscle.
Hyporeflexia: Diminished function of the reflexes.
Hypomobile: An abnormal limitation of normal motion.
Hypermobile: An abnormally large amount of motion.
Orthotics: The use of orthopedic devices for correcting deformity or malalignment.

Likewise, complaints of feeling "worse" after therapy may indicate that the exercise and/or treatment protocol was too intense. When applicable, these remarks should be noted in the patient's medical file.

The temptation often exists to focus on observable signs, such as swelling, discoloration, decreased ROM, and the reported symptoms of pain, numbness, and so on. Although the short-term objective of any given treatment session is to provide symptomatic relief, the long-term goal of proper healing and return to a normal lifestyle will not be met until the underlying pathology is identified and managed (Fig. 3–2). If we again consider the case of the patient who complains of pain during internal shoulder rotation, no permanent relief will be realized until the underlying biomechanical dysfunction is remedied. As we will see in the following sections, symptomatic treatments are required in the early treatment phases, but only as a transition to curative treatments.

A vast array of conditions may be identified during the evaluation process. Table 3–3 presents tools that are commonly used to identify these problems and common methods of measurement and provides an overview of the information

TABLE 3–4 Contraindications to the Use of Evaluative Tools

Tool	Contraindication
Subjective information	None.
Range of motion	Acute unstable injuries to ligaments, tendons, or bones.
Swelling or edema	None.
Strength	Acute unstable injuries to ligaments, tendons, or bones. Recent repairs of ligaments or tendons.
Weight-bearing status	None.
Atrophy or hypertrophy	None.
Pain	Caution should be exercised not to use a functional activity to assess pain that may compromise unstable or recently repaired tissues.
Deep tendon reflex	Recently repaired tendon.
Sensation	*Dementia* or disorientation.
Joint mobilization	Acute unstable injuries to ligaments, tendons, or bones. Recent repairs of ligaments or tendons, severe osteoporosis.
Balance and proprioception	Any contraindication to weight bearing on one leg.
Flexibility	Acute injuries to musculotendinous tissues.
Posture	None.
Special tests	Acute unstable injuries to ligaments, tendons, or bones. Recent repairs of ligaments or tendons.
Biomechanical analysis	Any analysis that would directly stress unstable or recently repaired structures.
Function	Any functional task that would directly stress unstable or recently repaired structures.

Dementia: The progressive loss of cognitive and intellectual functions without impairment of perception or consciousness. Symptoms include disorientation, memory impairment, impaired judgment, and impaired intellectual ability.

discerned from the measurements. The use of valid and reliable tools, correct measurement techniques, consistency during re-evaluation, and proper documentation of the results contribute to the accumulation of documented evidence of the patient's progress. These tools are not appropriate for every condition, and the patient may have one or more contraindications to their use (Table 3–4).

The patient's mental and emotional state should also be assessed. The patient should be educated regarding the nature of the injury, the treatment plan, and the goals. To maximize participation, the patient must be able to understand and comprehend the nature of the injury, the treatment plan, the treatment goals, and the expectations for recovery. The patient's motivational level must be assessed as well. Whereas some patients need to be held back because of their high motivation, others have to be continuously motivated to progress through their treatment plan. Patients who consistently lack motivation or display behavioral signs of disinterest in their recovery may need the assistance of a mental health care provider.

The information collected during evaluation and the treatment sessions should be identified and recorded in the patient's file using measurable and objective terms so that the patient's progress toward recovery can be documented over time. Although each treatment session should begin with a patient interview, a full re-evaluation of the patient's condition should be conducted at regular intervals (e.g., at the end of a goal period). Ongoing re-evaluation allows the patient's current state to be compared with baseline information. A determination can then be made as to whether the patient has improved as expected or if the treatment plan must be modified because of a lack of patient progress.

CASE STUDY 1

Recognition of the Problems

The following problems have been identified based on the information presented in the case study scenario:
1. Decreased ability to function without pain (i.e., ascending and descending stairs 5/10; sitting longer than 30 minutes yields 1/10 pain; inability to play soccer)
2. Poor patellar mobility and tracking secondary to muscular weakness and soft tissue adhesions, including the presence of a keloid
3. Increased swelling of the right knee as compared with the uninvolved knee
4. Decreased range of motion of the right knee
5. Decreased flexibility of the quadriceps, hamstrings, and calf muscles on the involved side as compared with the uninvolved side
6. Improper biomechanics of the right foot (pathological subtalar pronation)

Commentary

- The pain ratings given by the patient are important because pain indicates pathology and affects the individual's quality of life. Even though this patient is active, attention must be paid to the functional limitations affecting her daily life and work. Her relatively sedentary occupation contributes to her discomfort. Certainly she spends more time per week sitting at her desk, sitting in meetings, and going up and down stairs than she does exercising. Pain experienced during palpation should not be used to determine improvement in the patient because the amount of pressure applied to the area is not well controlled.

- The finding of joint effusion is significant. Accumulation of 20 to 30 mL of fluid within the knee joint capsule may cause inhibition of the vastus medialis, suggesting alteration of patellofemoral biomechanics leading to chronic inflammation.

- The ability to restore ROM this long after surgery may appear to be futile, but scar and tissue remodeling can remain active for 12 to 24 months. The chronic pain and swelling could indicate that the inflammation and remodeling phase is still active, increasing the possibility of restoring the tissue. Keep in mind that scarring, decreased patellar mobility, and muscle tightness negatively affect ROM. The loss of even a few degrees of ROM is problematic because of the biomechanical changes at the patellofemoral joint. This can lead to other biomechanical changes in both lower extremities caused by a length discrepancy that is created when the patient is weight bearing.

- Keloid formation along the incision on her patellar tendon and the findings of a hypomobile patella, decreased ROM, and chronic swelling may be indicative of *hypertrophic* scarring of the infrapatellar area. Abnormal patellofemoral joint biomechanics and patellofemoral pain are the most common complications after an accelerated ACL rehabilitation program. Normal tissue biomechanics must be restored before normal joint biomechanics can return and pain be decreased.

- Decreased flexibility of the quadriceps and hamstrings may cause increased stress on the knee joint capsule, retinaculum, and patellofemoral joint. The most common compensatory motion caused by tightness of the gastrocnemius and soleus is foot pronation, leading to increased tibial rotation and increased lateral forces on the patellofemoral joint.

- Even though the patient mentions that her knee "gives out," it is not listed as a problem because the results of all special tests were negative. In this case, the "giving out" sensation is most probably indicative of pain, quadriceps inhibition, or muscle weakness and will be resolved as these individual problems are addressed. If the patient continues to report this problem after strength has returned and swelling has decreased, ligamentous stability should be re-evaluated and/or the patient referred back to the physician.

Prioritization of the Problems

Prioritizing the patient's problems assists the clinician in developing the logical order of treatment. Determining the logical order of treatment requires an understanding of pathophysiology, the events associated with each stage of the healing process, and the beneficial effects (and the potentially hazardous effects) that

---

Hypertrophic: Increased in size.

each modality has on the injury response process. Prioritizing the problems based on their cause-and-effect relationship to the patient's chief complaints lends itself to developing an orderly treatment sequence, defining the focus of *self-treatment,* and maximizing the use of available treatment time. This method also helps prevent mistakes and allows the patient to return to the preinjury lifestyle in the safest, most expedient manner.

Multiple chief complaints and the conditions identified are likely to be interrelated. The key to resolving the patient's functional deficit is to identify the problem(s) that triggers the other signs and symptoms. A question that can be used in prioritizing the treatment plan is "What other signs and symptoms will be reduced if this problem is resolved?"

Consider a patient who cannot bear weight secondary to pain, decreased ROM, and swelling in the left ankle. Which one of these problems should receive the highest treatment priority? If our treatment approach focused solely on pain, the patient would still be unable to walk properly because of the swelling, decreased joint ROM, and a lack of strength. Indeed, a treatment approach of this nature would more than likely aggravate the remaining problems. The ROM exercises could not be adequately conducted because of the patient's pain and joint swelling, leaving swelling reduction as our highest treatment priority.

Recall that swelling places mechanical pressure on the nerve endings, inhibits blood flow to and from the area, and expands the tissues in the area. A treatment plan that emphasized edema reduction would decrease pain and increase ROM, opening the way for the return of normal gait. Because pain itself is so debilitating, reducing symptomatic pain must be emphasized as well. The treatments used to reduce swelling (e.g., ice, compression, and elevation) are likely to have a direct effect on suppressing pain transmission by lessening the pressure on nerve endings (compression and elevation) and slowing nerve conduction velocity (ice). The physician may also prescribe prescription or over-the-counter pain medication.

Once the inflammatory process has been controlled, swelling is reduced, and limited pain-free motion has been restored, functional exercises should be initiated. The ROM exercises, stretching, balancing, proprioception, and strengthening protocols would be introduced into the treatment plan, followed by functional exercises leading to normal gait and a return to the preinjury activity level.

CASE STUDY 1

Prioritization of the Problem

The patient's problems ranked in terms of treatment priority are:
1. Improper foot biomechanics
2. Decreased flexibility and range of motion of the quadriceps, hamstrings, and calf muscles
3. Swelling of the right knee
4. Hypomobile scar formation

Self-treatment: Treatment or rehabilitation performed by the patient without direct supervision including home treatment programs.

5. Poor patellar tracking
6. Pain during stair climbing, sitting, and contraction of the right quadriceps
7. Inability to play soccer

Commentary

Correcting the biomechanical causes for the patient's pain and dysfunction takes the highest priority in this treatment program. The patient may be excessively pronating to compensate for the lack of dorsiflexion arising from tightness of the calf muscles. The decreased flexibility of the muscles will put increased stress on the patellofemoral joint and contribute to decreased ROM of the knee and ankle. To prevent further compensation in the kinetic chain, the gastrocnemius and soleus flexibility must be increased.

If, after normal gastrocnemius-soleus flexibility is restored, the clinician feels that the hyperpronation of the feet is contributing to the pathology, a trial use of orthotics would be warranted. Treating the symptoms of pain and swelling without addressing the possible causes will provide only temporary relief of the symptoms. The plan must contain therapeutic exercises and the correction of biomechanical problems in the patient.

The patient's effusion causes pain and inhibition of the quadriceps. Eliminating the swelling will improve the quadriceps tone, ability to improve strength, and the ability to control the patella as it tracks through the femoral groove, aiding in the restoration of normal biomechanical function. If the therapy does not eliminate the swelling, the patient should be referred back to the physician.

The hypomobile tissues are important in the overall health of the patellofemoral joint. Before the quadriceps can properly track the patella through active muscle contraction, the patella must be able to move freely. Hypomobility of the scar and subcutaneous tissues as well as of the peripatellar tissues hinders normal tracking and places pathological stresses on the joint. Along with restoring normal movement, the clinician must emphasize neuromuscular reeducation of the muscle group to provide active control.

The pain and dysfunction caused by tendinitis are primary contributors to the patient's problems, and some clinicians may rank these as the highest priority. In this case, we chose to focus on eliminating the stresses that cause the inflammation and will purposefully avoid strengthening exercises through painful arcs of motion; strengthening will occur only within the patient's pain-free ROM.

The functional problems of this patient have not been given the highest treatment priority. The treatment is prioritized to eliminate and correct those problems that contribute to the symptoms. We would expect to see decreased symptoms as the patient's problem list decreases in magnitude and number.

Goal Setting

Clear, concise, and measurable goals translate the prioritized problem list into a well-structured treatment plan. Short-term (1 to 14 days) and long-term (more than 14 days) goals guide the rehabilitation program by establishing timelines, identifying outcomes, and measuring the effectiveness of the treatment protocol. The patient's ability to meet the established goals indicates that the program may advance to the next stage, whereas a lack of progress may indicate that the treatment approach needs to be modified. When used as an *outcome measure*, the patient's ability to meet the treatment goals can be used as the basis for research on treatment efficacy.[1] Properly written and documented goals are also used for insurance and legal purposes and demonstrate the criteria used to decide when to discharge the patient from care.[2]

Treatment goals are an estimation of where the clinician expects the patient's progress to be at a specific point in time and should be consistent with the patient's priorities, lifestyle, and (when feasible) expectations.[3] The patient and, when applicable, the patient's family should be encouraged to participate in setting the treatment goals. Patient compliance with the protocol and the program's effectiveness are increased when the goals are fully understood and agreed on by all involved.[4,5] Perhaps the most important reason to establish treatment goals is that of motivating the patient. Each goal that is met marks another milestone on the road to recovery.

Goals should be stated in objective terms that describe the quality and quantity of the desired outcome. Whenever possible, the short- and long-term treatment goals should be objectively measured. Not only should the question "Has this goal been met?" be answered with a "Yes" or "No" response; the magnitude of the goal should be described as well. Suppose that you are going to take an examination on your knowledge and skill on writing patient goals and you must obtain a score of 73 to pass. A qualitative measure of your success would be a grade of "Pass" or "Fail" when your exam was returned. Although this scoring system informs you (and your instructor) if you scored above or below the passing point, it doesn't let you know by how much. If the examination is returned with a grade of 99 or 66, you can easily determine if you reached your goal of passing the exam and by what magnitude you exceeded or fell short of the passing point.

Consider the two goals presented in Table 3–5: a loosely defined goal, "To increase active dorsiflexion," and a more measurably stated goal, "To increase active

TABLE 3–5 Measurable Goals

Problem	The patient has an inversion ankle sprain. Active range of motion produces 2° of dorsiflexion and the patient cannot ambulate with a normal gait.
Nonobjective goal	To increase active dorsiflexion.
Objective goal	To increase active dorsiflexion to 10°.
Re-evaluation	The patient has 8° of active dorsiflexion.
Assessment	The patient has met the nonobjective goal of increasing active dorsiflexion but has not met the objectively stated goal. Because a minimum of 10° of dorsiflexion is required for normal gait, we can assume that the patient has an altered gait.

Outcome measure(s): Data used to evaluate the efficacy of a treatment program or protocol.

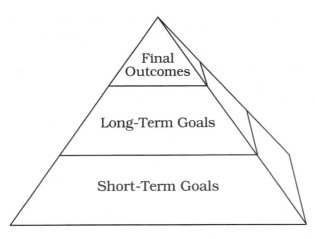

FIGURE 3–3 **The Goal Pyramid.** The patient's final outcomes (agreed on by the patient and clinician) are used to form the long-term goals. Short-term goals are then established to assist in fulfilling the long-term goals.

dorsiflexion to 10°." In our first example the patient may show improvement by increasing active dorsiflexion from 0° to 8°, but because 10° of dorsiflexion is required for a normal gait, the patient probably will not demonstrate a normal walking gait. Noting that the patient has increased active dorsiflexion to 8° documents improvement in the range of motion and the fact that the patient must still gain 2° of dorsiflexion to achieve the treatment goal.

Developing Written Goals

The clinician should start by taking all of the prioritized problems from the PSA and, in an orderly fashion, formulate the final treatment outcome, a list of long-term goals, and the list of short-term goals, realizing that one short-term goal may apply to more than one long-term goal (Fig. 3–3). The final step is to determine what goals should be reasonably accomplished in the given time frame.

Goals should be written using the ABCD format, stated in terms of what will be accomplished in the estimated time period rather than what limitations will still be present (e.g., "Shoulder elevation = 140°" versus "Shoulder elevation lim-

TABLE 3–6   **The ABCD Goal Writing Structure**

Segment	Purpose	Example
Audience	Person who will perform the task	"The patient will." "The patient and coach will modify practice to . . ." "The patient and employer will alter . . ."
Behavior	Description of task to be performed using action verbs	"The patient will **demonstrate** 90° of knee flexion."
Condition	Definition of tools or devices used in obtaining the goal	"The patient will balance for 30 seconds using **one hand for support.**"
Degree	Quality with which the task will be performed, usually described in numerical terms	"The patient will demonstrate **90° of knee flexion.**"

Source: Adapted from Kettenbach, G: Writing SOAP Notes, ed 2. FA Davis, Philadelphia, 1996.

TABLE 3–7 **Feasible Goals**

Problem	The patient has degenerative disk disease of the lumbar spine.
Nonfeasible goal	The patient will be pain-free.
Feasible goal	The patient's symptoms will be controlled with therapeutic exercise so that he or she is able to return to full function.
Assessment	With a chronic condition such as degenerative disk disease, the patient will most likely have a continuation of the symptoms or have intermittent symptoms. A feasible goal is to control the patient's symptoms to the point at which the individual can function within the limits of pain.

ited 30°") (Table 3–6). This serves to motivate the patient and also keep the clinician focused on how the plan must be altered to facilitate the patient's progress. Last, to avoid confusion, the goals should be written in precise versus general terms for each problem. For example, a general short-term goal stating that "All ROM will increase 50°" may not be clear if some motions are decreased by only 30° while others are decreased greater than 50°.

Long-Term Goals

Long-term goals provide direction to the treatment plan by identifying and quantifying the final outcomes of the treatment plan and are often used as outcome measures. In most cases the long-term goal is to return the patient to the preinjury level of function, but this is not always feasible (Table 3–7). Although long-term goals are subject to modification throughout the treatment process, they are revised less often than short-term goals. Last, but most important, the long-term goals should identify the patient's needs as the focus of the treatment rather than the individual pathologies afflicting the person.

Although every attempt should be made to make long-term goals measurable, they should also be functional. Goals such as "To return to full competition in college football" or "To return to the preinjury level of activity at the sawmill" define the final outcome of the patient's therapy, and their use should be encouraged. Because long-term goals attempt to describe the final outcome of the treatment, the number of long-term goals should be less than the number of short-term goals.

CASE STUDY 1

Long-Term Goals

At the time of discharge, the following long-term goals will be achieved:
1. The patient will be able to perform normal ADLs (e.g., climbing stairs, prolonged sitting) without pain.
2. The patient will be able to fully return to soccer and resume other recreational activities.
3. The patient will display equal strength in the right leg relative to the left leg.
4. The patient will display equal ROM in the right leg relative to the left leg.

5. The patient will demonstrate a pain-free, noncompensatory gait.

Commentary

Long-term goals 1 and 2 reflect the patient's expected treatment outcomes as derived from the patient interview. In this case, the patient's problem list and current level of functional activity make these goals realistic. If the patient were suffering from more severe trauma or significant disease, the long-term goals would have to be altered.

The remaining goals describe the functional behaviors that would be necessary for the patient to return to full athletic activity (goal 2). Each of these long-term goals will be addressed by one or more short-term goals. Notice that not all of the patient's problems are specifically cited in the long-term goal list. These issues, such as swelling, are addressed by the short-term goals.

Short-Term Goals

Short-term goals describe the functional progression that the patient will obtain in a specific time frame. The short-term goals usually focus on the specific problems identified during the evaluation that, if met, will achieve the long-term goals. The length of time set for the accomplishment of short-term goals depends on the specific condition at the time of the evaluation. In general, the time established for meeting the short-term goals is the time that the clinician feels is needed to produce a measurable change in the patient's condition.

The short-term goals serve as measuring sticks for the treatment plan. During the re-evaluation, the clinician should be able to determine that goals are being met and progress is being made. If short-term goals are not being met, the clinician needs to re-evaluate the treatment program and change it accordingly.

CASE STUDY 1

Short-Term Goals

The following short-term goals have initially been established for this patient:
1. The patient's hyperpronation will be controlled through stretching the calf muscles.
2. The patient's edema will be decreased by 0.5 cm around the joint line.
3. Medial patellar glide will improve to two out of four patellar quadrants.
4. The patient's flexibility will increase to:

Quadriceps:	Knee flexion will increase to 140°.
Hamstrings:	Knee extension will increase to −5°.
Calf Muscles:	Dorsiflexion will increase to 15°.

5. The range of motion of the knee will be from 0° to 140°.
6. Quadriceps can contract during exercise without pain.

7. The patient will be compliant and independent in a home exercise program.
8. The patient will not participate in soccer at this time.

Commentary

A 2-week period of short-term goals is initially set because it will take this long to appreciate changes in the condition of this patient. This patient has a chronic problem that will take months to fully resolve, not days or weeks. Goals have been set that can either be measured or easily answered as met or not met. The goals are a reasonable expectation of what the patient's condition should be after a 2-week period. All the goals represent progress in the condition and, if met, will signify that the plan is working.

To obtain a normal gait pattern, the patient's hyperpronation must be controlled. The physical evaluation findings indicate tightness of the calf muscles that prohibits an appropriate amount of dorsiflexion. Orthotics can be used to assist in restoring normal biomechanics. Decreasing the amount of swelling within the joint capsule can prevent inhibition of the vastus medialis oblique, further improving biomechanics by assisting in terminal knee extension and patellar tracking. Flexibility and ROM for the entire lower extremity will be emphasized.

Decreasing the adhesions associated with functional shortening of the lateral patellar retinaculum and the presence of the keloid scar will increase medial patellar glide. This goal will probably not be achieved during the 2-week time frame, and we would expect to see improvements in patellar mobility as the amount of swelling is decreased and the strength of the VMO increases. Exercises will have to be conducted to improve patellar tracking. The pain associated with contraction of the quadriceps should be decreased as patellar tracking is improved.

These goals are relatively in view of the short time frame. With this in mind, the patient must remain compliant with her home treatment program and stay within her prescribed limits of physical activity.

Goal 8, "The patient will not participate in soccer at this time," is different from the others in that it describes a behavior the patient must avoid. In this case, the rest from the aggravating activity is important for the rest of the treatment plan to be effective. Note that this is not written as a negative goal; it simply states the patient's current functional deficit. The last goal of independence in a home program will be essential for this patient to return to full function.

Treatment Planning

Once the patient's problems have been determined and prioritized and the appropriate goals have been established, the planning of the treatment follows naturally. The planning of the treatment is the application of your knowledge of the physiological effects of the therapeutic modalities and exercise to resolve the problems and to achieve the goals established for the patient's rehabilitation. The stage of

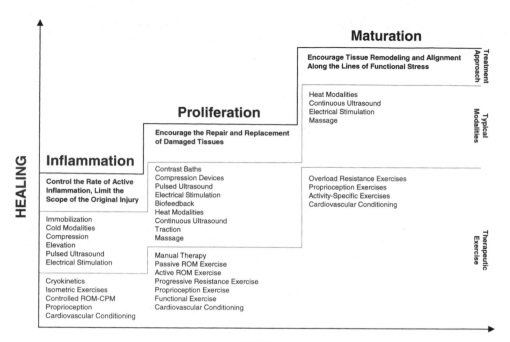

FIGURE 3–4 **Modality Boilerplate.** Each stage of the injury response has specific treatment goals that best respond to certain modalities and/or therapies. When the patient is in the "overlap" phase between two plateaus, the modalities and therapeutic exercises from the advanced stage on the right are commonly followed by the modalities of the lesser stage on the left. For example, a patient may use a hot whirlpool and perform active range-of-motion exercises followed by the use of an ice pack. CPM = continuous passive motion. (Adapted from Buxton, BP: Physiological considerations of healing. In Anderson, MK and Martin, M. (eds): Quick Reference Guide in Athletic Training. Williams & Wilkins, Baltimore, 1998, p 57).

the healing process and the choice of therapeutic techniques largely determines what modality types will be used to address the therapeutic problem (Fig. 3–4).

The decision process regarding the type of modality to use (e.g., heat, cold, electrical) is based on the tissue characteristics, their *conductive properties,* the stage of the healing process, the depth to which the particular modality penetrates, and the desired physiological responses for the stage of inflammation (Fig. 3–5). Once the type of modality to use has been determined, the optimum method of application is determined based on physical characteristics of the surface area being treated. For example, if a chronic lateral ankle sprain is being treated and there is little or no swelling, the modality of choice would probably be heat. In this scenario, the physical characteristics of the lateral ankle (an irregular surface) would most likely call for the use of a warm whirlpool rather than a moist heat pack.

A common frustration is that in many cases there is no one "best" choice of modality. Often the final decision of what modality to use is based on personal

Conductive properties: The ability of a tissue to transfer heat (from a high temperature to a low temperature) or electrical energy.

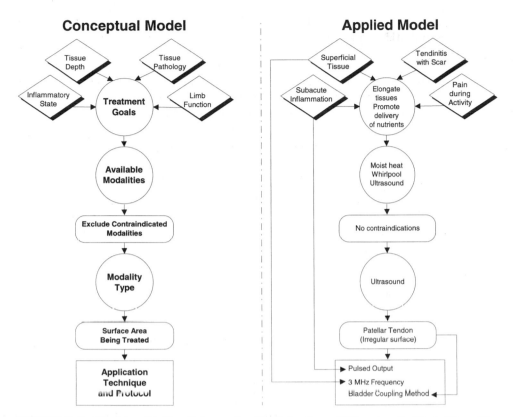

FIGURE 3–5 **Decision-Making Scheme for the Selection of Therapeutic Modalities.** The model on the left shows the factors used when deciding what therapeutic modality to use. First the treatment goals are considered along with the types of tissues that are injured and the current inflammatory state. Contraindicated modalities are excluded from the modalities available to the clinician and the most appropriate modality type is selected. The contour and size of the body area are then considered in deciding the best application technique. Note that often more than one modality can be considered the best to use.

comfort, past experience with the modality, and patient input. However, this situation can also work to your advantage. If satisfactory results are not being obtained from one modality, the treatment protocol can easily be modified to incorporate an alternate modality.

CASE STUDY 1

Treatment Planning

The following treatment approaches have been selected to meet the short-term goals:
1. Orthotics to Control Hyperpronation

   THEORY

   Permanent control of foot motion is needed to decrease recurrent stress on the patellofemoral joint.

2. Ultrasound Application to the Scar Tissue
Output of 3 MHz; 8 minutes; high intensity.

THEORY

Ultrasound will be applied with an output frequency of 3 MHz because of the superficial nature of the tissues involved in this condition. This modality will heat the tissues and, when followed by manual stretching and joint mobilization, will encourage the elongation of the involved tissues and lead to a reduction in scar tissue adhesion. The concern of the increased inflammation associated with heating could be addressed through the use of ice packs after the treatments.

3. Mobilization of Scar Tissue

THEORY

Scar mobilization and cross-friction techniques aid in restoration of tissue mobility. These should be performed immediately after ultrasound while the tissue temperatures are still elevated.

4. Patellar Mobilization

THEORY

Increase patellar motion through stretching of *peripatellar* tissues before performing ROM and neuromuscular reeducation techniques.

OPTION

Ultrasound, 3 MHz, continuous output for 8 minutes at the maximum intensity tolerated by the patient performed over the lateral retinaculum while the mobilization is being performed. Keeping the patient's tissues stretched while mobilizing them may be more effective than mobilization alone. These parameters would be effective in increasing the tissue temperature over an area this size based on the effective radiating area of the ultrasound head.

5. Electrical Stimulation
Output of 50 Hz, with a carrier frequency of 2500 Hz and a duty cycle of 25 percent. Electrodes are placed on the femoral triangle and the distal quadriceps.

THEORY

Electrical stimulation will help restore normal neuromuscular activity within the involved muscles and assist in regaining strength. The patient would be encouraged to voluntarily contract the muscle during stimulation to maximize motor unit recruitment. Parameters given are consistent with maximal recruitment of the quadriceps mechanism.

6. Flexibility Exercises: Quadriceps, Hamstrings, and Gastrocnemius-Soleus Muscle Group
Minimum of 30 seconds, 5 repetitions each.

THEORY

Increasing the flexibility will improve the normal mechanics about the joint and decrease abnormal stress on the joint capsule. Flexibility techniques could

Peripatellar: Around the patella.

range from various positions and self-stretching to contract-relax stretching with the clinician. Any technique should produce a gentle stretch in the involved muscle but not cause pain in the patellofemoral joint.

OPTION

A 10-minute warm-up on a stationary bicycle could be used to physiologically elevate tissue temperatures before stretching as long as the patient did not have symptoms while on the bike.

7. Range of Motion Exercises for Active Knee Flexion and Extension

THEORY

Use of active assisted ROM and passive ROM is needed to restore normal joint biomechanics. A low-load prolonged stretch should be used with all stretches. Prone hangs could be used to improve extension. Weights placed on the foot during the prone hang should be gauged to provide a strong stretch, yet not cause a reflex contraction of the hamstring. Moist heat can be used to promote hamstring relaxation. Continuous passive motion machines would not be beneficial with this patient. As the knee reaches the terminal degrees of full extension it becomes more difficult to maintain the alignment of the knee joint with the axis of the machine and provide effective stretching.

8. Biofeedback for Active Exercise
Placed over the VMO used in a step-up mode set at 80 percent of the maximal voluntary contraction.

THEORY

True neuromuscular reeducation can be achieved with voluntary contractions, whereas electrical stimulation produces an involuntary contraction. The biofeedback unit can be used to emphasize voluntary contraction of the VMO. Initially, the biofeedback unit can be used with quadriceps setting, adductor sets, straight-leg raises with hip flexion, adductor straight-leg raises, and then continue to be used as the patient is progressed to closed- and open-chain strengthening, such as mini-squats, step exercises, leg presses, and open kinetic chain quadriceps strengthening through a pain-free arc.

9. Strengthening of the Hip, Hamstring, and Gastrocnemius-Soleus Muscle Group

THEORY

The patient's plan should include strengthening the entire lower extremity. These exercises can be performed immediately as long as they do not create pain at the patellofemoral joint. The clinician should keep in mind that this patient may not have fully recovered her strength from ACL reconstruction surgery and needs to continue strengthening the entire lower extremity.

10. Cardiovascular Exercise

THEORY

The patient is very active and must maintain her cardiovascular fitness. An upper body ergometer could be used. The patient could also attempt free-style swimming for cardiovascular endurance as well as for strengthening of the lower extremity.

11. Ice

THEORY

The patient's program may create inflammation in the patellofemoral joint. Application of ice would be effective because the affected tissues are superficial.

12. Patellar Tape or Brace

THEORY

A brace or tape may physically or proprioceptively assist in controlling the patella, although there is debate regarding the efficacy of this approach. Bracing may be more realistic with this patient. Use of tape or brace would be required for at least a few weeks.

13. Home Exercise Program: Scar Massage, Patella Mobilization, Flexibility Exercises, and Ice

THEORY

Initially, these exercises and modalities are needed to accomplish our goals. Because this patient is very active, the program may also include ROM and strengthening. When increasing the home program beyond three exercises or modalities, the clinician should use the best judgment based on the time available to the patient to perform the exercises, the motivation of the patient, and the activity level of the patient.

Considerations of the Healing Stage

Each stage of the injury response process entails special needs that must be addressed during treatment. Although the time needed to reach each stage of the healing process fluctuates from case to case, the process of healing and the associated treatment strategy follow an orderly, predictable sequence (see Fig. 3–4).

A common trait among these treatment approaches is the need to maintain, and in some cases improve, the patient's cardiovascular level. Except in conditions in which cardiovascular exercise is impractical or medically contraindicated, some form of cardiovascular endurance exercise should be incorporated into either the patient's clinical or home treatment plan. Patients who are suffering from lower-extremity injuries may be able to exercise with an upper body *ergometer* or perform pool or wheelchair exercises. In cases in which the upper extremity is injured, stationary bike exercises, pool exercise, or jogging may be used for cardiovascular maintenance.

Active Inflammatory Stage

In the hours and days after the onset of acute trauma or after surgery, the aim of the treatment approach is to control, but not eliminate, the amount of active inflammation and to contain the scope of the original injury by reducing secondary hypoxic injury and controlling edema and spasm. Cold modalities are used to re-

---

Ergometer: A device used to measure the amount of work performed by the legs or arms.

duce the amount of secondary hypoxic injury, reduce pain, and eliminate spasm. Compression devices and elevation are used to encourage venous and lymphatic return, and immobilization devices are used to limit the limb's ROM. Electrical stimulation may assist in decreasing vascular permeability, limiting the amount of edema formed, and help to reduce pain.

Exercise may take the form of gentle, pain-free ROM and possibly isometric exercises within the patient's pain tolerance. In some acute injuries or postsurgical conditions, a physician may prescribe continuous passive motion exercises to maintain joint mobility. Obtaining this motion should not come at the expense of compromising tissue integrity. Cardiovascular maintenance programs should be implemented as soon as possible into the rehabilitation scheme for athletes and other physically active individuals.

Proliferation Phase

The proliferation stage overlaps portions of the inflammatory and maturation stages. During the proliferation stage of the injury response process, the goal is to assist the body in delivering nutrients and materials necessary to repair the injured tissues and in removing the inflammatory debris. This goal is met by increasing blood flow to and from the injured tissues.

Range of motion is needed to stretch the tissues, to prevent functional shortening of the fibers, and to encourage the alignment of collagen along the lines of stress. Low-intensity tension is placed on the structures to slowly increase their tensile strength and to assist in the formation of proprioceptive nerves. Proprioceptive activities and muscle reeducation exercises are begun to help protect the limb during the ADLs. Newly formed capillary buds are fragile, and care must be taken not to damage them through excessive joint movement or increased tension.

Early in the proliferation stage, these needs may still conflict with the residual effects of acute inflammation. As the signs and symptoms of acute inflammation are resolved, the patient should report decreased pain. Edema may continue to clog the delivery of fresh blood and the modalities used during this stage may tend to increase edema, so a balance must be maintained among the treatment approaches. A common example of this is the use of heat before rehabilitation exercises, followed by ice application afterward.

Maturation Phase

During the maturation phase, therapeutic modalities are used to increase tissue extensibility and to control postexercise inflammation because the tissue is still remodeling to form a strong, permanent repair. Usually, this scar tissue does not have the same functionality as the tissue it replaces, so the fibers must be arranged along the lines of functional stress to prevent the scar from creating limitations in ROM or strength.

Proprioceptive activities and muscle strengthening are used to protect the limb during exertion. These exercises should follow a functional progression from that of ADLs to sport- or work-specific activities (e.g., walking, jogging, running in a straight line, running in all forms, and cutting).

Self-Treatment

Although the treatment and rehabilitation activities conducted by the clinician guide the patient back to health, ultimately, the patient's compliance with the rehabilitation scheme determines the return to full, unaltered activity in the least possible time. A strong argument can be made that the time spent **between** treatment visits is the most important factor in determining the return-to-activity time frame. A kind of "protective custody" is formed when the clinician is working directly with the patient. In this situation, the clinician ensures that the patient complies with the prescribed routines. However, once the patient leaves this structured care, his or her behavior will either reinforce or hinder the healing process.

Most rehabilitation plans contain home treatment components in which the patient self-administers therapeutic treatments (e.g., an ice pack), performs exercise routines (e.g., straight-leg raises), and adheres to modified activity (e.g., the use of crutches). Noncompliant patients reduce their actual therapeutic activities to the time spent with the clinician and can actually do harm to their condition by not following the prescribed protocol (e.g., not using crutches as prescribed, going dancing 2 weeks after anterior cruciate ligament reconstruction). Compliance with the full scheme of the rehabilitation program can be increased by educating the patient about the nature of the injury being treated, the benefits to be seen from complying with the home treatment program, and the potential consequences of straying from the plan.

To help maintain compliance, self-treatment plans should include no more than three treatments or exercises at any one time. The patient should be instructed on how to perform the self-treatments and exercises before being allowed to leave the treatment facility. These instructions should be given to the patient in writing, and illustrations that depict the exercises to be performed are also helpful.

Evaluation of the Treatment Plan

The re-evaluation of the patient serves as an evaluation of the treatment plan. The clinician assesses the findings of the re-evaluation to determine if the plan has been successful in guiding the patient toward achieving the long-term goals. The short-term goals can be used to determine progress toward achieving the long-term goals. If the short-term goals are met, the clinician re-establishes new short-term goals and makes any necessary adjustments to the plan. If the goals are not met, the clinician must identify the reason(s) for the deficiency. Possible reasons include goals that were too ambitious, lack of compliance by the patient, a plan that is too conservative, or something that was missed in the evaluation and not properly addressed in the plan. After establishing why the goals were not met, the clinician must re-establish short-term goals and a new treatment plan based on the re-evaluation of the patient.

CASE STUDY 1

Changes in the Program

1. Ultrasound can be used before the scar massage and patella mobilization until the tissue extensibility is restored and the scar massage and patellar mobilization are discharged from the program.
2. Modalities other than ice may be used to treat the patellar tendinitis. Phonophoresis and iontophoresis are two options.

3. Electrical stimulation and biofeedback may be discharged as the patient demonstrates control of the patella during functional activity.
4. Strengthening exercises are progressed based on the clinician's judgment. Using pain-free exercise as a guide, any strengthening exercise may be performed throughout the rehabilitation.
5. Range-of-motion exercises would be eliminated as full motion is restored. The patient would be encouraged to continue active-assisted ROM.
6. As soon as the patient could tolerate standing on one leg without symptoms, proprioception exercises would be added to improve function in the surgically reconstructed leg. These may not be performed until some of the more pertinent problems have been resolved.

    The patient would be taken through a functional progression of running, agility training, and sport-specific skills to return to full activity. This regimen may not actually be performed in private clinics because of insurance industry restrictions. In this case, the clinician must educate the patient on the exercise progression during discharge planning and remain in verbal contact with the patient.

WORKPLACE INFLUENCES

The clinical setting where the treatment is provided influences the patient's treatment plan. Possible clinical settings where a patient may be treated include acute care hospitals, subacute settings, home care, outpatient rehabilitation, and the athletic training room. The focus of treatment and the criteria for discharge vary from setting to setting. In many instances, a patient is discharged from one rehabilitation setting to enter a different setting. For example, an athlete who receives hospital-based therapy after surgery is then discharged to the college's athletic training staff.

    The treatment plan is affected by both internal and external factors. Internal factors such as the experience and expertise of the staff and the type of equipment available to the clinician affect the formation of the plan. External forces affecting the treatment plan include time and financial constraints imposed by insurance companies, the time the patient is able to dedicate to the supervised and home therapeutic program, the support the patient receives from friends and family, and the patient's motivation.

    The treatment plan for the patient hospitalized in the **acute care setting** will focus on stabilizing the patient and preparing him or her for discharge to subacute care or to the home for home care or outpatient rehabilitation. In light of this, the goals of treatment are more immediate, focused on what needs to be accomplished in days versus weeks or months. The evaluation and treatment plan focuses on areas such as wound healing, restoration of ROM, and maximal independence in *transfers* and mobility.

    A patient who is medically stable but requires skilled care and further rehabilitation may be discharged to a **subacute care facility,** such as a skilled nursing facility or rehabilitation hospital. As in the acute care setting, the treatment plan

---

Transfers: Assisted patient mobility, such as moving from a wheelchair to a bed.

continues to focus on attaining maximal functional independence for the patient so that he or she may go home. The focus of the plan will be developing the ROM, strength, and mobility required to allow the patient to perform activities of daily living with the least amount of assistance at home.

Because it is more cost-effective than inpatient care, **home rehabilitation** is becoming increasingly popular. This is an ideal alternative for the patient who no longer requires inpatient care but cannot attend outpatient rehabilitation. Patients may lack the resources to get to the outpatient setting or may lack the physical mobility required to travel to and from the clinic. If the patient will not be able to attend outpatient rehabilitation, the goals and plan for the patient will be more long-term in their scope, similar to those of outpatient settings. The plan will need to focus on the maximal relief of symptoms and restoration of function. If the patient will eventually attend outpatient rehabilitation, the home rehabilitation plan will focus on permitting the patient to travel to the clinic.

Outpatient rehabilitation focuses on obtaining maximum patient independence. Areas that enter into the treatment plan are relief of symptoms, restoration of range of motion, strength, balance, and return to ADLs. Although the goals and plan focus on these areas, the ultimate goal is the restoration of function.

Historically, patients may have received outpatient rehabilitation until all aspects of their condition had been alleviated or they had plateaued. With restrictions placed on the amount of outpatient rehabilitation by the insurance industry, new factors have entered into the planning process for a patient's condition. The clinician must be aware of time constraints that may enter into the patient's treatment planning. For example, an insurance company may establish a limit of 60 consecutive days of treatment, regardless of the severity of the injury. With lesser injuries, the treatment goal is to return the patient to normal activity, but in instances of greater pathology, the focus may be for the patient to recover to the point at which self-treatment could be conducted in a safe manner.

The **athletic training room** presents some unique circumstances for the clinician when planning the treatment. The patients are a specific group of athletes who are the sole responsibility of the clinicians. The patients in this case tend to be in better physical condition, younger, and oriented to heavy exercise. The clinicians may be able to treat the patients not only on a daily basis but sometimes multiple times during the day. All of the above allows clinicians to be more aggressive with their goal setting and planning. As the circumstances are unique, clinicians must keep in mind that the expectations for return to activity are also unique. The patients in this setting will be returning to activities that place them under great physical stress and require psychological confidence, and these factors must be considered by the clinician when formulating a treatment program.

DOCUMENTATION

Medical records serve a wide range of purposes (Table 3–8). In the context of this text, treatment documentation serves a valuable purpose in the planning and evaluation of the treatment protocol by providing a method to determine the effectiveness of the protocol. In addition, records describe the quantity and quality of the services provided by the facility. Many different documentation methods

TABLE 3–8 **Purpose of Medical Records**

Serve as a communication tool among healthcare providers
Document treatment and/or rehabilitation progression
Assist in the continuity of care given
Provide a basis for developing future treatment and/or rehabilitation plans
Serve as a legal document to show that the medical staff provided reasonable care
Provide a database for research

are available, and desktop computers are playing an increasing role in this area (Table 3–9).

The evaluation findings and the treatment plan should be documented as specifically as possible so that continuity of care can be established in the event that more than one clinician is treating the patient. Even seemingly minor changes in a modality's application parameters can produce drastically different physiological effects. A lack of continuity of treatment is a pitfall that may delay the patient's rehabilitation progress. One measure that assists in avoiding this situation is good documentation of the evaluation and treatment of all care given.

All medical records are considered to be confidential documents, and to be released to outside individuals (e.g., a physician, college athletic recruiter, military), written permission must be obtained from the patient. The release-of-information form should explicitly state to whom the information is being released and for what purposes it will be used. If this information is being released on the grounds of obtaining a college athletic scholarship, professional sports contract, or other employment, a disclaimer is needed stating that the information will be used

TABLE 3–9 **Types of Medical Records**

Document	Purpose
Medical history	Details prior medical conditions. Identifies conditions that contraindicate the use of certain modalities, although the patient should be specifically questioned before applying any device (e.g., a person with a history of cardiovascular disease requiring medication would be excluded from full-body warm whirlpools).
Preparticipation physical examination	Used with athletes to identify the status of any existing condition and to determine the current status of pre-existing conditions.
Consent forms	Indicates that the patient (or the parent[s] if the patient is under the age of 18 years) has granted permission to be treated. Consent forms do not protect the clinician from liability stemming from acts of negligence.
Injury reports	Used in athletics to document the onset of an acute injury or the aggravation of a chronic condition.
Referral forms	Allows for feedback from the physician regarding the level of activity and prescribed course of rehabilitation.
Treatment and rehabilitation notes	Provides an ongoing record and documentation of the patient's adherence to, and progress with, the treatment plan.

as part of the decision-making process and may be used in determining the individual's final disposition. The confidentiality of medical records applies to the spoken word as well. Last, as with all medical forms, if the patient is under the age of 18 years, permission must also be granted by the parent(s) or *legal guardian.*

Well-documented records can assist in proving that the staff exercised reasonable care in the management of an injury. If a liability case were to come to trial, the medical staff may use these records to refresh their memories when testifying about the case, and the documents themselves may be admitted as evidence.[6]

Although the primary role of documentation is to improve patient care by ensuring treatment continuity among caregivers, medical records are also potential business documents. Insurance companies may review these documents to determine if reimbursement for the services is warranted. When the bill for service appears excessive or the amount of care provided seems prolonged, the documentation may undergo peer review for determination of reimbursement.

In the case of possible excessive billing, the documentation is compared with the billing during the treatment session. The documentation must be clearly and concisely written so that someone reviewing the chart can gain a full understanding of the care provided in order to make a fair determination of the reimbursement. When the amount of care provided seems prolonged, the reviewer will use the documentation to determine if care was truly needed or if it was unnecessarily extended.

LEGAL CONSIDERATIONS IN PATIENT CARE

The legal issues associated with the medical care and treatment of patients are a growing concern. During treatment and rehabilitation, the clinician's legal duty is to prevent further injury or harm to the patient by performing the tasks at hand in a professionally accepted manner. Courts have ruled that reasonable facilities and equipment, as well as qualified personnel, are necessary to provide proper medical coverage.[7]

Clinicians must be intimately familiar with the effects and side effects of the devices being used, and caregivers should be able to recognize those physical conditions that prohibit the use of various therapeutic modalities and therapeutic exercise. In addition, to ensure the proper application of therapeutic modalities, clinicians must know the characteristics, maintenance requirements, and safety considerations of the devices being used.

Scope of Practice

The legal boundaries that limit the manner in which clinicians may practice, or the scope of practice, is established on a state-by-state basis through processes such as licensure, registration, or certification. Although there are differences in the scope of practice from one profession to another, there are also discrepancies in the scope of practice for a single profession among states.[8]

Legal guardian: An individual who is legally responsible for the care of a minor.

Generally, state practice acts make provisions for students to practice those skills that they have been taught, so long as these techniques are delivered under the immediate supervision of a licensed practitioner. However, both the student and the student's supervisor can be held liable for negligent acts performed by the student under the *doctrine* of **respondeat superior** or **vicarious liability.** Supervisors can also be held legally accountable for the acts of their employees, their own failure to supervise, or acts that exceed the profession's scope of practice.[9]

A professional responsibility is to become knowledgeable about the practice acts relative to your state and your profession. This information can usually be obtained through your professional organization or through state governmental agencies.

Informed Consent

Except in cases of emergency care and treatment, patients must grant their consent to be treated. Otherwise, an act of criminal *battery* may have been committed. Before beginning the treatment, patients should be educated about the modality or exercise, the sensations to be expected during the treatment, and any adverse warning signs. The patient should also be fully informed about any potential hazards associated with the use of the device and any residual side effects (Table 3–10).

All facilities should have an informed consent form signed by the patient on file. If the individual is under the age of 18, the patient's parent(s) or guardian must grant consent. This document not withstanding, patients have the right to refuse any particular form of treatment or modality.

Negligence

Patients have the right to receive safe and proper treatment without exposure to undue hazards. This implies that care is provided in a professionally competent and accepted manner. This standard includes not only the physical act of applying

TABLE 3–10 **Informed Consent for Rehabilitation**

Description of the modality or exercise
An overview of how the device works
Benefits provided by the device (physiological responses)
Expected normal sensations
Adverse sensations to be reported
Potential hazards associated with the device
Residual effects

Doctrine: A statement of fundamental government policy.
Battery: The unwanted touching of one person by another.

therapeutic modalities and implementing rehabilitation routines but also the devices being used must be in safe operating condition and the facility free of foreseeable hazards.

Negligent Delivery of Treatment

Negligent behavior occurs when a healthcare practitioner departs from the standard of care imposed by society.[6] If a clinician, or a student serving under the direction of the professional staff, performs unnecessary or detrimental acts, he or she could be found liable for failure to use *due care* under the law of negligence.[7] Negligence may be classified into two types on the basis of behavior: (1) omission and (2) commission.

Omission occurs when an individual fails to respond to a given situation when a response is necessary to limit or reduce harm. Consider the following example: a patient goes to the physician with complaints of an injury. If the physician fails to evaluate, treat, or refer the injury, an act of omission may have occurred. In this case, the negligent act stems from the physician's failure to properly respond to a medical condition.

Commission occurs when an individual acts on a situation but does not perform at the level that a reasonable and prudent person would. In the rehabilitation process, an act of commission could occur if a clinician treats lower leg pain with ultrasound and the injury turns out to be a fracture. In this example, negligence occurred because the individual responded to an injury but with an improper technique.

Negligent Care of Facilities

The design of the rehabilitation facilities must guarantee that patients receive treatment in the safest environment possible. Ensuring safety is an ongoing process involving thorough planning, evaluation, and maintenance. Injury sustained through improper or unsafe facilities can result in charges of negligence being brought against the staff, the facility, or the institution. Of special concern regarding the facility's physical design are the hydrotherapy area and areas where electrical modalities are used (Table 3–11).

Knowingly using an unsafe therapeutic modality reflects negligent behavior on the part of the clinician. All therapeutic equipment must be inspected and calibrated by a qualified service technician at the intervals recommended by the manufacturer. The inspection or service date, the technician, and the services performed should be documented and kept on file.

Proper care is the primary factor for maintaining the equipment in safe working order. Wear and tear through normal use are to be expected, and proper care of the equipment will keep this to a minimum. Logical precautions, such as avoiding spills into the equipment, proper positioning of electrical cords, and regular inspection of plugs, assist in maintaining the longevity of equipment.

Due care: An established responsibility for an individual to respond to a given situation in a certain manner.

TABLE 3–11   **Considerations for Safe Facilities**

- All electrical modalities should be connected to a ground fault interrupter. Whirlpools and jacuzzis must be connected to these devices.
- Patients must not be permitted to turn whirlpools or jacuzzis on or off while they are in the water. Ideally, the switches should be located so that they cannot be reached from these tubs.
- All modalities should be inspected and calibrated by a licensed professional at intervals prescribed by the manufacturer.
- Flooring should be made of a nonslip material.

SUMMARY

To properly develop a patient's treatment plan requires knowledge and skill from the areas of evaluation, pathology, pathomechanics, therapeutic modalities, therapeutic exercise, goal setting, and patient motivation. The PSA describes a method of identifying and prioritizing the patient's list of symptoms, setting goals, and developing the treatment plan.

The type of environment in which the care is given will influence the treatment plan. In those settings where the patient has a limited number of visits, increased emphasis must be placed on self-treatment.

CASE STUDY 2

Scenario

A 62-year-old man sprained his left ankle 2 days ago while participating in a doubles match in a club tennis tournament. He was evaluated by his primary physician and given a diagnosis of a grade I lateral ankle sprain. He has been referred to you for evaluation and treatment of his injury. The following information has been obtained from the patient and the patient's medical records.

Chief complaint: He reports that he has pain on weight bearing, located along the lateral aspect of the left ankle.

History: The patient reports that he rolled onto the outside of his left foot during the last set of his match. He was able to finish the match, but once he cooled down, the pain increased and the ankle began to swell. The patient has a history of bilateral ankle sprains.

Diagnostic tests: X-rays showed an old avulsion fracture of the lateral malleolus; otherwise, the images are unremarkable.

Activity: He has advanced to the next round of the doubles tennis, which is to be held in 5 days. He reports that he is teamed with his business partner and it would be very disappointing for him not to be able to finish the tournament.

General medical: The patient has a history of peptic ulcers and has insulin-dependent diabetes.

Contraindications to modality use: The patient has diabetes. Caution must be used with heat modalities if sensory exam of feet is not normal.

Medications: Insulin. The doctor prescribed acetaminophen for the pain because the patient does not tolerate nonsteroidal antiinflammatory drugs as a result of his peptic ulcer.

Patient goals: To play in the tennis tournament in 5 days. Pain-free ADLs.

Evaluation findings:

Function:	The patient cannot walk without pain.
	The patient cannot play tennis.
Observation:	The patient ambulates with an *antalgic gait.*
	Swelling is present along the distal aspect of the lateral malleolus.
	The rest of the foot and ankle, including the skin, is in good condition with no signs of ulceration.

Weight-bearing status: Full weight bearing

ROM:

	Left	Right
Dorsiflexion (knee extended)	7°	15°
Dorsiflexion (knee flexed)	10°	15°
Plantarflexion	32°	37°
Inversion	5°	15°
Eversion	3°	5°

Swelling:

	Left	Right
Figure eight technique	21.25 in.	19.5 in.
Base of the fifth metatarsal	12.25 in.	12.0 in.

Strength:
  Dorsiflexors: 5/5, but painful
  Plantarflexors: 5/5
  Invertors: 5/5
  Evertors: 5/5, but painful

Balance:

	Left	Right
One-leg stance for 20 seconds	2 deviations	0 deviations
Base of the fifth metatarsal	12.25 in.	12.0 in.

Pain rating: 2/10 with level walking
Special tests: All tests for laxity negative
Palpation: Pain over the anterior talofibular ligament
Sensation: Intact for light touch and hot and cold discrimination throughout both feet

Case Study 2: Recognition of the Problems

The following problems have been identified based on the information presented in the case study scenario.

1. Decreased function secondary to pain, including the ability to participate in tennis

---

Antalgic gait: A gait resulting from pain on weight bearing. The stance phase of gait is shortened on the affected side.

2. Decreased ROM of the left ankle
3. Swelling of the left ankle
4. Decreased balance and proprioception of the left ankle

Commentary

- The pain rating given by the patient is not abnormal, considering that he sustained a grade I lateral ankle sprain that morning. It is significant that he does have pain with weight bearing and must compete again in 5 days. Under many circumstances, treatment of this injury would be to simply have the man rest for a few days, but because he is involved in a tournament, it is prudent to attempt to return him to safe activity. The physician and rehabilitation clinician must explain the ramifications and risks to the patient so that he may make a reasonable decision as to continuing to participate.
- The ROM restrictions are limited, probably because of the pain and swelling. Someone participating in an activity that involves running should have at least 15° of dorsiflexion to maintain a normal biomechanical pattern without compensation.
- The swelling is minimal at this time, but it may reduce the overall motion in the ankle. Also, the patient does have some balance difficulties that may be affected by the swelling disrupting the joint receptors responsible for proprioception. Although inhibition of the quadriceps has been shown with knee joint effusions, no definitive relationships have been made between swelling in the ankle joint and inhibition of the musculature.
- Assessing the strength of the dorsiflexors and evertors reveals strong contractions that produce pain within the joint. Although pain is elicited, it does not arise from the musculature; therefore, a strength rating of 5/5 is given.
- The disruption in the patient's balance is a key factor in his return to activity in a safe and timely manner. The clinician should challenge the patient's balance and proprioception with functional activities related to tennis before clearing him to play.
- Although it does not seem to be a problem in this patient, the clinician must remain aware of the patient's diabetes and the effect of treatment on this condition. The evaluation of the patient revealed insulin-dependent diabetes that is seemingly well controlled. The skin is intact and sensation is normal. Under these circumstances, the patient should not have any contraindications to treatment.

Case Study 2: Prioritization of the Problems

1. Swelling of the left ankle
2. Decreased ROM of the left ankle
3. Decreased balance and proprioception of the left ankle
4. Decreased function secondary to pain, including the ability to participate in tennis

Commentary

Most of the patient's problems are related to acute swelling within the ankle joint, increasing pain, decreasing ROM, and decreasing ability to bear weight without pain. By addressing the swelling as the highest priority, the clinician should attempt not only to reduce the swelling but also to inhibit any new swelling.

The decreased ROM is certainly a significant deterrent to the patient's ability to play tennis in 5 days. For the patient to return to safe activity, ROM must be restored to permit an adequate amount of ankle plantarflexion and dorsiflexion. Strength and flexibility will most likely be restored to normal as the swelling and pain are reduced. A reassessment of the strength and flexibility of the left ankle can be conducted as pain and swelling decrease.

Balance and proprioception are essential to all athletic activity. In the case of this patient, balance is required because he will be called on to quickly stop, start, and change direction. Proper proprioceptive ability is needed for the patient's muscles to protect the joint from potentially injurious forces.

The ability to balance is essential to any activity, either walking or running. This patient's balance is even more essential because he will be called on to stop and start quickly as well as to change directions. The clinician must be careful to respect any pain that the patient has while performing balance exercises. These exercises cannot be performed at the expense of any harm they may do to the injury.

The inability to function in a safe, pain-free manner is the biggest problem facing the patient and clinician because of the time constraints in this scenario. By addressing these problems, the rehabilitation will lead to a return to safe function.

Case Study 2: Long-Term Goals

At the time of discharge the patient will:
1. Regain a normal gait pattern within 5 days
2. Be able to play in a tennis match using a protective support in 5 days

Commentary

Although the long-term goals for this patient are described within a 5-day time frame, the goals are reasonable and obtainable. However, the clinician must carefully evaluate the patient at the end of 5 days to verify that it is safe for him to compete. If the long-term goals are not met, the rehabilitation clinician, physician, and patient must be prepared to withhold participation.

The ability to return to competition does not imply that the patient is totally healed. After the match, the patient will need to resume therapy so that the rehabilitation program can be completed.

Case Study 2: Short-Term Goals

The following short-term goals have been established for this patient:
1. Swelling will decrease to within 1/4 inch relative to the right ankle within 3 days.
2. The patient will be able to walk without pain (0 to 1/10) within 3 days.
3. The patient's ROM in the left ankle will be 10° of dorsiflexion, 35° of plantarflexion, 8° of inversion, and 4° of eversion within 4 days.
4. The patient will be able to display equal balance between the left and right ankle within 4 days.
5. The patient will not participate in tennis at this time.

Commentary

A 3-day period was established for obtaining the first short-term goal. Referring back to the commentary for prioritizing the problems, you will note that swelling must be reduced before any improvement can be effected in the remaining problem areas. If the first goal is met early, the remaining time frames can be accelerated. The fifth goal is different from the rest in that it describes a behavior that is to be avoided. In this situation, the patient must avoid placing harmful stresses on the involved joint.

Case Study 2: Treatment Planning

The following treatment approaches have been selected to meet the goals for this patient:

1. Intermittent Compression with Elevation
Sixty minutes. Pressure setting of 60 mm Hg with an on-off cycle of 30 seconds "on" to 15 seconds "off."

THEORY

Intermittent compression, in combination with elevation, assists in the venous and lymphatic return of edema. Reducing the edema will decongest the area and allow nutrients and oxygen to reach the damaged tissues. Initially the clinician will use this as the primary focus of the treatment to control and decrease the edema. As the edema becomes stabilized, this intermittent compression may be used post-treatment to control the edema.

2. Retrograde Massage
Effleurage strokes from the toes to the lower leg to "milk" edema proximally. "Uncorking" the leg proximal to the ankle would precede the effleurage strokes.

THEORY

Effleurage massage will aid the venous and lymphatic system in transporting edema proximally. Movement of this material out of the injured area will decrease pain and help to improve ROM.

3. Range of Motion and Flexibility Exercises

THEORY

The patient will need specific exercises to promote increased ROM to achieve functional limits. *Cryokinetics* may initially be used to speed the reacquisition of motion.

4. Resistance Exercises

THEORY

The patient will need to maintain strength in the injured area and return the surrounding musculature to proper function. He may start out with *isometric*

Effleurage: Massage using long, deep strokes.
Cryokinetics: A treatment technique that involves moving the injured body part while it is being treated with cold, thus decreasing pain while increasing range of motion.

contractions and progress to *isotonic contractions* or resistance tubing as tolerated.

5. Balance Exercises

THEORY

The patient demonstrated balance deficits during the initial evaluation that will decrease optimal function. The patient can use a balance system or one-leg stance exercises, progressing from stable to less stable surfaces as tolerated.

6. Maintain Cardiovascular Conditioning

THEORY

Cardiovascular and musculoskeletal endurance must be maintained so that the patient is ready to return to strenuous physical activity.

7. Progressive Return to Activity

THEORY

The capability of the injured ankle to withstand progressively more difficult stresses must be addressed to allow the patient to return to activity in a safe manner. The functional progression would include jogging, running, and progressively harder agility, as well as sport-specific drills to tax the injured area.

8. Ice, Compression, and Elevation
Twenty minutes after exercise and during home treatments.

THEORY

Cold will decrease the metabolic rate in the treated tissues, helping to limit further damage secondary to anoxia and will assist in decreasing pain. The patient will be educated about how to apply a compression wrap and instructed to keep his leg elevated as much as possible, including at work, at rest, and during sleep.

9. Home Exercise Program: ROM, Strengthening, Balancing Exercises, and Ice with Elevation

THEORY

To achieve the goals in a short time, the patient must have an inclusive home program addressing the areas of deficits. Patient compliance is imperative because of the goal of return to activity in 5 days.

CASE STUDY 3

The scenario, recognition, and prioritization of problems and the short- and long-term goals of the patient in this case study are introduced in this section. Each of the remaining chapters in this book concludes with a discussion regarding how

Isometric contractions: Muscle contraction without appreciable joint motion.
Isotonic contractions: Muscle contraction through a range of motion against a constant resistance.

the various modalities could be incorporated into the patient's treatment and re-habilitation plan, although not all of the modalities described in this text would be applicable to this case.

Scenario

A 16-year-old basketball player has been referred to you by his primary care physician for evaluation, treatment, and rehabilitation. The patient was involved in a motor vehicle accident and has been given a diagnosis of a cervical strain and sprain. The following information has been obtained from the patient and the patient's medical records.

Chief complaint: The patient reports pain and muscle spasm in his cervical musculature that limit his motion. Basketball practice is scheduled to begin in 1 week.

History: While driving with his father 4 days ago, they were rear-ended by another driver. He was in the passenger seat and was wearing his seat belt. He was taken to the emergency room from the accident scene and released home that night. The next day he followed up with his family physician and was referred to you.

Diagnostic tests: X-rays taken at the emergency room were negative.

Activity: The patient is a student at the local high school and a point guard on the school's basketball team. He should start for the varsity team this year.

General medical conditions: The patient suffers from asthma; otherwise, he is healthy.

Medications: The patient uses an inhaler for his asthma. Muscle relaxants have been prescribed for his cervical injury.

Contraindications to modality use: None.

Contraindications to therapeutic exercise: None.

Patient goals: To be able to sleep through the night and begin basketball practice as soon as possible.

Evaluative findings:

Function:	The patient cannot play basketball because of pain and spasm.
	The patient cannot sleep through the night undisturbed by pain.
Observation:	The patient wears a soft cervical collar for com-fort.
	The patient has a guarded posture.
Active ROM (C-spine):	Flexion: 50 percent
	Extension: 40 percent
	Right rotation: 50 percent
	Left rotation: 50 percent
	Right-side bending: 25 percent
	Left-side bending: 50 percent
Strength:	Testing of all cervical musculature elicits pain—no grades given because of pain.
Passive ROM:	Flexibility of cervical musculature cannot be assessed due to pain and guarding.
Pain rating:	Pain with right-side bending is 7/10.
	Patient reports constant pain of varying intensity with all ADLs.

Upper quarter screen:	Deep tendon reflexes are 2/2 bilaterally.
	Sensations are intact to light touch bilaterally.
	Result of manual muscle test is 5/5 throughout.
Special tests:	Cervical compression: No *radicular pain;* increased cervical pain
	Cervical distraction: No radicular pain; increased cervical pain
Palpation:	Increased tone is present in the left upper trapezius due to muscle spasm.
	Trigger points are palpated in both upper trapezius muscles, with the left more tender than the right.

Case Study 3: Recognition of Problems

The following problems have been identified with this patient:

1. Inability to play basketball.
2. Inability to sleep undisturbed secondary to pain.
3. Decreased cervical ROM.
4. Inability to assess strength and flexibility of the cervical musculature because of pain.
5. Pain is rated 7/10 during right-side bending.
6. Increased tone because of muscle spasm of the left upper trapezius.
7. Patient wears a soft cervical collar for comfort.

Commentary

- The inability to function is the result of the pain, spasm, and loss of ROM of the cervical muscles. Although all of these are significant problems, the chief reason why someone seeks and needs rehabilitation is to reduce pain and restore function.
- The decreased cervical ROM is most likely a result of pain and spasm versus true joint restriction of the connective tissues about the joint. In an otherwise healthy 16-year-old patient, you would not see changes in the joint structures so quickly after an injury of this type.
- The inability to complete any portion of the patient assessment should be noted, and the reason for the omission should be explained. This documentation serves as a reminder to assess these at a future date and informs other clinicians who are not familiar with the patient's history that these tests were not performed. By noting that these examinations were not conducted, other clinicians will not assume that areas were not assessed or were assessed and were normal.
- The increased muscle tone of the trapezius is caused by the pain-spasm-pain cycle and is typical after acute musculoskeletal injury, secondary to a reflexive protective mechanism. Although this mechanism is protective during the acute stages of an injury, the clinician must work to relieve the pain-spasm-pain cycle so that healing may take place. The spasm will restrict blood flow and the delivery of nutrients and oxygen to the injured tissues and surrounding areas.

Radicular pain: Radiating pain arising from a spinal nerve root and affecting the corresponding dermatome.

- The soft cervical collar is not a problem itself; it is a reasonable treatment option at this time. Although this collar serves an important protective purpose, it does not allow normal function.

Case Study 3: Prioritizing the Problems

The prioritized problem list for this patient is:
1. Pain is rated 7/10 during right-side bending.
2. Increased muscle tone secondary to muscle spasm of the left upper trapezius.
3. Decreased cervical ROM.
4. Inability to assess strength and flexibility of the cervical musculature because of pain.
5. Inability to play basketball.
6. Inability to sleep undisturbed because of pain.
7. Patient wears a soft cervical collar for comfort.

Commentary

This patient's pain and spasm are given the highest priority because they cause the patient's restricted motion. The pain-spasm cycle is a protective response that, when prolonged, can delay the return of the patient to full activity. The decreased cervical ROM will limit the ability of the patient to perform ADLs, will prohibit him from competing in basketball, and will hinder rehabilitation exercises. The clinician must use modalities and exercise to reduce the pain-spasm cycle and increase blood flow to the area.

Assigning a low priority to the functional problems should not be interpreted as indicating that these concerns are trivial. These functional problems are a result of the patient's other problems. By correcting the problems of pain, spasm, ROM, and any inadequacies of strength and flexibility, the clinician will be able to return the patient to functional activity.

The wearing of the soft cervical collar is not of great concern at this time. Although a patient should not be allowed to rely on this orthosis, it is prudent to allow him to wear it for comfort. He should be weaned from it as tolerated.

Case Study 3: Long-Term Goals

The following long-term goals have been established for this patient:
1. The patient will return to full activity playing basketball.
2. The patient will be able to sleep undisturbed without use of the cervical collar.
3. The patient will have normal ROM, flexibility, and strength.
4. The patient will be symptom-free.

Commentary

The long-term goals have been established for a 3-week period. The goals address basic ADLs such as sleep as well as more strenuous activities (e.g., sports, fitness, and work). Note that the patient will have normal ROM, flexibility, and strength. This goal is certainly feasible in this period and essential if this patient is to return to activity, predisposing himself to further injury.

Case Study 3: Short-Term Goals

The following short-term goals have been established for this patient:
1. The patient's pain with right-side bending will be reported as 3/10 or less.

2. The patient's muscle spasm will decrease to the point at which the cervical collar will be worn only at night.
3. The patient's cervical ROM will improve to:

    | Flexion: | 75 percent |
    | Extension: | 60 percent |
    | Right rotation: | 75 percent |
    | Left rotation: | 75 percent |
    | Right-side bending: | 50 percent |
    | Left-side bending: | 75 percent |

4. The clinician will be able to assess the strength and flexibility of the patient's cervical musculature.
5. The patient will be able to sleep throughout the night undisturbed by pain.
6. Patient will not participate in basketball at this time.
7. Patient will be compliant and independent in a home exercise program.

Commentary

A 1-week period for attaining the short-term goals is initially set. In a young, active, otherwise healthy person this period should be adequate to note changes in the patient's condition. Because this patient has a short time frame before the start of basketball season, the clinician will want to evaluate the patient more frequently so that changes can be expediently made to the rehabilitation program.

The first three goals are set to measure the efficacy of the program in relieving the patient's pain and spasm. Goal 4 is information that could not be determined during the initial evaluation because of the patient's pain.

The goals concerning sleep and the use of the collar are reasonable. If they are met, the patient will be less dependent on the collar and function better. The patient should not be participating in basketball because he is likely to aggravate the injury and may be at risk for reinjury.

The final goal is always important because we should always strive to make our patients independent through compliance with their home program, which will expedite the rehabilitation process.

Case Study 3: Treatment Planning

The treatment plan for this case study is presented in Chapters 4 through 7. The plan outlined in each chapter focuses on modalities discussed in that chapter. Although the various chapters present a wide range of treatment strategies, this is not to imply that all of these modalities would be used during the same treatment session. Care must be taken to avoid overtreating the patient, especially when the patient is billed per modality used.

All of the possible treatment approaches are not necessarily presented, and your instructor may describe other treatment plans or challenge you to devise your own strategy.

The following would also be incorporated into the patient's treatment plan:

1. Cardiovascular Exercise
Stationary bicycle riding for 30 minutes, maintaining the patient's heart rate at 122 to 163 beats per minute.

THEORY

Cardiovascular exercise would be incorporated early to maintain the patient at a high level of conditioning. The patient must maintain his heart rate in the target range to achieve aerobic conditioning. The patient could progress to other forms of cardiovascular conditioning as his healing permits.

2. Weaning from the Cervical Collar

THEORY

The patient should be allowed to wear the cervical collar as needed as long as he does not become dependent on it. He should be encouraged to wean himself from its use, wearing it less during waking hours, only at night for sleep, and then not at all as long as he can sleep undisturbed and perform normal ADLs without increasing his symptoms.

3. Strengthening Exercises
Progressive resistance exercises (PREs) for the lower extremities, upper extremities, and spinal musculature as the patient's cervical ROM becomes normal and there is no pain with ADLs.

THEORY

Strengthening of the injured area and maintaining peak muscular strength are needed so that the patient may return to full activity in the shortest possible time. Exercise for the lower extremities could be started almost immediately; PREs for the upper extremities and spine should be started after the pain begins to subside and the ROM begins to increase.

4. Progressive Return to Basketball
The patient would first progress through individual basketball drills and then to one-on-one drills. After successful completion of these, he could progress to scrimmaging and then full competition.

REFERENCES

1. Deyo, RA and Carter, WB: Strategies for improving and expanding the application of health status measures in clinical settings: A researcher-developer viewpoint. Med Care 30:MS176, 1992.
2. Menard, MR and Hoens, AM: Objective evaluation of functional capacity: Medical, occupational, and legal settings. J Orthop Sports Phys Ther 19:249, 1994.
3. Wilson, BM: Promoting compliance: The patient-provider relationship. Adv Ren Replace Ther 2:199, 1995.
4. Northern, JG, et al: Involvement of adult rehabilitation patients in setting occupational therapy goals. Am J Occup Ther 49:214, 1995.
5. Nelson, CE and Payton, OD: A system for involving patients in program planning. Am J Occup Ther 45:753, 1991.
6. Pozgar, GD: Legal Aspects of Health Care Administration, ed 3. Aspen Publications, Rockville, MD, 1987.
7. Drowatzky, JN: Legal duties and liability in athletic training. Athletic Training 20:10, 1985.
8. Morin, GE: An overview of selected state licensure athletic training laws. Journal of Athletic Training 27:162, 1992.
9. Gieck, J, Lowe, J, and Kenna, K: Trainer malpractice: A sleeping giant. Athletic Training 19:41, 1984

CHAPTER 4

Thermal Agents

This chapter contains information regarding those modalities that rely on electromagnetic properties to elicit various responses in the body's systems. The chapter is broken down into two sections, cold and heat, with specific modalities covered according to their various local effects.

Thermal agents transfer energy to or from the tissues. This transfer of energy may be based on a temperature gradient, as with ice or heat, or the conversion of electromagnetic energy, as with the diathermies (see Appendix B). Compared with the extreme range of temperatures found on the electromagnetic spectrum, there is relatively little difference between the upper and lower temperature limits of thermal treatments. Within our tissues, the 65°F that form the upper and lower limits of heat and cold modalities elicit a wide range of cellular and vascular events (Box 4–1).

COLD MODALITIES

Cold is a relative state characterized by decreased molecular motion. The term **cryotherapy** is used to describe the application of cold modalities that have a temperature range between 32°F and 65°F. During cryotherapy, heat is removed from the body and absorbed by the cold modality, causing the body to respond with a series of local and systemic responses. The magnitude of these effects is related to the temperature of the modality, the duration of the treatment, and the surface area exposed to the treatment. The local effects of cold application include vasoconstriction and decreased metabolic rate, decreased inflammation, and decreased pain (Table 4–1).

To obtain therapeutic benefits, the skin temperature must be decreased to approximately 57°F for the optimal decrease in local blood flow to occur and to approximately 58°F for analgesia to occur.[1–3] The application of cold to the skin activates a mechanism that is thought to conserve heat in the body's core, triggering a series of metabolic and vascular events that produce the beneficial effects of

BOX 4–1 **Heat as a Physical Entity**

Temperatures, their perception, and their effects are relative. If the temperature outside is 60°, we think, "It's cold," if it was 80° yesterday; "It's warming up," if it was 40° yesterday; or "I wish the weather would change," if the previous day's temperature was also 60°. This concept also holds true for the application of thermal modalities. The classifications of "heat" and "cold" are based on the physiological response elicited by the temperature. When the temperature of an object is measured, the speed of molecular movement is being quantified. Increased speed of molecular motion is measured as an increase in temperature.

The basic principle behind any thermal modality is to transfer heat across a temperature gradient (that is, one object is warmer than the other). Heat, a form of energy, is lost from the warmer object and moved into the cooler object. The greater the temperature gradient, the more quickly energy is transferred.[4] When a moist heat pack is placed on a patient, energy is transferred away from the pack and absorbed by the tissues. Likewise, when a cold pack is used, the heat is drawn away from the tissues and delivered to the pack.

Heat is measured in **calories,** which describe the amount of energy needed to raise the temperature of 1 gram of water by 1°C. Some objects require less energy per unit of mass to raise their temperature than others. This ability, **thermal capacity,** is measured by the number of heat units required to raise the temperature of a unit of mass by 1°C. Iron, for example, requires less energy to raise its temperature than water. If an equal mass of these two substances were to be heated with an equal amount of energy, the iron would reach the terminal temperature faster than water. Likewise, the water would cool to its original temperature faster than the iron.

An object's ability to transmit thermal energy is measured in terms of **specific heat.** The specific heat of an object is determined by the ratio of its thermal capacity to that of water, which has been given the baseline thermal capacity of 1. In comparing the specific heat of the three states of water, ice has a specific heat of 0.5, water 1.0, and steam 0.48.

cryotherapy. A moderate correlation ($r = 0.65$) exists between the skin temperature and *intra-articular* temperature, but the skin temperature must be decreased a minimum of 36°F to produce intra-articular temperature changes within the knee.[5,6] As the temperature of the skin overlying a joint decreases, the temperature within the joint decreases proportionally (e.g., decreasing the skin temperature 10°F would result in a 6.5°F decrease in the intra-articular temperature).[7]

TABLE 4–1 **Local Effects of Cold Application**

Vasoconstriction
Decreased rate of cell metabolism resulting in a decreased need for oxygen
Decreased production of cellular wastes
Reduction in inflammation
Decreased pain
Decreased muscle spasm

Intra-articular: Within a joint.

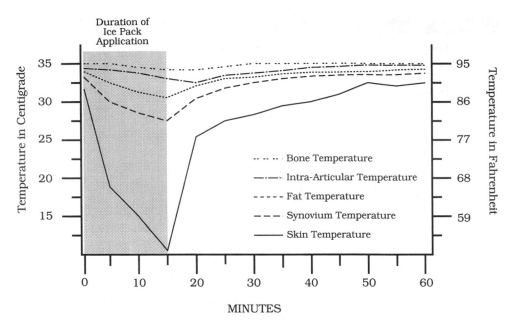

FIGURE 4–1 **Depth of Penetration during the Application of an Ice Pack.** Using electrodes implanted in a dog's knee, this figure indicates the rate, magnitude, and duration of temperature decrease in subcutaneous tissue. (From Bocobo et al,[8] p 183, with permission.)

This principle can be applied to the application of heat modalities: Increased skin temperature results in increased joint space temperature (although, as we will see, the effects of heat do not penetrate as deeply as those of cold).

During treatment, the most rapid and significant temperature changes occur in the skin and *synovium,* with the magnitude of this response varying among the different methods of cold application (Fig. 4–1). Using probes implanted in dogs' knees, intra-articular temperatures have been measured to drop 36.4°F during ice immersion.[8] In humans, intra-articular temperatures may drop as much as 16.9°F during the application of an ice pack to the knee.[9]

If the temperature of circulating blood is decreased by 0.2°F, the *hypothalamus* responds by initiating several systemic effects (Table 4–2). A systemic vasoconstriction occurs and the heart rate is decreased in an attempt to localize the cold. If the proportion of the body area being cooled is sufficient, the heart rate is reduced in an attempt to maintain the body's core temperature by limiting the rate at which cool blood is circulated. If the core temperature continues to decrease toward the point of *hypothermia,* shivering and increased muscle tone assist in keeping the body heat inward. This severe response is normal when the human body is exposed to extremely cold environments (e.g., falling into a near-frozen lake). It is **not** a common response in therapeutic cold application.

Cold modalities may be used effectively during all stages of the inflammatory response. Indications for the use of cold include acute injury or inflammation, pain,

---

Synovium: Membrane lining the capsule of a joint.
Hypothalamus: The body's thermoregulatory center.
Hypothermia: Decreased core temperature.

TABLE 4–2   **General Systemic Effects of Cold Exposure***

> General vasoconstriction in response to cooling of the posterior hypothalamus
> Decreased respiratory and heart rates
> Shivering and increased muscle tone

*These systemic effects primarily occur when the entire body is exposed to cold temperatures. Therefore, we would expect them to occur during a full-body cold immersion rather than during the application of an ice pack.

muscle spasm, and restoration of range of motion (Table 4–3). Primary contraindications for the use of cold are conditions in which the body is unable to cope with the temperature because of allergy, hypersensitivity, or circulatory insufficiency.

Effects on the Injury Response Process

Cold modalities are perhaps the most versatile of therapeutic modalities. The body's response to cold elicits a wide range of cellular, vascular, and nervous system responses that regulate the inflammatory response, decrease pain and muscle spasm, and limit the scope of the original injury. Cold may be safely applied to most orthopedic injuries and other conditions throughout the healing process.

TABLE 4–3   **General Indications and Contraindications for Cold Treatments**

Indications

Acute injury or inflammation
Acute or chronic pain
Small, superficial, first-degree burns
Postsurgical pain and edema
Use in conjunction with rehabilitation exercises
Spasticity accompanying central nervous system disorders
Acute or chronic muscle spasm
Neuralgia[76]

Contraindications

Cardiac or respiratory involvement.
Uncovered open wounds.
Circulatory insufficiency.
Cold allergy.
Anesthetic skin.
Advanced diabetes.
Raynaud's phenomenon: Although this is usually a benign condition, Raynaud's phenomenon may be a symptom of an underlying disease state, most commonly systemic sclerosis.[77]

Raynaud's phenomenon: A vascular reaction to cold application or stress that results in a white, red, or blue discoloration of the extremities. The fingers and toes are the first to be affected.

Cellular Response

The most beneficial effect of cold application during an acute injury is the decreased need for oxygen in the area being treated.[4,10] A cold environment decreases cellular metabolic rate, consequently decreasing the amount of oxygen required by the cells to survive. During a 20-minute treatment, cell metabolism decreases by 19 percent.[2] By reducing the number of cells killed by a lack of oxygen, the degree of secondary hypoxic injury is limited. Because fewer cells are damaged from secondary hypoxic injury, reduced amounts of inflammatory mediators are released into the area, containing the scope of the injury (see Chap. 1).

Blood and Fluid Dynamics

Because cold application decreases the rate of cell metabolism and reduces the tissue's need for oxygen, it would seem to follow that blood flow to the treatment area would be lessened. Despite this seemingly sound logic, the effects of cold application on blood flow have been (and still remain) a topic of much investigation.

Vasoconstriction occurs because of the stimulation of local nerve receptors, triggering a response from the sympathetic nervous system instructing the vessels to constrict. As the molecular motion of the blood and tissue fluids slows, their viscosity increases. The reduction in blood flow occurs too late in the injury response process to affect the hemorrhaging process, but it may prevent hematoma formation.[4,11]

Lewis[12] performed studies in 1930 on the dynamics of blood flow during cold treatments. When the fingers were immersed in cold water, alternating periods of cooling and warming were seen in the skin. Termed the **hunting response,** it appeared that blood vessels underwent a series of vasoconstriction and vasodilation in an attempt to adapt to the temperature. However, the hunting response has been identified only in selected areas of the body (e.g., fingers, nose).[13]

Later, Knight[4] examined the reputed increase in blood flow as the result of **cold-induced vasodilation.** His work suggested that the degree of vasodilation only lessened the amount of initial vasoconstriction. Despite the vasodilation, there was still a net vasoconstriction when compared with the vessel diameter before treatment (Fig. 4–2).

The effect of cold application on blood flow has been measured using *impedance plethysmography,* and most studies indicated that cold application causes decreased blood flow,[2,13,14] but the results are not universally conclusive.[15] A 20-minute cold pack application appears to decrease soft tissue blood flow 26 percent and skeletal blood flow 19 percent[2] and reduces the amount of edema in traumatized ankles.[14] Because of the effects associated with rubbing the skin, ice massage may increase blood flow, at least in the skin.[15] All studies do agree, however, that reactive vasodilation did not occur during a 20-minute period of cold application. Any increase in blood flow appears to be transitory and related to another mechanism, such as increased heart rate or stroke volume, as the vessel diameter does not appear to change.[13]

Impedance plethysmography: A determination of blood flow based on the amount of electrical resistance in the area.

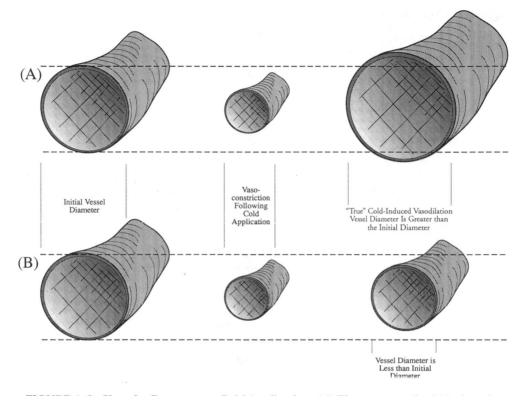

FIGURE 4–2 **Vascular Response to Cold Application.** (*A*) The concept of cold-induced vasodilation. After the application of therapeutic cold there is an immediate vasoconstriction. This is followed by vasodilation, resulting in a larger diameter than before the ice application. This event has not been substantiated. (*B*) Vascular reaction as suggested by Knight.[9] After the initial vasoconstriction there is a dilation of the vessel, but its diameter is still reduced in comparison to the original diameter.

    Evidence supporting the beneficial effects of cold in reducing the collection of edema is not as great as once thought, and the mechanisms that would encourage venous and lymphatic return are unclear.[15] It stands to reason that the vasoconstriction described for arteries would apply to both the venous and lymphatic vessels. The same mechanism that limits blood flow to the region, vasoconstriction, would also hinder drainage from the area and could actually cause an initial increase in limb volume.[16] However, a study using an animal model suggested that cold application does not decrease the cross-sectional diameter of arterioles but, surprisingly, increased the diameter of venules.[17] Increasing the diameter of the veins not only decreases the fluid's resistance to flow but also increases the surface area needed to reabsorb the edema. This effect has also been substantiated in clinical studies.[14]

    Despite the relatively contradictory and confusing findings relative to the application of cold on an injured body part, the primary benefit of its use, especially in the treatment of acute injuries, is the reduction of cell metabolism. Likewise, the effects of compression and elevation in limiting the formation of edema have been substantiated as well. These three elements together prevent further hypoxic injury (see section on Effects of Immediate Treatment, p 118).

Effects on Inflammation

Changes in cellular function and blood dynamics serve to control the effects of acute inflammation. Cold application suppresses the inflammatory response by:

- Reducing the release of inflammatory mediators[10,11]
- Decreasing prostaglandin synthesis[10]
- Decreasing capillary permeability[10]

The secondary formation of edema and hemorrhage is reduced because of an inhibitory effect on the mediators and decreased capillary permeability.

As described by the injury response cycle (see Fig. 1–2), limiting the amount of inflammation inhibits the effects of the remaining components. Limiting inflammatory mediators reduces the degree of hemorrhage and edema; lessening the mechanical pressure on nerves decreases pain. As muscle spasm and edema are reduced, there is less congestion in the area, and the amount of secondary hypoxic cell death is limited.

Muscle Spasm and Function

Cold reduces muscle spasm in two ways:

1. It decreases pain by reducing the threshold of afferent nerve endings.
2. It decreases the sensitivity of muscle spindles.

A drop of 9°F in surface skin temperature reduces the sensitivity of muscle spindles. The drop in muscle spindle activity, combined with the decreased rate of afferent nerve impulses, inhibits the stretch reflex mechanism and results in decreased muscle spasm.[11,18] A short-term break in the pain-spasm-pain cycle may result in long-term relief of muscle spasms secondary to decreasing the amount of mechanical pressure placed on the nerves and other tissues.

This mechanism also affects the limb's muscular ability. Decreased nerve conduction velocity, decreased sensitivity of muscle spindles, and increased fluid viscosity lead to a decreased ability to perform rapid muscle movements. After a 20-minute cold application, the quadriceps femoris muscle group produces decreased concentric and eccentric strength and decreased isokinetic strength, power,[19–23] and endurance[19–22] for up to 30 minutes after the termination of treatment.

Pain Control

Cold application affects pain perception and transmission by interrupting pain transmission, decreasing nerve condition velocity, reducing muscle spasm, and reducing or limiting edema. By stimulating the large-diameter neurons, cold inhibits pain transmission, acting (in terms of the gate control theory) as a *counterirritant*.[24] The sensory events associated with the application of a cold modality stimulate the large-diameter nerves to decrease the transmission and perception of pain.

Physiologically, the transmission of noxious impulses is reduced by lowering the excitability of free nerve endings, resulting in an increased pain threshold. Small-diameter, myelinated nerves are the first to exhibit a change in their con-

---

Counterirritant: A substance causing irritation of superficial sensory nerves so as to reduce the transmission of pain from underlying nerves.

duction velocities. The last to respond to cold temperatures are unmyelinated, small-diameter nerves. This sequence of nerve fiber activation can provide an explanation for the sequence of sensations that accompany cryotherapy.

Cold decreases the speed of nerve conduction by slowing communication at the synapse. In certain cases, this can lead to *neurapraxia* and *axonotmesis*.[25,26] During normal treatment duration and intensity, nerve conduction velocity displays the greatest decrease immediately after the application of ice.[27] If the tissue temperature continues to decrease (i.e., a constant cold temperature is used) or if the treatment continues for extended periods, the nerve conduction rate will drop to a point at which nerves can no longer transmit impulses.[28] Cold-induced nerve palsy has been reported after the treatment of injuries to the anterior compartment of the lower leg.[29,30]

Because cold disrupts muscle spasm, pain is reduced by alleviating the mechanical stimulation placed on the nerve receptors in the area of spasm. A brief disruption in pain may break the injury response cycle and allow tissue healing and repair to proceed unhindered.[10]

Despite its ability to interrupt the transmission and perception of pain, cold application does not appear to significantly inhibit joint proprioception. After standard cold treatments of the knee, lower leg, and ankle, proprioception, balance, and agility are not significantly altered relative to the same, uncooled body parts.[31,32]

Sensations Associated with Cold Application

The terms traditionally used to describe the sensations accompanying cold application are cold, burning, aching, and *analgesia*.[33,34] *Numbness* is a result of decreasing the nerve conduction velocity and increasing the threshold required to fire the nerves.[10] Not all people experience the same sensations during cold application. Eighteen to 21 minutes of cold application are needed before numbness (anesthesia) occurs, and true analgesia is seldom achieved.[35]

Although these reactions are most pronounced during ice immersion, they may also occur during other methods of cold application, and the affective response during the initial treatment period may deter patient compliance. Educating the patient about the sensations to be expected during the treatment tends to make cold application, especially cold immersion, more tolerable.[36,37] Also, repeated exposures to cold treatments can decrease the sensory and affective response to cold application.[38]

Frostbite

When frozen water is used as a means of cold application, there is little chance of frostbite occurring under normal conditions.[18,28] Picture in your mind these

---

Neurapraxia: A temporary loss of function in a peripheral nerve.
Axonotmesis: Damage to nerve tissue without physical severing of the nerve.
Analgesia: Absence of the sense of pain.
Numbness: Lack of sensation in a body part.

forms of ice application: an ice bag, ice massage, and ice immersion. During the course of each of these treatments, water is present. An ice bag fills with water as it melts, ice massage leaves a trail of water with each stroke, and water is the medium used during an ice immersion.

The presence of water indicates that ice is melting and therefore that the temperature of the surface of the ice is 32°F. Frostbite occurs when the skin temperature falls below freezing. When the subcutaneous temperature falls below 55°F, tissue damage occurs. During the course of a 20-minute treatment, cold modalities that have water present cause a decrease in subcutaneous tissue temperatures of 9° to 18°F, a range well within the limits of safety.[18]

After 5 minutes of cold application, the skin should be marked by *hyperemia,* indicating that the circulatory system is continuing to deliver warm blood, even though the skin temperature has dropped substantially. If the area displays signs of *pallor,* the circulatory system has been unable to maintain tissue temperatures within normal physiological limits. In this case, the superficial vasculature has constricted to conserve heat in the underlying tissues. If the tissues become *cyanotic,* the treatment should be discontinued.[28]

If the treatment is applied below the recommended temperature, if the duration of the treatment exceeds the recommended time, or if the patient suffers from severe circulatory insufficiency or decreased sensation, the risk of frostbite (or cold injury) increases (Box 4–2). Prolonged exposure to intense cold decreases circulation throughout the body. Blood traveling through the veins cools the incoming arterial blood and acts to increase the amount of systemic vasoconstriction and to further lower the heart rate. If the treated area is highly ischemic, warm blood cannot reach the tissues.

The risk of frostbite is present when using reusable cold packs. These devices contain water mixed with antifreeze and are stored at temperatures below freezing. Because the surface temperature of the pack may be below freezing, a medium such as a wet towel must be placed between the pack and the skin.

Effects of Immediate Treatment

Immediate treatment—rest, ice, compression, and elevation (RICE)—serves to counteract the body's initial response to an injury. Rest limits the scope of the original injury by preventing further trauma. In acute trauma, "rest" may take the form of immobilizing the body part, the use of crutches, or other methods of avoiding additional insult to the injured tissues.

The function of ice application during immediate treatment is to decrease the cell's metabolism and therefore decrease the need for oxygen in the injured area. This effect reduces the amount of secondary hypoxic injury by enabling the tissues in the injured area to survive on the limited amount of oxygen they are receiving. Crushed ice is the ideal form of cold application during immediate treat-

---

Hyperemia: A red discoloration of the skin caused by increased blood flow. The skin turns white when pressure is applied.
Pallor: Lack of color in the skin.
Cyanosis (cyanotic): A blue-gray discoloration of the skin caused by a lack of oxygen.

BOX 4–2   Signs and Symptoms of Frostbite

Even the most minor case of frostbite is accompanied by extreme pain. This pain is so severe that patients who have normal sensory function will not allow the treatment to continue. The primary concern is for patients who have sensory and/or circulatory impairment or those on whom reusable ice packs are applied.

The first physical sign of frostbite is the fading of the redness normally associated with cold application. This color is replaced by a waxy white sheen. If frostbite is allowed to continue, the skin will blister or molt and lead to an obvious buildup of edema.

During any physical procedure, the circulation to the extremities can be checked by monitoring the flow of blood to the nailbeds. Gently squeezing the nail removes the blood, making it turn white or pale. When the force is removed, the original color should return. If it fails to return, circulatory impairment should be suspected.

If frostbite is suspected, immediately remove the patient from the source of the cold. Rewarm the body part by immersing it in water at 100°F, and refer the patient to a physician for follow-up evaluation.

ment because it produces the most rapid and significant temperature decrease relative to other forms of cold application, and it conforms well to the body part being treated.[39,40] Ice application may also provide a secondary benefit in the immediate treatment of an injury through the reduction of pain. Because of the other factors surrounding the injury (e.g., the severity of the injury or the person's emotional state), the effects of ice on limiting pain cannot be accurately predicted for every case.

Compression decreases the pressure gradient between the blood vessels and tissues. This discourages further leakage from the capillary beds into the interstitial tissues while also encouraging increased lymphatic drainage. Compression wraps are best applied so that a pressure gradient is formed between the distal end of the wrap and the proximal end. The wrap should be applied from distal to proximal end, gradually decreasing the pressure with each turn. Wraps applied with even pressure throughout their length are often counterproductive because they form a kind of tourniquet, inhibiting flow both to and from the area.

Compression may be applied to an injured area through three different techniques:[41]

1. **Circumferential compression** provides an even pressure around the entire circumference of the body part. The cross-sectional area remains circular, but the diameter of the body part decreases. Common forms of circumferential compression are elastic wraps and pneumatic or water-filled sleeves. This type of compression is best suited for evenly shaped body areas, such as the knee or thigh.
2. **Collateral compression** produces pressure on only two sides of the body part, so that the cross-sectional area deforms elliptically. The soft tissues are compressed between the device and the bone. A common form of collateral compression is found in air-filled stirrup braces.
3. **Focal compression,** applied with U-shaped "horseshoe" pads, provides direct pressure to soft tissue surrounded by prominent bony structures (e.g.,

the lateral ligaments of the ankle or the acromioclavicular joint). The pad is placed over the area so that it is in contact with the injured soft tissue while avoiding the bone. A circumferential or collateral compression wrap is then used to apply pressure (Fig. 4–3).

Using an elastic wrap to secure the ice bag to the body part produces a significant reduction in subcutaneous tissue temperatures as compared with the use of an ice bag alone, so long as the wrap is not placed between the ice pack and the skin.[42,43] The combination of ice and compression results in reduced cell metabolism deeper within the tissues, helping to limit the scope and severity of secondary hypoxic injury. An additional benefit arising from the use of an elastic wrap over the injured area is increased joint proprioception secondary to stimulating the afferent receptors in the skin and superficial subcutaneous tissues.[44] This effect can serve to protect injured joints by assisting the body's awareness of the joint's position.

Compression and **elevation** act to decrease the hydrostatic pressure within the capillary beds and to encourage absorption of edema by the lymphatic system. This effect is greatest when the extremity is at 90° perpendicular to the ground; however, this position is not necessarily practical. The limb should be elevated as high as possible while still maintaining a comfortable position. Mechanical implements such as split-leg tables can effectively raise the lower extremity to a 45° angle, at which point the effect of gravity is 71 percent of that in the vertical position (see Fig. 1–6).

Cryokinetics

As its name implies, **cryokinetics** involves the use of cold in conjunction with movement ("cryo" equals cold plus "kinetic" equals motion) and is used to im-

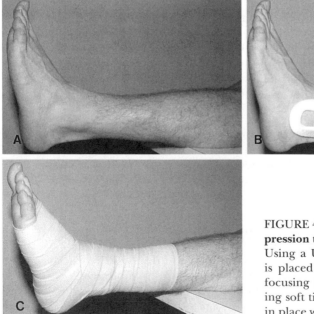

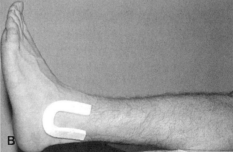

FIGURE 4–3 **Application of Focal Compression to the Lateral Ankle Ligaments.** Using a U-shaped "horseshoe," the pad is placed around the lateral malleolus, focusing the pressure on the surrounding soft tissue. The horseshoe is secured in place with an elastic wrap.

prove motion by eliminating or reducing the element of pain. Early, safe, pain-free motion through the normal range results in a more pronounced macrophage reaction, quicker hematoma resolution, increased vascular growth, faster regeneration of muscle and scar tissue, and increased tensile strength of healed muscle.[9]

Cryokinetics may be initiated in cases in which the underlying soft tissue and bone are intact and in which pain is limiting the amount of functional movement. Although cryokinetics is useful in increasing range of motion, care must be taken to prevent the masking of pain.

HEAT MODALITIES

Heat, the increase in molecular vibration and cellular metabolic rate, is commonly classified into three major categories based on its source:

1. Chemical action associated with cell metabolism
2. Electrical or magnetic currents as those found in diathermy devices
3. Mechanical action as found with ultrasound (see Chap. 6)

The application of therapeutic heat to the body is referred to as **thermotherapy,** and the methods of heating are classified as being superficial or deep (Table 4–4). Superficial heating agents must be capable of increasing the skin temperature within the range of 104°F to 113°F to produce therapeutic effects.[45] The transfer of heat to underlying tissues occurs via conduction, but superficial heating agents are limited to depths less than 2 cm (Box 4–3).

The effects of heat on metabolic rate, blood and fluid dynamics, and inflammation are generally opposite to those of cold (Table 4–5). Both heat and cold applications decrease pain and muscle spasm by altering the threshold of nerve endings. Systemically, local heat application results in increased body temperature, pulse rate, and respiratory rate and decreased blood pressure (Table 4–6). The use of heat is indicated in the subacute and chronic inflammatory stages of injury (Table 4–7).

Because the effects of heat application are essentially opposite to those of cold, its use in the treatment of acute injuries should be avoided. Applying heat to an active inflammatory cycle will increase the rate of cell metabolism and accelerate the amount of hypoxic injury.

TABLE 4–4 Classification of Heating Agents

Superficial Heat	Deep Heat
Infrared lamps	Microwave diathermy*
Moist heat packs	Shortwave diathermy
Paraffin baths	Ultrasound (see Chap. 6)
Warm whirlpool and/or immersion	

*Approved only for research purposes.

BOX 4–3 The Transfer of Thermal Energy

"Heat" is not an actual form of energy; rather, it is a term used to describe certain forms of energy transfer. Within the range of thermal therapeutic modalities, heat transfer involves the exchange of *kinetic energy* between two or more objects (e.g., a hot pack and the skin). For this exchange to occur, one fundamental condition must be met: one object must have a higher temperature than another object. Energy carriers then transmit energy from the high temperature area to the cooler object.[5] This transfer of energy occurs via: conduction, convection, radiation, or evaporation.

Conduction involves the transfer of heat between two objects that are in physical contact with each other. Kinetic energy is exchanged through the collision of molecules, moving the energy from an area of high temperature to an area of lower temperature. This concept can be illustrated by heating one end of a metal rod. The heat is gradually passed from one end of the rod to the other until the rod has an equal temperature along its length. Examples of therapeutic modalities that operate by way of conduction include moist heat packs and ice application. Within the body, the transfer of energy from one tissue layer to another occurs by way of conduction.

Some materials are better conductors of heat than others. Consider wooden and metal picnic tables that have been sitting in direct sunlight and have the same temperature. If you placed one hand on the wooden table and the other hand on the metal table, the metal table would feel "hotter" more rapidly. Even though you are touching two objects with equal temperatures, the greater ability of metal to conduct heat (compared to wood) warms your hand more rapidly.

Convection involves the transportation of heat by the movement of a medium, usually air or water. Of the three *states of matter,* gases are the poorest conductors of heat, whereas liquids are good conductors and solids, generally speaking, are better conductors. Adding motion to gases and liquids, such as circulating air or water, increases their ability to transport heat. The actual transfer of energy from the medium to the body still occurs through conduction; the delivery of the energy occurs by movement of the media. The circulation of the medium results in the cooling of one object and the subsequent heating of another object. Whirlpools are the most common example of therapeutic modalities that use convection.

Radiation is the transfer of energy without the use of a medium, and the heat gained or lost through radiation is termed **radiant energy.** Infrared energy is emitted from any object having a temperature greater than absolute zero. *Divergence* of the energy radiated may occur, resulting in a reduction of the energy received by an object in its path. All thermal therapeutic modalities provide radiant energy. Infrared lamps, for example, deliver most of their energy through radiation. Even modalities that deliver their energy to the body through conduction, such as moist heat packs, lose some of their energy through radiation. This effect can be illustrated by placing your hand just above a moist heat pack. The heat you feel is being lost from the pack via radiation.

Heat loss can also occur through **evaporation.** The change from the liquid state to the gaseous state requires that thermal energy be removed from the body. The heat absorbed by the liquid cools the tissue as the liquid changes its state into gas. Vapocoolant sprays are an example of a modality that operates by evaporation.

Kinetic energy: The energy an object possesses by virtue of its motion.
States of matter: Physical matter can take three forms: solid, liquid, and gas. Using H_2O as example, we see the three states of matter as ice, water, and steam.
Divergence: The spreading of a beam or wave.

TABLE 4–5   **Local Effects of Heat Application**

Vasodilation
Increased rate of cell metabolism
Increased delivery of leukocytes
Increased capillary permeability
Increased venous and lymphatic drainage
Edema formation
Removal of metabolic wastes
Increased elasticity of ligaments, capsules, and muscle
Analgesia and sedation of nerves
Decreased muscle tone
Decreased muscle spasm
Perspiration
Increased nerve conduction velocity

TABLE 4–6   **Some Systemic Effects of Heat Exposure***

Increased body temperature
Increased pulse rate
Increased respiratory rate
Decreased blood pressure

*These systemic effects primarily occur when the entire body is exposed to warm temperatures. Therefore we would expect them to occur during a full-body warm immersion rather than during the application of a moist heat pack.

TABLE 4–7   **General Indications and Contraindications for Heat Treatments**

Indication

Subacute or chronic inflammatory conditions
Reduction of subacute or chronic pain
Subacute or chronic muscle spasm
Decreased range of motion
Hematoma resolution
Reduction of joint contractures

Contraindications

Acute injuries
Impaired circulation
Poor thermal regulation
Anesthetic areas
Neoplasms

Neoplasm: Abnormal tissue, such as a tumor, that grows at the expense of healthy tissue.

Effects on the Injury Response Process

Despite the fact that heat and cold produce many of the same outcomes, decreased pain, for example, the timing of when to begin using heat modalities is much more critical. A primary effect of heat modalities is an increase in cell metabolism and the rate of inflammation. If heat is applied too soon in the injury response process, the increased cell metabolism causes an increase in the number of cells injured or destroyed because of hypoxia. Increasing the inflammatory rate could possibly extend the acute and subacute inflammatory stages.

Cellular Response

The rate of cell metabolism increases in response to the rise in tissue temperature. For each increase of 18°F in skin temperature, the cell's metabolic rate increases by a factor of two to three.[46] As the cell's metabolic rate increases, so does its demand for oxygen and nutrients. As with all living organisms that consume energy, the amount of waste excreted from the cell increases as its activity increases.

There is a reciprocal relationship between tissue temperature and the rate of cell metabolism. Not only does increased temperature cause an increase in cellular metabolic rate, but an increase in cellular metabolic rate also causes tissue temperature to rise. As with all heat applications, increased cellular metabolic rate causes arteriolar dilation and increased capillary flow. This supports the therapeutic properties of exercise.

Blood and Fluid Dynamics

The body responds to the rise in tissue temperature by dilating local blood vessels, the amount of vasodilation being greater in superficial vessels than in the deeper vessels. Increased capillary flow results in an increased supply of oxygen, nutrients, and antibodies to the affected area.

The amount of edema is increased, but the capability of removing it is greater. Increased capillary pressure forces edema and harmful *metabolites* from the injured area. Increased capillary permeability aids in the reabsorption of edema and the dissolution of hematomas. These wastes can drain into the venous and lymphatic systems. If venous and lymphatic return is not encouraged, further edema occurs.

Effect on Inflammation

The local application of heat accelerates inflammation. Soft tissue repair is facilitated through an accelerated metabolic rate and increased blood supply. Blood flow must be increased to encourage the removal of cellular debris and to increase delivery of the nutrients necessary for the healing of tissues.[47] Increased oxygen delivery stimulates the breakdown and removal of tissue debris and inflammatory metabolites. Nutrients are delivered to the area to fuel the

---

Metabolite: A by-product of metabolism.

cells, and there is also an increase in the delivery of leukocytes, encouraging phagocytosis.

Muscle Spasm and Tissue Elasticity

Increased temperature reduces the primary and secondary muscle spindles' sensitivity to stretch, decreasing the amount of muscle spasm present (see Box 1–3). Increasing blood flow and reducing local muscle metabolites further alleviate spasm.[5] Most muscular tissues are not directly heated by superficial heating agents.

Range of motion is subsequently improved by increasing the extensibility of collagen and the viscosity and plastic deformation of tissues.[48] This effect alone is not sufficient to decrease contractures or increase the elasticity of healthy tissues. Neither anterior laxity of the knee (as measured by a KT-1000 arthrometer) nor hamstring flexibility has been shown to be affected by heat modalities alone.[49,50] Tension, in the form of gentle stretching, is necessary to elongate muscle and capsular tissues while the tissues are still within the therapeutic temperature range.

Pain Control

Mechanical deformation and/or chemical irritation of nerve endings stimulate pain transmission. In acute injuries, the primary cause of pain is the mechanical damage done to the tissue in the area. In the subacute and chronic stage of injury, ischemia and irritation cause chemical pain from certain chemical mediators. Mechanical pain is caused by increased tissue pressure (swelling) and the tension placed on nerves by muscle spasm. Increasing circulation to the area decreases congestion, allowing oxygen to be delivered to the suffocating cells. Increased circulation (blood flow to and away from the area) assists in washing out the pain-producing chemicals in the area.

Mechanical pain is decreased by reducing the pressure on the nerves, thus lessening the pain-spasm-pain cycle. By encouraging venous and lymphatic return through the use of elevation and muscle contraction, the swelling is removed, decreasing interstitial pressure.

An increase in temperature leads to a state of analgesia and *sedation* in the injured area by acting on free nerve endings. Nerve fibers are stimulated, blocking the transmission of pain with a counterirritant effect. This effect appears to last only as long as the stimulus of heat is applied, and when heat is removed, the pain symptoms quickly return.[25,51]

Dissipation of Heat in the Treatment Area

When therapeutic heat is applied to the body, there is a rapid rise in skin temperature. This rise occurs because energy is being absorbed faster than the cool blood delivered to the area can remove it. After approximately 10 to 15 minutes of exposure, the temperature gradient begins to even out. At this point, the body is able to counteract the energy being applied by supplying an adequate amount of blood to cool the area. At this time, the patient may claim that the modality has cooled down when, in fact, its intensity is unchanged (Fig. 4–4).

When a maximal vasodilation has occurred and the intensity of the treatment stays constant (or increases), the vessels begin to constrict. This phenomenon,

---

Sedation: The result of calming nerve endings.

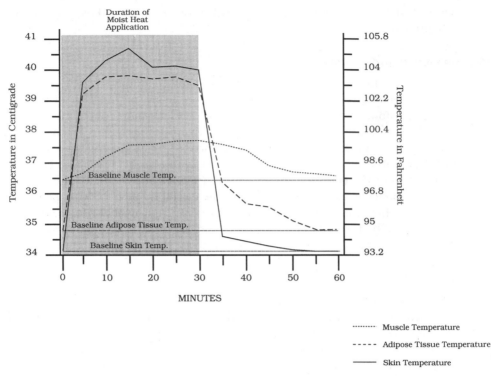

FIGURE 4–4 **Depth of Penetration and Duration of Superficial Heating.** During the application of superficial heat (moist heat pack), the skin temperature has the most significant temperature increase. Muscular temperature has the lowest temperature increase, but the increased temperature has the longest-lasting effects. (Adapted from Abramson, DI, et al: Changes in blood flow, oxygen uptake, and tissue temperatures produced by the topical application of wet heat. Arch Phys Med Rehabil 42:305, 1961.)

known as **rebound vasoconstriction,** occurs approximately 20 minutes into the treatment.[28] This is the body's attempt to save underlying tissues by sacrificing the superficial layer. If the intensity of treatment is too great or if the duration of exposure is too long, burns will result.

Mottling of the skin is a warning sign that tissue temperatures are rising to a dangerously high level. In this case, ghost-white areas and beet-red splotches mark the patient's skin. When mottling occurs, the treatment should be discontinued immediately.

The likelihood of rebound vasoconstriction increases with treatments in which the temperature and intensity are kept constant. Modalities such as infrared lamps and paraffin immersion baths maintain a constant intensity throughout the treatment. With modalities such as moist heat packs, the intensity of the treatment decreases with time because the modality loses heat during the application.

CONTRAST AND COMPARISON OF HEAT AND COLD APPLICATION

Cold modalities are more penetrating and their effects longer lasting than those of heat modalities. Heat causes a vasodilation that delivers cool blood to the area while the warmer blood is transported away. In contrast, cold application causes a vaso-

TABLE 4–8 **Comparison of Heat and Cold Treatments**

Effect	Cold	Heat
Depth of penetration	5 cm	1–2 cm (superficial agents) 2–5 cm (deep-heating agents)
Duration of effects	Hours	Begins to dissipate after the removal of the modality
Blood flow	Decreased (Vasoconstriction)	Increased (Vasodilation)
Rate of cell metabolism	Decreased	Increased
Oxygen consumption	Decreased	Increased
Cell wastes	Decreased	Increased
Fluid viscosity	Increased	Decreased
Capillary permeability	Decreased	Increased
Inflammation	Decreased	Increased
Pain	Decreased	Decreased
Muscle spasm	Decreased by reducing the sensitivity of muscle spindles and decreasing pain	Decreased by reducing ischemia and pain
Muscle contraction velocity	Decreased by reducing nerve conduction velocity and increasing fluid viscosity	Increased

constriction, resulting in a decreased amount of blood arriving to warm the area. This allows deeper tissues to be affected more by cold than by heat (Table 4–8).

After the removal of the modality, the effects of cold are longer lasting than those of heat. This is a result of the same mechanisms that account for the depth of penetration. After heat treatment, cool blood continues to flow to the area, decreasing the temperature. In contrast, the cool tissue temperature resulting from cold application causes the vasoconstriction of blood vessels and a decrease in the amount of blood delivered to the area, so that a longer time is needed for rewarming than for recooling.[52]

Both modalities effectively reduce pain perception by increasing the patient's pain threshold. Although patients prefer moist heat modalities, their effectiveness is short-lived after the treatment.[51]

The application of cold reduces the amounts of inflammatory mediators and cell by-products released into the area. These cellular wastes, including lactic acid and nitrogen, are insulting to the tissues and increase the amount of tissue damage and pain. When heat is applied during the proliferation stage of inflammation, the vascular response assists in removing cellular waste.

Use of Heat versus Cold

One of the questions most asked by students is "How do you know when to use heat and when to use cold?" There are no clear-cut answers to this question. Many texts and articles give definitive time frames, such as: "Use ice for the first 24 hours and heat for the next 48." Unfortunately, statements like this are incorrect and unjustified.

One of the first points made in this text was that the body heals an injury at its own rate. Not only does this rate vary from person to person but also it may vary from injury to injury in the same person. The patient's physical and psychological state, as well as the type and amount of tissue damaged, factor into the time frame required for healing.

The decision-making process is similar to the steps involved when a pipe ruptures in the basement of a house. Before bailing out the water and cleaning up the mess, you have to stop the leak. Likewise, before encouraging an increase in the rate of cell metabolism in an injured area, the active process of inflammation must be calmed down (Table 4–9).

Cold application is indicated under three conditions: (1) in the acute stages of the inflammatory reaction, (2) before range-of-motion exercises, and (3) after physical activity. When cold is applied as a form of immediate treatment or in the active inflammation stage, some form of ice pack should be used. When cold is being administered before rehabilitation exercises, a cold whirlpool or immersion should be used because of the latent cooling effects of these modalities.[39] Athletes and other highly motivated persons often return to physical activity before full healing of the tissues, thus perpetuating the inflammatory process. As a result, cold application is often used over an extended time frame in these persons as compared with the general population.

Heat application is indicated under these five conditions: (1) to control the inflammatory reaction in its subacute or chronic stages, (2) to encourage tissue healing, (3) to reduce edema and ecchymosis, (4) to improve range of motion before physical activity (e.g., participation in the sport) or rehabilitation, and (5) to promote drainage from an infected site.

A distinction should be made between using cold modalities for range-of-motion exercises and using heat modalities before competition. As you will recall, cold increases fluid viscosity and decreases the ability to perform rapid movements. During participation in a sport, athletes rely on the ability to move the extremities in a rapid, powerful manner. Heat is used for its ability to allow this type of movement. Ice is indicated after the activity to prevent reactivation of the inflammatory process. If motion is limited by pain, then cold should be used; if motion is limited by stiffness, heat would be the modality of choice.

The decision about when to use heat and cold should not be based on any predetermined time frame. This decision should be based on the desired physiological responses at any one point in time. When the desired goal is to limit or reduce the amount of inflammation, cold should be used. When the inflammatory

TABLE 4–9   **Deciding Whether to Use Heat or Cold**

Evaluate the patient to determine the answer to each of the following questions:
1. Does the body area feel warm to the touch?
2. Is the injured area still sensitive to light to moderate touch?
3. Does the amount of swelling continue to increase over time?
4. Does swelling increase during activity (joint motion)?
5. Does pain limit the joint's range of motion?
6. Would you consider the acute inflammation process to still be active?
7. Does the patient continue to display improvement with the use of cold modalities?
If all of the answers to these questions are "no," then heat can be safely used. As the number of "yes" answers increases, so does the indication to use cold.

response has subsided to the point at which tissue healing begins, heat is applied. When in doubt, use cold.

To a lesser degree, the patient's preference of modalities may be considered. Some patients prefer cold modalities, but more commonly they prefer heat. For many, the change from cold to heat is a milestone signaling that their healing process is progressing.

SUMMARY

The physiological effects of heat or cold application are the result of the body's attempt to adjust to the temperature. Several considerations must be made to determine which temperature must be used in the treatment of orthopedic injuries. Immediate treatment of injuries involves the use of ice, compression, elevation, and rest to limit the scope of the original injury. While the inflammatory process is in its active state or while the tissues are ischemic, cold application is used primarily to decrease the amount of secondary hypoxic injury by reducing the cells' needs for oxygen. Additional benefits are gained through cold application in the form of pain relief and decreased muscle spasm.

Heat application may be initiated when the inflammation process is in a more passive mode. The increased temperature accelerates the rate at which blood and nutrients are delivered to the injured tissues. The increased capillary pressure forces edema and metabolites from the area, and their removal from the area is augmented by increased capillary permeability. By decreasing the amount of mechanical pressure placed on nerve endings and supplying oxygen to the tissues, pain is reduced.

CLINICAL APPLICATION OF THERMAL MODALITIES

The following sections describe the most common methods of applying therapeutic cold and heat to the human body; any unique physiological effects (in addition to those described at the beginning of this chapter); the procedures used; and the indications, contraindications, and precautions to their use.

Cold Packs

Cold compresses may be delivered to the body through four techniques: (1) plastic bags filled with crushed or flaked ice, (2) reusable cold gel packs, (3) controlled cold therapy (CCT) units, and (4) chemical (or "instant") cold packs in which the sensation of cold is produced by a chemical reaction. Each method of cold pack application has its own advantages and disadvantages.

Clinicians often place some form of insulation between the cold pack and the skin, often performed with the well-meaning intent of preventing frostbite. With the exception of reusable cold packs, this technique often limits the effects of cold to the point where few or no therapeutic effects are gained from the treatment (Table 4–10). Cases that indicate the use of an insulating medium include those conditions in which the blood flow to the area is compromised, nerve or cold intolerance, and Raynaud's phenomenon. If the use of an insulating medium

TABLE 4–10 **Skin Temperatures Obtained during Ice Pack Application with and without Insulators***

Ice Pack and Insulator	Minimum Skin Temperature Obtained
None	37.8
Wet wrap	48.0
Frozen wrap	51.4
Dry wrap	67.1
Synthetic cast	67.5
Plaster cast	65.7
Dry towel	69.6

*The skin temperature should be decreased to approximately 57° for the benefits of cold application to be realized (Bugaj[1]).
Sources: Tsang et al[53]; Metzman, Gamble, and Rinsky[78]; Urban and Knight.[79]

is indicated, the treatment duration must be extended beyond the normal treatment time before the skin temperature is decreased to the desired therapeutic range. Ice applied over an elastic wrap would require a treatment duration of approximately 151 minutes to decrease the skin temperature to therapeutic ranges; when applied over a single layer of dry terry cloth toweling, a treatment duration of 109 minutes would be required.[53]

Without question, **ice bags** are the most commonly used modality in the treatment of acute injuries. They are easy, efficient, and safe to use. They require only plastic bags and either flaked or cubed ice. Ice bags, especially when filled with crushed ice, provide the quickest cooling of the skin and subcutaneous tissues.[39] A drawback of this method of cold application is that ice machines are expensive and their cost may be prohibitive in some situations.

Reusable cold packs contain a gel consisting of *silica,* water, and a form of antifreeze sealed in a plastic pouch. When not in use, these packs are stored in a cooling unit. Although a convenient method for cold application in the clinical setting, the effectiveness of reusable cold packs diminishes when they are stored in an ice chest for long periods.

Use of reusable cold packs significantly increases the possibility of frostbite. Because this method of cold application does not involve the true use of ice (i.e., frozen water), it may lower the skin temperature below the freezing point. To prevent frostbite, a medium such as one layer of wet toweling or a wet elastic wrap must be placed between the pack and the skin. The liquid medium helps to moderate the cold, but still provides an effective treatment.

Care must be taken to avoid overinsulating the area. One or two layers of wet toweling or a wet elastic wrap will serve as good protection against frostbite. Adding too much insulation will prevent the effects of the cold from reaching the skin. Regardless of the insulating medium being used, the patient's skin should be checked regularly for signs of frostbite (see Box 4–2).

Controlled cold therapy units combine static external compression and cold application (Fig. 4–5). The CCT's appliances are designed to contour with spe-

Silica: A finely ground form of sand capable of holding water.

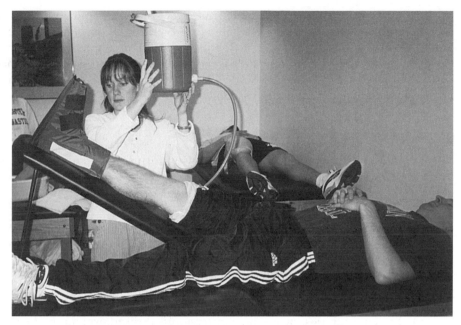

FIGURE 4–5 **Controlled Cold Therapy (CCT) Unit.** A mixture of water and ice is added to the cooler. Using detachable hoses, the appliance is filled with cold water, providing cold and compression to the injured body area.

cific body areas (e.g., the ankle, knee, and shoulder). The appliances are filled with chilled water to provide 40 mm Hg of circumferential compression that prevents the formation of swelling, decreases the amount of edema, and increases the effective depth of cold penetration (see Intermittent Compression Devices in Chap. 7).[54] These effects factored together lead to decreased pain, decreased recovery time, and increased range of motion after acute injury or surgery.[55–58]

Instant cold packs contain two chemicals separated from each other by a plastic barrier. When the seal between them ruptures, they are allowed to mix, causing a chemical reaction that produces cold. The degree of cold produced and the short duration of the reaction give them a workable life of only a few minutes. Instant cold packs are convenient in that they may be stored in a medical kit for emergency use. These packs can be used only once and must be properly disposed of after use.

When mixed, the chemicals contained in instant cold packs are extremely caustic to the skin. If a pack should develop a leak, discard it immediately and rinse the patient's skin with running water. For this reason, do not use instant cold packs on the face.

Effects on the Injury Response Cycle

The application of ice packs decreases tissue temperature, resulting in a decrease in cellular metabolic rate. Lowering the transmission rate of nerve impulses and increasing the pain threshold decrease muscle spasm. The decreased release of inflammatory mediators occurs as a result of the reduced rate of cell metabolism and reduced blood flow.

In acute injuries, the most beneficial effect of cold application is to reduce the need for oxygen. More cells are able to survive in the oxygen-starved environment because of their decreased metabolic rate. When coupled with compression and elevation, the edema in the area is reduced, and compression acts to have the effects of cold affect deeper tissues.[42] These factors limit the scope of the original injury and reduce the amount of secondary hypoxic injury.

Setup and Application

Before the application of each of the following forms of cold application, ensure that the patient is free of contraindications (see Table 4–3).

Ice Bags

1. Fill the bag with enough ice to last for the duration of the treatment, but avoid overfilling. If the bag becomes too full, it cannot be molded to the body part.
2. Remove excess air from the bag to allow the ice to conform to the body part being treated.
3. Many body parts will require more than one bag to fully cover the area.
4. In acute injuries, or when compression is desired, wet an elastic wrap and apply one layer around the injured area. This technique will result in a further decrease in subcutaneous tissue temperatures.[42] (Some clinicians keep a tub of cold "wet wraps" soaking in the refrigerator for this purpose.)
5. Apply the ice bags over the injured area. Secure in place with an elastic wrap.

Reusable Cold Packs

1. Select a pack large enough to cover the injured area, or use multiple packs.
2. Cover the area to be treated with a wet towel or wet elastic wrap. **At no time should a fully cooled reusable cold pack be allowed to come into contact with the skin.** Equally important, do not overinsulate the area. Too much toweling may decrease the heat flow from the skin to the point at which the treatment becomes ineffective.
3. Secure the pack in place with an elastic wrap.
4. Check the patient regularly for signs of frostbite.
5. The reusable cold pack may lose its effective treatment temperature after 20 minutes of use.[59]

Instant Cold Packs

1. Shake the bag so that the contents are evenly distributed.
2. Squeeze the bag to break the inner pouch.
3. Shake the bag to thoroughly mix the contents.
4. If indicated on the instructions of the particular brand of chemical cold pack you are using, place a wet towel between the pack and the skin.
5. Secure in place with an elastic wrap.

Controlled Cold Therapy Units

1. Fill the cold cooling unit with ice as indicated. Shorter treatment times require less ice than treatments having a longer duration.

2. Add cold water to the depth of the FILL mark.
3. Allow the water to chill for approximately 5 to 10 minutes.
4. Choose the appropriate appliance for the body part and size of the area being treated.
5. Fasten the distal strap snugly, but not tight enough to cut off blood flow.
6. Fasten the proximal strap loosely enough to allow for proper venous drainage. Overtightening the proximal strap can inhibit or block venous and lymphatic drainage.
7. Connect the appliance to the cooler using the hose(s) provided. If applicable, open the air vent on the top of the cooler to allow the fluid to flow into the appliance.
8. Elevate the cooler above the body part being treated. The height of the cooler determines the amount of pressure within the appliance; consult your unit's user manual.
9. If applicable, remove the air-bleed cap to allow any trapped air to be forced out of the appliance.
10. Disconnect the hose(s) from the appliance.
11. Draining the appliance or rechilling the fluid:
    a. Reconnect the appliance to the hose(s).
    b. Place the cooler at a level below the cuff.
    c. Allow the fluid to drain from the appliance.
    d. If the fluid is being rechilled, allow the fluid to remain in the cooler for 15 to 30 minutes; then repeat steps 7 through 10.

Duration of Treatment

Ice Bags, Reusable Cold Packs, and Instant Cold Packs

Treatment times range from 15 to 30 minutes and may be repeated as needed. Because of the lasting effects of cold treatments, applications should be no less than 2 hours apart. In the immediate care of injuries, keep the body part wrapped and elevated between treatments.

Controlled Cold Therapy Units

In addition to the preceding treatment regimens, CCTs may be applied continuously for 24 to 72 hours after acute injury or surgery.[6,55,57,58] The periods used to rechill the water provide sufficient time for the body part to rewarm.[59]

Precautions

- Some areas, such as the acromioclavicular joint, are not practical for wet wraps. A moist towel or thin sponge placed over the injured tissues may be substituted. The cold packs may then be held in place with dry wraps.
- The tension of the elastic wrap should be enough to provide adequate compression, but unwanted pressure should be avoided. This is especially true in cases where fractures are suspected. Check the distal extremity (fingers, toes) to ensure that adequate circulation is maintained.
- Check the patient for frostbite. Even though the chance of frostbite occurring with the use of ice bags is slim, patients with impaired circulation are

at a higher risk. The use of elastic wraps and cold further decrease skin temperature and require that the physiological reaction be more closely monitored.

- Application of ice packs over large superficial nerves (e.g., peroneal or ulnar nerves) has been reported to cause neuropathy in isolated cases. This risk increases when an elastic wrap is used to fixate the pack in place. If this is the case, care must be taken not to apply the wrap too tightly (less tension than usual should be used). Recheck the patient regularly for signs of nerve dysfunction, such as tingling in the distal extremity.

Indications

- Acute injury or inflammation
- Acute or chronic pain
- Postsurgical pain and edema

Contraindications

- Cardiac or respiratory involvement
- Uncovered open wounds
- Circulatory insufficiency
- Cold allergy and/or hypersensitivity
- Anesthetized skin

Ice Massage

Ice massage is an appropriate method of delivering cold treatments to small, evenly shaped areas. It is most effective in cases involving muscle spasm, contusions, and other minor injuries contained to a well-localized area. In many cases, the patient may administer self-treatment either in the clinical setting or as a part of the home treatment program (Fig. 4–6). This method of cold application is a convenient, practical, and time-efficient method of providing cold treatments in situations in which there is no ready access to an ice machine.

Effects on the Injury Response Cycle

In addition to the effects associated with the application of ice packs, the massaging action of this treatment assists in decreasing pain and muscle spasm. The sensation of movement stimulates large-diameter nerves, inhibiting the transmission of pain and in turn allowing for a break in the pain-spasm-pain cycle.

Ice massage is not the treatment of choice for acute injuries because no compression is available during the treatment, potentially increasing the amount of hemorrhage and edema. Subcutaneous tissue temperatures are not reduced at the same magnitude as other forms of cold application, an effect related to the decreased treatment duration and the movement of ice. The possibility of increased blood flow in the superficial tissues has also been suggested.[15] In the event that this is the only form of ice treatment available at the time of the injury, additional steps must be taken to limit the amount of swelling. The injured body part should

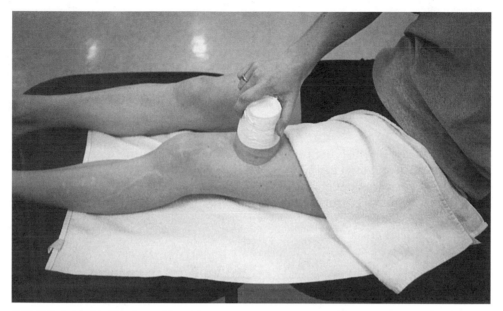

FIGURE 4–6 **Application of Ice Massage.** This form of cold application is convenient for self-treatment. A towel should be draped around the treatment area to absorb water run off.

be wrapped with an elastic bandage and elevated to reduce edema after the treatment.

Setup and Application

1. Ice cups are made by filling paper cups three-quarters full and storing them in a freezer.
2. The treatment area should be no larger than three times the size of the ice cup.
3. The body part to be treated is surrounded with toweling to collect water runoff.
4. The ice is slowly massaged over the injured area in overlapping strokes or circles.
5. The paper must be continually removed to prevent it from rubbing on the skin.

Duration of Treatment

The standard treatment time is 5 to 15 minutes, or until the ice runs out. If the purpose of the ice massage is to produce numbness, the treatment may be discontinued when the patient's skin is insensitive to touch. These treatments may be repeated as necessary.

Precautions

- In some injuries, the pressure of the massage may be contraindicated.

Indications

- Subacute injury or inflammation
- Muscle strains
- Contusions
- Acute or chronic pain

Contraindications

- Cases in which the pressure on the injury is contraindicated
- Suspected fractures
- Uncovered open wounds
- Circulatory insufficiency
- Cold allergy and/or hypersensitivity
- Anesthetized skin

Ice Immersion

Ice immersion (ice slush or ice bath) involves placing the body part into a mixture of ice and water having a temperature range of 50°F to 60°F. This type of treatment is useful for those injuries involving a relatively small, irregular surface (Fig. 4–7).

This is a very uncomfortable method of cold application, especially when the fingers or toes are immersed. A higher degree of pain is experienced because of the increased surface area exposed to the cold. When the fingers or toes are immersed, they are exposed to cold across their circumference and at the distal end. Because their diameter is small, the effects of cold penetrate to bone level. Another factor that may account for the increased pain experienced is stimulation of the lumina in the nailbed. This is a hypersensitive area that may be overstimulated by the presence of cold. You can test this hypothesis on yourself by simply applying pressure with your thumbnail on the white crescent in your opposite thumbnail. When the fingers or toes are not the target of the treatment, the use of a *Neoprene* covering makes this treatment more tolerable (Fig. 4–8).[37,60]

Repeated exposure to ice immersion decreases the amount of discomfort associated with this treatment method.[38] The affective response to the pain associated with this treatment, and perhaps explaining to the patient the types of sensations to be expected as well, can reduce the perceived level of discomfort.[36,37]

Despite the discomfort associated with this treatment, ice immersion allows for circumferential cooling and simultaneous range-of-motion exercise. The use of toe caps, gradually decreasing the temperature of the immersion, and communicating with the patient can make this treatment more tolerable and maximize its therapeutic potential.

Effects on the Injury Response Cycle

The effects of ice immersion are as described in the general effects of cold application. The intensity of cold is greater with ice immersion because of the large

---

Neoprene: A synthetic rubber material.

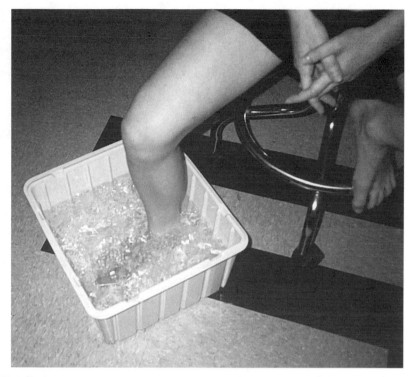

FIGURE 4–7   **Ice Immersion.** This form of cold application is used when treating relatively small, irregularly shaped areas. Because the limb is placed in a gravity-dependent position, this is not a recommended method of immediate treatment (see text).

surface area being treated. Therefore, the resultant drop in skin and subcutaneous temperature is more pronounced than with other forms of cold application.[7] As long as a proper rewarming period is provided (e.g., 20 minutes), ice immersion does not appear to negatively affect joint proprioception during activity.

The use of ice immersion places the limb in a dependent position, increasing the hydrostatic pressure within the capillaries.[61] This encourages the leakage of fluids into the interstitial space, resulting in increased edema. The use of active range-of-motion exercises during the immersion will aid venous return. After the treatment of acute or subacute injuries, the limb should be wrapped and elevated to encourage venous and lymphatic drainage.

Ice immersion can be used in conjunction with electrical stimulation as a form of immediate treatment. Although the effects of electrical stimulation in acute injuries are debatable (see Chap. 5), the limb should be wrapped and elevated after the treatment.

Setup and Application

1. Prepare a bucket, tub, or any other container with cold water and ice. The temperature used will depend somewhat on the person's ability to tolerate the cold. Generally, patients who have had repeated exposure to this treat-

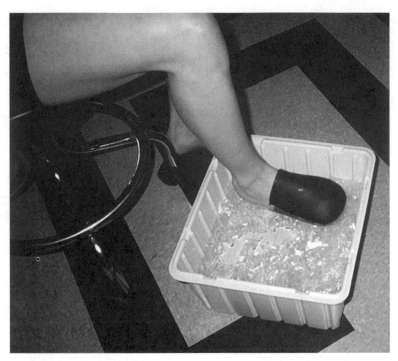

FIGURE 4–8 **Neoprene Toe Cap.** Covering the toes or fingers with an insulating material makes ice immersion more tolerable.

ment can tolerate a lower temperature. Another approach is to start the patient at a tolerable temperature and to add ice as the treatment progresses.

2. The temperature of the treatment is related to the size of the body area being treated (Fig. 4–9). To prevent hypothermia as the size of the area being treated (the proportion of the total body area) is increased, the temperature of the water is increased.

3. Colder treatment temperatures may be tolerated if the fingers or toes are insulated from the water by Neoprene toe caps.

4. If not contraindicated, active range-of-motion exercise should be encouraged.

Duration of Treatment

This treatment is continued for 10 to 20 minutes. Lower treatment temperatures require a shorter duration. This treatment may be repeated as needed, with proper rewarming time allotted between treatments.

Precautions

- Ice immersion is the most uncomfortable of all the cold treatments. Take care that patients do not become unconscious during the treatment.
- Avoid having the patient continually immerse and withdraw the body part from the immersion. During the initial minute or so, the cold will cause a burning or aching sensation. To lessen the discomfort, explain to the pa-

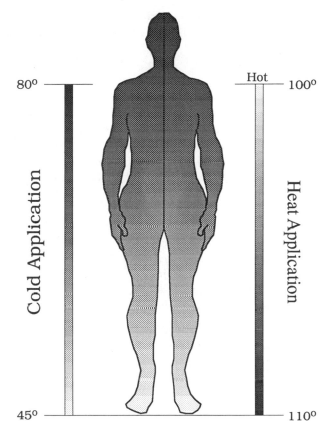

FIGURE 4–9 **Relationship between Treatment Temperature and the Percentage of the Body Immersed.** During cold immersion, the temperature of the water increases as the percentage of the body immersed increases. During hot immersion, the temperature of the water decreases as the percentage of the body immersed increases.

tient that the treatment will be uncomfortable for a few minutes, but numbness will soon follow. If the limb is repeatedly removed and then reimmersed, it only increases the duration of pain.

- Because the limb is placed in a gravity-dependent position, it should be wrapped and elevated after the treatment.
- Care should be taken when relatively subcutaneous nerves (e.g., ulnar nerve as it crosses the elbow) are immersed. Because of the chance of cold-induced nerve palsy, slightly increase the temperature of the immersion, and check the patient regularly.

Indications

- Acute injury or inflammation
- Acute or chronic pain
- Postsurgical pain and edema

Contraindications

- Cardiac or respiratory involvement (see p. 113)
- Uncovered open wounds
- Circulatory insufficiency
- Cold allergy and/or hypersensitivity

- Anesthetized skin
- **Absolute** inability to tolerate the cold temperature

Cryostretch

The effects of cold application and passive stretching are combined in the cryostretch technique, leading to its alternate name, "spray and stretch." A vapocoolant spray is used to rapidly decrease the temperature of the skin and decrease pain transmission. This is combined with simultaneous passive stretching to relieve local muscle spasm (Fig. 4–10) to effectively reduce the amount of pain and spasm associated with strains and trigger points. A chart of trigger point pain patterns is presented in Appendix A.

Cryostretch has traditionally been performed with ethyl chloride because of its ability to quickly evaporate and cool the superficial tissue. Ethyl chloride possesses many inherent dangers: It is highly flammable; it acts as a general anesthetic if inhaled; and because it decreases the skin temperature so drastically, there is a high potential for frostbite. Because of these risks, ethyl chloride has been replaced by fluoromethane spray, which is less volatile and has a safer cooling effect.[62]

Effect on the Injury Response Cycle

The effect of cold sprays is limited to that of a counterirritant. The evaporation of the coolant on the skin causes cooling in a manner that elicits a localized in-

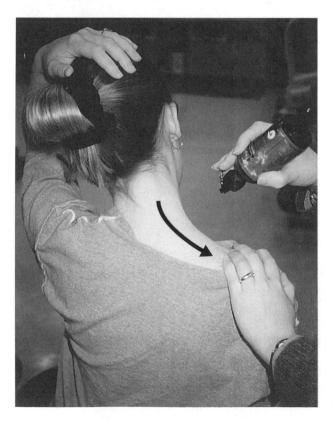

FIGURE 4–10 **Spray and Stretch.** Treatment of the upper trapezius for muscle spasm.

flammatory response. In turn, this stimulus "masks" the previous pain by reducing the intensity and speed of pain transmission. Vapocoolant sprays do not cause the cellular and vascular responses associated with other forms of cold application.

The passive stretching assists in breaking the pain-spasm-pain cycle by lengthening the muscle fibers. This combination of pain reduction and soft tissue stretching makes this a particularly effective method of trigger point therapy.

Setup and Application

1. Position the patient so that the muscle group being treated may be easily stretched.
2. The nozzle of the bottle should be approximately 12 inches from the skin. The spray should strike the skin at an acute angle of about 30° to 45°.
3. Spray the entire muscle length in a sweeping manner. The spray should be in one direction only. The speed of the sweep should allow the tissue to become covered, but not frosted.
4. Apply pressure to passively stretch the muscle group. Come to, but do not exceed, the point of pain.
5. Allow the tissue to rewarm.
6. Continue for two or three more sweeps with increasing stretch on the muscle. Allow the tissue to rewarm between each sweep.
7. Repeat until the desired amount of stretch has occurred.
8. The cryostretch treatment may be followed by a moist heat treatment or massage.

Duration of Treatment

The treatment proceeds through three or four sweeps, with sufficient time for the tissue to rewarm between sprays. Treatments are given once a day.

Precautions

- Cold sprays are capable of causing frostbite if improperly used.
- If ethyl chloride is used, be aware that:
  - It is extremely flammable. Avoid using it around possible sources of ignition, including smoking and electrical sparks.
  - Ethyl chloride is a local anesthetic. However, if the fumes are inhaled, it very quickly becomes a general anesthetic.[63]
- The use of vapocoolant sprays in the treatment of acute injuries is generally based on tradition rather than on fact. Although the evaporation of the liquid rapidly cools the skin and produces temporary pain relief, the other physiological effects of cold application are not achieved.

Indications

- Trigger points
- Muscle spasm
- Decreased range of motion

Contraindications

- Allergy to the spray
- Acute and/or postsurgical injury
- Open wounds
- Contraindications relating to cold applications
- Contraindications relating to passive stretching
- Use around the eyes. When treating the upper extremity, torso, or neck, protect the patient's eyes from the spray.

Whirlpools

Whirlpools are an effective method of applying heat or cold to irregularly shaped areas. Energy is transferred to or from the body by means of convection. The presence of water creates a good supportive medium for active range-of-motion exercises. During slow-moving exercises, the buoyancy of the limb assists motion. When exercises are performed more rapidly, the water creates a resistance to movement. The agitation and aeration of the water, provided by the turbine, provides a massaging effect resulting in sedation, analgesia, and increased circulation.

Whirlpools use a turbine to regulate the water flow and the amount of air introduced into the flow (aeration). Water is introduced through an inlet on the turbine's stem, where the motor forces it back into the tub, causing agitation of the water (the "whirlpool" effect). Air is also introduced into the stream, causing bubbles to circulate in the tank. The agitation and aeration are controlled by separate valves and can be adjusted to produce a wide range of effects (Fig. 4–11).

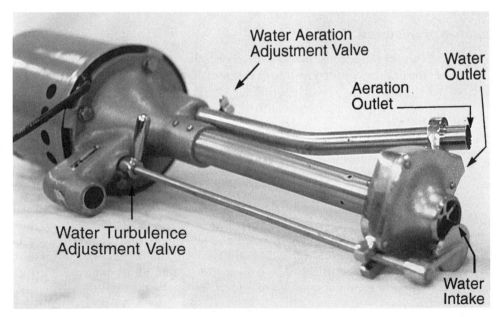

FIGURE 4–11 **A Whirlpool Turbine.** Note the position of the turbulence and aeration valves and the water intake port. The water is driven through the turbine and returned to the tub under pressure. The aeration outlet is in front of the water outlet, forcing bubbles to flow in the water.

There is a significant relationship between the temperature of the water and the proportion of the body area being treated. In cold whirlpool treatments, the temperature of the water is increased as the body area being treated increases. In this case, the body may be placed in a state of hypothermia if too large of a body area is cooled too rapidly.

During hot whirlpool treatments the temperature of the water is decreased as the total body area immersed increases (see Fig. 4–9). When the temperature of the water is equal to or greater than the body temperature, heat loss can occur only through evaporation and respiration. If the patient's core temperature is increased too greatly, *hyperthermia* may result. This fact should be remembered if the patient is receiving a near-total body immersion. In this case, the person can lose heat only through the head and through breathing, increasing the risk of heat stress (Box 4–4).

Because the limb is placed in a gravity-dependent position, venous return is not promoted, and the agitation and increased water temperature further increase the volume of the extremity being treated.[61] Cold whirlpool treatments are not recommended for the care of acute injuries in which edema is still forming (e.g., if no other form of cold application is available). If this method of acute injury management is unavoidable, the turbine should be set on "low" or not be turned on during treatment. A compression wrap should be applied and the body part should be elevated after the treatment.

If open wounds are being treated or are present on the immersed extremity, the tank should be cleaned with an appropriate disinfectant before and after the treatment. The tank is filled with water and a disinfectant is added. After the treatment, the tank should again be drained and cleaned. Only stainless steel tubs should be used for wound cleansing and/or debridement, because tile tubs or spa-type whirlpools may harbor germs and are much more difficult to clean properly.[64]

Effects on the Injury Response Cycle

The effects of hot and cold whirlpools are as described in the relevant sections at the beginning of this chapter. Most notably, hot whirlpools promote muscle relaxation and cold whirlpools decrease muscle spasm and muscle spasticity. Cold whirlpools administered at a temperature of 50°F for 20 minutes result in the same amount of intramuscular cooling as found with ice packs. However, unlike ice packs, with which intramuscular temperature begins to increase immediately after removal of the modality, the intramuscular temperature of limbs treated in a cold whirlpool continue to cool for 30 minutes following the treatment. This effect is beneficial when used before rehabilitation exercises.[39] An additional effect of the turbulence from the flowing water is the creation of a sedative and analgesic effect on sensory nerves.

Setup and Application

1. Instruct the patient not to turn the whirlpool on or off or touch any electrical connections while in the whirlpool or while the body is wet.

Hyperthermia: Increased core temperature.

BOX 4–4 **The Hydrotherapy Area**

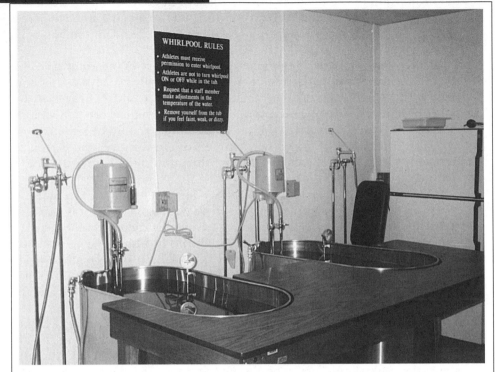

WHIRLPOOL RULES

• Athletes must receive permission to enter whirlpool.

• Athletes are not to turn whirlpool ON or OFF while in the tub.

• Request that a staff member make adjustments in the temperature of the water.

• Remove yourself from the tub if you feel faint, weak, or dizzy.

Of special safety concern is the hydrotherapy section of the athletic training room. It is here, perhaps more than in any other portion of the facility, that the greatest potential hazards exist. Of foremost concern is electrical safety. As described previously, all whirlpools (or similar devices) must be connected to a certified ground fault interrupter (see Box 4–5 and Fig. 4–12). Whirlpool outlets should be located high enough above the floor to avoid any accidental contact with water. Likewise, whirlpool cords should be secured so that they do not touch the floor.

Ideally, the ON-OFF switches controlling the whirlpool motors should be located so that an athlete who is in the tub cannot reach them. If the whirlpool has this switch mounted on the motor, athletes are not to turn the unit on or off while in the water. It is a good practice to post signs stating rules for the use of these devices in the hydrotherapy area.

The hydrotherapy area itself should be in full view of the clinical staff. Because of the noise associated with this modality, this area is normally "glassed off" from the rest of the athletic training room. The floor should be made of a nonslip surface and should be gently sloped toward one or more floor drains. The room itself should be well ventilated.

2. Fill the whirlpool to a depth sufficient enough to cover the area being treated. Most turbines have a minimum depth. Be sure the amount of water is enough to run the motor safely.

3. Add a whirlpool disinfectant according to the manufacturer's directions.

4. If wounds are present on the body part being treated, add a disinfectant such as povidone, povidone-iodine, or sodium hypochlorite to the water.

BOX 4–5   Ground-Fault Interrupters

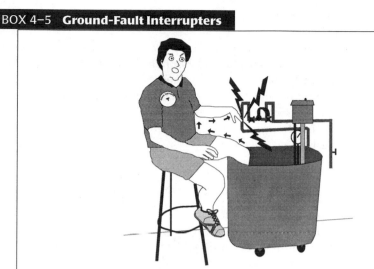

Ground-fault interrupters (GFIs or GFCIs for ground-fault circuit interrupters) are used to guard against hazardous currents by continuously monitoring the amount of current entering a circuit compared with the amount of current leaving it (see Fig. 4–12). If there is a discrepancy of more than 5 mA, current leakage has been detected, and the GFI will halt the flow of electricity to the unit in as little as 1/40 of a second.[80]

Always seeking the course of least resistance, electrical currents tend to stay within the insulation of the path formed by the circuit, but because of condensation, microscopic imperfections in the circuitry, or even dust, some current leakage inevitably occurs. Only two leads are required to complete an electrical circuit; however, most outlets contain a third conductor that leads to the ground. As this name implies, the grounded wire literally leads to a pipe or other conductor that is buried in the ground. Normally when current leaks into the chassis, it will follow the ground wire back to the earth. This leakage is termed a "ground fault" and occurs to some degree in all electrical equipment.

Any leaked current must find an alternate path back to the ground. Ideally, this route is through a grounded circuit, but if the circuit is not properly grounded or the leakage is too great, the current must find an alternate route back to the ground. A person who is in contact with an ungrounded device while touching a grounded source (e.g., a whirlpool and a pipe) can easily form this alternate route for the current to take. In this case, the current would leak from the chassis of the ungrounded device and flow through the person to the ground, producing potentially fatal results.

Ground-fault interrupters must be distinguished from standard circuit breakers. While GFIs stop the current flow at very low amperages, standard circuit breakers require a much larger discrepancy (up to 25 A) to be activated. Circuit breakers are not adequate for use in athletic training rooms, physical therapy clinics, or hospitals, especially in hydrotherapy areas. The 1991 National Electric Code requires the use of GFIs in all healthcare facilities that use therapeutic pools.[81] A GFI may be housed in either the wall outlet or in the circuit breaker box. In either case, GFIs are easily recognizable by their TEST and RESET buttons. Each GFI should be tested at regular intervals, with monthly intervals being considered ideal. Each testing date should be documented.

In the event that the GFI trips itself, disconnect the patient from the unit, and turn off the power to the unit. Check all connections, restart the equipment without the patient being in contact with it, and ensure that a ground fault did not occur. Depress the RESET button on the GFI and reinitiate the treatment. If the GFI trips again, disconnect the unit, label the unit and the outlet "Out of Order," and call for service.

5. Adjust the temperature for the type of effect desired and for the proportion of the body being treated.
6. If an extremity is being treated, place the patient in a comfortable position using either a high chair or a whirlpool bench. If the entire body is being immersed, use a whirlpool stool or sling seat.
7. Turn the turbine on and adjust the turbulence. With subacute injuries, do not focus the turbulence directly on the affected area.
8. Patients receiving full-body treatments, whether hot or cold, must be monitored continuously.

Cleaning the Whirlpool

1. Drain the whirlpool after treatment.
2. Refill the tub with enough water to safely operate the turbine.
3. Add a commercial disinfectant, antibacterial agent, or chlorine bleach to the water, using the concentration indicated on the packaging.
4. Run the turbine for at least 1 minute to allow the cleaning agent to cycle through the internal components.
5. Drain the whirlpool and scrub the interior with a cleaner, paying close attention to the external turbine, thermometer stem, drains, welds, and other areas that could retain germs.
6. Thoroughly rinse the tub.
7. Clean the exterior surface with a stainless steel (or appropriate) cleaner.

Duration and Frequency of Treatment

Initial whirlpool treatments are given for 5 to 10 minutes. The duration of treatments may be increased to 20 to 30 minutes as the program progresses. Treatments may be given once or twice a day.

Precautions

- The whirlpool must be connected to a ground-fault circuit interrupter (Box 4–5 and Fig. 4–12).
- Instruct the patient not to turn the whirlpool motor on or off while in the water. Ideally, the switch to the motor should be out of the patient's reach.
- Patients who are receiving whirlpool treatments should be in view of a staff member at all times.
- Because of the discomfort associated with cold immersions, the treatment may be started at a comfortable, yet cool, temperature. Decrease the temperature gradually during the treatment by adding cold water.
- The combination of increased circulation and placement of the extremity in a gravity-dependent position tends to increase edema.
- Range-of-motion exercises will increase blood flow in the deep muscle layers.
- Do not run the whirlpool turbine dry.
- The flowing water may nauseate some patients, especially those prone to motion sickness.[63,64]

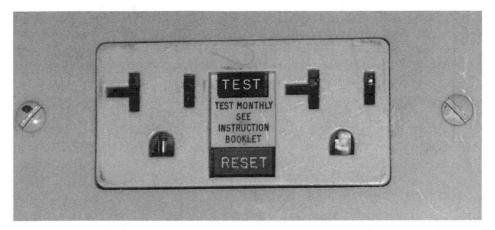

FIGURE 4–12 **A Ground-Fault Circuit Interrupter Mounted in a Standard Outlet.** The "Test" and "Reset" buttons are unique to ground-fault circuit interrupters. These devices should be tested at regular intervals. Note that some ground-fault interrupters are located in circuit breaker boxes.

- Patients who are under the influence of drugs (including alcohol) or those who have seizure disorders or heart disease are at risk of losing consciousness during treatment, especially when hot whirlpools are used.[62]

Indications

- Decreased range of motion
- Subacute or chronic inflammatory conditions
- *Peripheral vascular disease* (use a neutral temperature)
- Peripheral nerve injuries (avoid the extremes of hot and cold)

Contraindications

- Acute conditions in which water turbulence would further irritate the injured areas or in which the limb is placed in a gravity-dependent position.
- Fever (in hot whirlpool).
- Patients requiring postural support during treatment.
- Skin conditions in spa-type tubs. Otherwise, follow the cleaning instructions noted on page 146.

Peripheral vascular disease: Actually a syndrome describing an insufficiency of arteries and/or veins for maintaining proper circulation (also known as PVD).

Contrast Baths

A contrast bath consists of alternating immersion in warm and cold water. Either stationary water or tandem whirlpools may be used for this application. This action results in a kind of vascular exercise, causing a cycle of vasoconstrictions and vasodilations of the blood vessels in the area. This "pumping" action stimulates peripheral blood flow and aids in venous and lymphatic return. Contrast baths are an effective method of making the transition from cryotherapy to thermotherapy. This treatment may also increase circulation in the *contralateral* limb.[65]

Contrast baths are most commonly indicated in subacute or chronic conditions for the removal of edema and/or ecchymosis. The most effective time ratio between hot and cold has not been determined, but the most commonly used ratios are 3:1 and 4:1 (i.e., 3 and 4 minutes in the hot immersion to 1 minute in the cold).

The treatment may end after either the hot or the cold immersion, depending on the stage of the injury, the desired effect of the treatment, and the patient's activity plans after the treatment. When a state of vasoconstriction is desired, the treatment is terminated after a cold immersion. If vasodilation is desired, the treatment is terminated after a warm immersion. In subacute conditions, it is generally beneficial to finish the treatment with a cold immersion. In chronic conditions, the bout is most often ended after the warm immersion.

Effects on the Injury Response Cycle

The exact effects on cellular responses from contrast baths are not clear. Theoretically, the cellular metabolic rate increases or decreases in response to the temperature of the treatment; however, contrast baths do not appear to significantly influence subcutaneous tissue temperatures at depths greater than 1 cm.[40] As a consequence, the series of vasodilations and vasoconstrictions increases circulation in both the treated and the opposite extremity. The resulting influx of new blood assists in removing edema by unclogging the vasculature, increasing joint range of motion, and decreasing pain.

Setup and Application

1. Position the tubs as close together as possible without touching. ("Tubs" refers to either immersion buckets or whirlpool tanks.) The patient should be able to remove the body part from one tub and immediately immerse it in the other.
2. Fill one tub with water in the range from 105° to 110°F and the other with water between 50°F and 60°F.
3. Position the patient on a chair or bench in a manner requiring a minimal amount of motion from tub to tub. A clock or watch should be available to time the treatment segments.
4. In most cases, heat treatments are given first.

Contralateral: Pertaining to the opposite side of the body. The left side is contralateral to the right.

5. Have the patient alternate between the treatments according to the protocol being applied.
6. As with all hot or cold treatments, the patient should be monitored.
7. The treatment ends after the hot immersion if relaxation and vasodilation are desired or after the cold immersion if vasoconstriction is desired.

Duration of Treatment

Contrast baths are given for 20 to 30 minutes and may be repeated as needed.

Precautions

- The same care taken with whirlpool treatments should be applied to contrast baths.

Indications

- Ecchymosis removal
- Edema removal
- Subacute or chronic inflammatory conditions
- Impaired circulation (monitor the patient closely)
- Pain reduction
- Increasing joint range of motion

Contraindications

- Acute injuries
- Hypersensitivity to cold
- Contraindications relative to whirlpool use
- Contraindications relative to cold applications
- Contraindications relative to heat applications

Moist Heat Packs

The moist heat pack is a canvas pouch filled with silica gel or a similar substance capable of absorbing a large number of water molecules. This pack is kept in a water-filled heating unit that is maintained at a constant temperature ranging between 160°F and 170°F (this temperature range also assists in killing any bacteria that may collect in the heating unit). These packs are capable of maintaining a workable therapeutic temperature for 30 to 45 minutes after removal from the heating unit.

Moist heat packs are a superficial heat modality, transferring energy to the patient's skin by way of conduction. Each subsequent underlying tissue layer is heated through conduction from the overlying tissue. Using the triceps surae muscle group as a model, temperatures at 1 cm deep within the tissues are elevated by 38.5°F (±30.7°F) compared to only 17.6°F (±21.2°F) at a depth of 3 cm.[66]

The layering around the hot pack (see Setup and Application) serves as insulation between the pack and the skin. When the pack is placed on the skin, there is little compression of the protective covering, allowing air pockets to form within the layering, which provide additional insulation. If the hot pack is compressed, such as when the patient is lying on it, the layering is moved together and the air is forced out of the spaces. This decreases the available insulation and increases the amount of energy being transferred, increasing the possibility of the patient suffering burns. Lying on the hot pack also decreases capillary flow, further increasing the possibility of burns occurring.

Moist hot packs are suitable for use over localized areas or on areas that normally cannot be treated by immersion in water (the neck, for example). The wide array of sizes and styles of moist heat packs make them acceptable for use over the lumbar spine (medium or large size), the cervical spine (cervical pack), the shoulder (medium size), and the knee (medium size). The effectiveness of the moist heat pack is diminished when used over irregular areas such as the ankle or fingers.

Effects on the Injury Response Cycle

The specific effects of moist heat packs are the same as described for heat in general. When compared with dry heat, moist heat is considered a more comfortable method of application and may have greater benefit in reducing pain. Dry heating agents, such as an electrical heating pad, do not increase the skin temperature as rapidly as moist agents, allowing fresh blood to keep the tissue temperatures relatively low during normal therapeutic treatment durations. However, because electrical heating maintains a constant temperature during the treatment, over time the chance of burns increases.

The application of moist heat results in a rapid increase in the surface temperature of the skin. Vasodilation of the vessels produces an influx of blood to the area in an attempt to cool the tissues. The vasodilation, increased blood flow, and increased pulse rate associated with thermotherapy occur only while the hot packs are in contact with the body.[15]

During the course of the treatment, there is an increase of approximately 39.2°F in the tissues 1 cm beneath the skin,[18] and the effects may penetrate to depths of 3 cm, but not in therapeutic dosages.[66]

Superficial muscle layers (e.g., those less than 1 cm deep) can be directly heated by the heat packs, resulting in relaxation of the affected tissues. Relaxation of muscles or muscle layers that are more deeply situated results from soothing of the superficial motor and sensory nerves. When treating obese individuals, the clinician may find that hot packs are less effective in raising subcutaneous tissue temperature because the adipose tissue layer serves as insulation.

Setup and Application

1. Cover the pack with a commercial terry cloth covering, or fold a terry cloth towel so that there are five or six layers of towel between the pack and the skin.
2. Place the pack on the patient in a comfortable manner. If having the patient lie on the pack is unavoidable, additional toweling should be placed between the patient and the hot pack.
3. When treating an infected area, completely cover the skin with sterile gauze. After the treatment, dispose of the gauze in a biowaste container and wash the hot pack's covering according to the universal precautions.

4. Check the patient after the first 5 minutes for comfort and mottling. Recheck the patient regularly, and adjust the toweling if needed.
5. Some clinicians replace the hot pack every 8 to 10 minutes to maintain high treatment temperatures,[18] but properly heated packs contain sufficient energy for a 30-minute treatment.[67] If hot packs are replaced during the treatment, extra caution must be taken to check for burns arising from increased temperatures and rebound vasoconstriction.
6. After the treatment, return the moist heat pack to the heating unit and allow it to reheat for a minimum of 30 to 45 minutes before reuse.

Duration of Treatment

Moist heat packs are commonly used in treatment bouts of 20 to 30 minutes. The treatments may be repeated as needed, but sufficient time should be allowed for the skin to cool before the next treatment is given.

Precautions

- Do not allow the moist heat pack to come into direct contact with the skin because burns may result.
- If the packs are changed during the course of the treatment, additional care must be taken to prevent burns.
- Infected areas must be covered with sterile gauze or another type of material to college seepage.

Indications

- Subacute or chronic inflammatory conditions
- Reduction of subacute or chronic pain
- Subacute or chronic muscle spasm
- Decreased range of motion
- Hematoma resolution
- Reduction of joint contractures
- Infection (see procedures in Setup and Application of moist heat packs)

Contraindications

- Acute conditions: This modality will increase the inflammatory response in the area.
- Peripheral vascular disease: The heat cannot be dissipated, thus increasing the chance of burns.
- Impaired circulation.
- Poor thermal regulation.

Paraffin Bath

A paraffin bath contains a mixture of wax and mineral oil in a ratio of seven parts wax to one part oil (7:1). Melted paraffin is kept at a constant temperature of 118°F to 126°F for upper extremity treatments (Fig. 4–13). Temperatures for

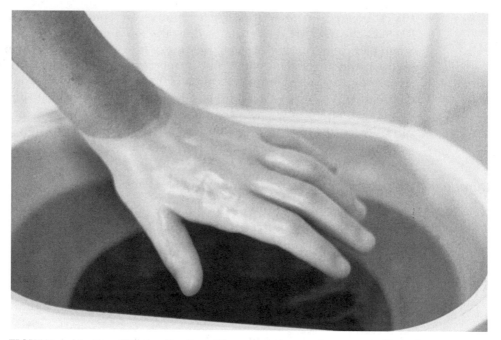

FIGURE 4–13 **Paraffin Application.** The normally translucent paraffin mixture turns a dull white when it dries.

treatments given to the lower extremity are decreased (113°F to 121°F) because the circulation is less efficient.[28] Because of its low specific heat (0.5 to 0.65), paraffin can provide approximately six times the amount of heat as water. Consequently, the paraffin feels cooler and is more tolerable than water at the same temperature (see Box 4–1).

Paraffin is a superficial agent used for delivering heat to small, irregularly shaped areas, such as the hand, fingers, wrist, and foot. Although its use in sports medicine is limited, it is an effective method for delivering heat, and this form of thermotherapy may increase intra-articular temperature as much as 6.3°F.[8] The application of paraffin is beneficial in chronic conditions in which range of motion is not an essential part of the treatment protocol, such as arthritis or chronic inflammatory conditions.

Effects on the Injury Response Cycle

In addition to the standard effects of heat application, paraffin increases perspiration in the treated area and softens and moisturizes the skin.

Setup and Application

There are several methods of paraffin application, each with its own advantages and disadvantages. The more common methods, immersion and glove, are discussed in this text. In addition to providing heat to the area, the paraffin wax may act as an insulator if it is allowed to dry on the skin. With this in mind, the amount of heat delivered can be adjusted by increasing or decreasing the wax layers. During immersion baths, the amount of insulation is increased with the number of layers added.

Preparation for Treatment

To avoid contamination of the mixture, the body part to be treated should be thoroughly cleaned and dried before treatment.

Immersion Bath

This is the best method for raising tissue temperature. However, the chance of burns is increased, so the patient must be closely monitored.

1. Thoroughly clean the body part being treated.
2. The patient begins by dipping the body part into the paraffin and removing it. Allow this coat to dry (it will turn a dull shade of white).
3. Dip the extremity into the wax 6 to 12 more times to develop the amount of insulation necessary. Allow the wax to dry between dips.
4. The patient then places the body part back into the paraffin for the duration of the treatment.
5. Instruct the patient to avoid touching the sides and bottom of the heating unit because burns may result.
6. Instruct the patient who is receiving an immersion treatment not to move the joints that are in the liquid. The cracking of the wax will allow fresh paraffin to touch the skin, increasing the risk of burns.
7. After the treatment, scrape off the hardened paraffin and return it to the unit for reheating, or discard it.

Pack (Glove) Method

The glove method is the safest but least effective method for delivering heat to the body with paraffin wax. This method is recommended for those patients who are in the subacute stage of healing or have a vascular or nerve condition that would predispose them to burning. The body part may also be elevated during this form of paraffin application.

1. Thoroughly clean the body part being treated.
2. Begin the treatment by immersing the extremity in the wax so that it becomes completely covered. Remove the body part and allow the wax to dry.
3. Continue to dip and remove the body part in the wax 7 to 12 times.
4. After the final withdrawal from the wax, cover the extremity with a plastic bag, aluminum foil, or wax paper. Then wrap and secure a terry cloth towel around the area.
5. If indicated, the body part may be elevated.
6. Following the treatment, remove the towel and inner layering. Scrape off the hardened paraffin and return it to the bath for reheating, or discard it.

Duration of Treatment

Paraffin treatments are given for 15 to 20 minutes and may be repeated several times daily.

Precautions

- The sensation of the paraffin is misleading as to the actual temperature of the treatment. The temperature of the paraffin is sufficient to cause burns, but its specific heat and thermal capacity requires a longer period of time to transfer the energy (see Chap. 2).

- Avoid using paraffin with athletes who are required to catch or throw a ball (e.g., basketball players, wide receivers) or workers who are required to maintain a good grip (e.g., carpenters) after the treatment. The mineral oil in the paraffin mixture tends to make the hands slippery, making the task of catching a ball or holding onto a hammer difficult.

Indications

- Subacute and chronic inflammatory conditions
- Limitation of motion after immobilization

Contraindications

- Open wounds: Wax and oil would irritate the tissues.
- Skin infections: The warm, dark environment is excellent for breeding bacteria.
- Sensory loss.
- Peripheral vascular disease.

Infrared Lamp

Infrared generators provide radiant energy for superficial heating of the skin. They are considered radiant modalities because no medium is required to transmit the energy. There are two types of infrared generators, near infrared (luminous) and far infrared (nonluminous). The treatment energy is produced by passing an electrical current through a carbon or tungsten filament. The intensity of the treatment is controlled by adjusting the current flow through the filament or by changing the distance between the lamp and the tissues.

Luminous generators produce some degree of visible light, placing them on the "near" end of the infrared spectrum (Appendix B). Because visible light is present, some of the treatment energy is reflected by the surface of the skin. Nonluminous generators do not produce visible light, placing them on the "far" end of the infrared spectrum.

Nonluminous infrared radiation is less penetrating than luminous, with effects at 2 mm and at 5 to 10 mm beneath the surface of the skin. Because nonluminous infrared is less penetrating, the skin being treated will feel warmer than with a luminous generator.

With the wide range of heating modalities available for use, infrared generators are not common in clinical settings. Infrared radiation was once thought to assist in the healing of open wounds, such as turf burns. This practice actually deters the healing process because it dehydrates the tissues.[68]

Effect on the Injury Response Cycle

Infrared radiation heats the skin almost exclusively. Deeper tissues are heated by conduction to depths up to 1 cm. The primary physiological effects occur almost entirely in the superficial skin. Hyperemia occurs as a result of increased capillary flow and increased capillary pressure.

Setup and Application*

1. Warm up the lamp if necessary.
2. To prevent the concentration of heat, clean the area of any sweat, dirt, or oils, and remove any jewelry.
3. Position the patient in a comfortable manner. Drape the body part so that only the area to be treated is exposed.
4. If a moist heat treatment is desired, place a damp terry cloth towel over the area.
5. Place the lamp so that the source of the heat is approximately 24 inches away from the patient. Adjust the lamp so the energy will strike the tissues at a right angle (see the Inverse Square Law and the Cosine Law in Appendix B).
6. To prevent burns, instruct the patient not to move.
7. Check the patient's comfort periodically. The intensity of the treatment may be adjusted by moving the lamp toward the skin (increasing the temperature) or away from the skin (decreasing the temperature).
8. Instruct the patient to summon assistance if the intensity of the treatment becomes too great.

Duration of Treatment

The treatment time is 20 to 30 minutes and may be given as needed.

Indications

- Subacute or chronic inflammatory conditions.
- Skin infections.
- Peripheral nerve injuries before electrical stimulation: Another modality should be considered if the patient lacks temperature perception.

Contraindications

- Acute conditions
- Peripheral vascular disease
- Areas with sensory loss or scarring
- Sunburns

Shortwave Diathermy

A deep-heating modality, shortwave diathermy (SWD), uses energy that is similar to broadcast radio waves but has a shorter wavelength. The energy delivered to the body

---

*Consult the user's manual of your particular modality.

is actually a high-frequency alternating current but lacks the properties needed to depolarize motor or sensory nerves. The Federal Communications Commission has reserved the frequencies of 13.56, 27.12, and 40.61 MHz for medical use. One of two therapeutic diathermies, SWD is more prevalent in the treatment of musculoskeletal injuries than its counterpart, microwave diathermy (Box 4–6 and Fig. 4–14).

High-frequency electromagnetic energy (greater than 10 MHz) passing through the patient's body is absorbed by the selected tissues. The friction caused by the movement of ions produces the heating effect. Free ions within the treatment field are attracted to the pole having the opposite charge and are repelled from the pole having the like charge. Some molecules have ions that are capable of moving only within the cell membrane, causing a *dipole* action in which the ions within the membrane align themselves along the charges (Fig. 4–15).[69] The heating effect occurs as a result of friction between the moving ions and the surrounding tissues.

Structures with high water content, such as adipose tissue, blood, and muscle, are selectively heated at depths of 2 to 5 cm. Local tissue temperature may reach 107°F, but the subcutaneous fat layer dissipates a significant portion of the energy. This leads to a secondary heating of the superficial muscle layer by heat conducted from the adipose tissue.[46] The amount of intramuscular temperature increase compares favorably with that seen during ultrasound application, producing an increase of more than 7°F.[70,71] Because of the relatively large area affected by diathermy, the deep-heating effects are longer lasting than those experienced with ultrasound.[71] However, SWD is less effective on those persons who have a large amount of subcutaneous fat.

BOX 4–6 Microwave Diathermy

Microwave diathermy (MWD) is a deep-heating modality that converts high-frequency electromagnetic energy into heat. The Federal Communications Commission has reserved 915 Hz and 2450 Hz for the medical use of MWD. Although MWD is similar to SWD, there are differences between the two.

Electrical fields are predominant with MWD, in contrast to the magnetic fields that predominate in SWD. Heating occurs through a dipole response created within the cell membrane. The rotation of these molecules causes friction, resulting in heat production. Because of the spreading of the radio waves and absorption of the energy, superficial tissues tend to be heated more than deeper tissues. Although MWD produces biophysical effects similar to those of SWD, the treatment is more superficial because the microwave radiation cannot penetrate the fat layer to the same extent as shortwave radiation. Because the energy is collected by the adipose tissue, the effects occur at about one-third the depth of SWD effects.

The indications and contraindications for the use of MWD are similar to those for SWD. However, there can be **no** metal within the treatment field (4 feet from the pads, drums, or coils). This not only includes not only metal on the patient but implanted metal (plates, screws, intrauterine devices, and so forth) as well.

The commercial availability of MWD is low in the United States. Microwave radiation possesses an inherently high risk because it tends to be reflected and scattered into the surrounding environment and has been associated with an unacceptably high incidence of miscarriages among female therapists who regularly operate these units.[82]

Dipole: A pair of equal and opposite charges separated by a distance.

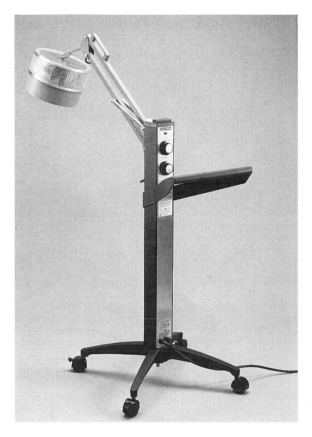

FIGURE 4–14 **Shortwave Diathermy Induction Coil Drum.** (The Auto*Therm, courtesy of Mettler Electronics Corp., Anaheim, CA.)

Shortwave diathermy can be delivered in either continuous or pulsed forms. Continuous SWD produces the greatest increase in subcutaneous temperatures, but its use is generally limited to chronic conditions. The generator's output may also be pulsed, allowing this form of SWD to be used on some acute and subacute conditions. The amount of heating that occurs is based on the total amount of power (measured in watts) and the ratio between the length of the "on" pulse and the duration of the "off" cycle. Thermal effects are obtained when the total amount of energy delivered to the patient's body is greater than 38 watts. When the output is less than 38 watts, the treatment effects are nonthermal, a technique known as pulsed radio frequency energy.

Two types of SWD units are commonly used: (1) the condenser unit and (2) the conduction unit. A condenser field SWD unit places the patient in the actual electrical circuit, whereas the use of an induction field places the patient in the electromagnetic field produced by the equipment.

Condenser Unit

Application of SWD by way of a condenser unit places the patient within the actual circuit of the machine's energy. Two insulated plates are placed on either side of the site being treated. The flow of electromagnetic energy passes

(A) Tissue Ions Before Application of Electromagnetic Energy

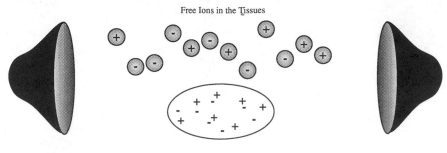

Free Ions in the Tissues

Ions within the Cell Membrane

(B) Ionic Reaction to Electromagnetic Energy

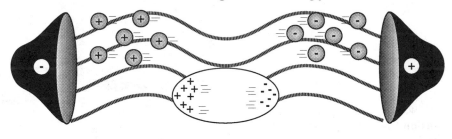

Dipole Action

FIGURE 4–15 **Dipole Response to an Electromagnetic Field.** (*A*) Tissue ions before the application of electromagnetic energy. (*B*) Ionic reaction to electromagnetic energy. The ions move toward the pole having the opposite charge.

through the tissues, which act as electrical resistors and produce frictional heating.

Heating occurs at depths of 2.5 to 5 cm but is uneven because of differences in the resistance to energy transportation of various tissue types (Fig. 4–16). When condenser plates or pads are used, heating tends to occur in the subcutaneous tissues and the superficial muscle layer.

Induction Unit

The induction method of SWD does not place the patient directly in the unit's circuit. Tissues are affected by radiation emitted from the electromagnetic field created by the electrode. The effects of the induction method may heat tissues up to 5 cm beneath the skin, but the primary temperature increase occurs in the superficial and middle muscle layers (see Fig. 4–16).

The tissues are placed in the electromagnetic field by the use of an insulated cable electrode. The cable may be wrapped around the extremity (Fig. 4–17) or coiled flat like a pancake and placed on the skin. Another method of SWD has the cable in a self-contained drum (see Fig. 4–14).

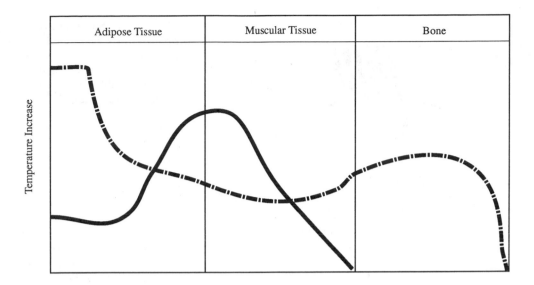

Shortwave Diathermy: Condenser Method

Shortwave Diathermy: Induction Method

FIGURE 4–16 **Comparison of the Heating Effects of Shortwave Diathermy Delivered by the Condenser Method and Induction Method.** The condenser method of application results in superficial heating of the adipose tissue layer and the bone/muscle interface. The induction method results in the muscle belly being primarily heated. (Adapted from Paetzold, J: Physical Laws Regarding the Distribution of Energy for Various Frequency Methods Applied in Heat Therapy. Ultrasonics in Biology and Medicine.) Thomas Publishing Co., Springfield, IL, 1967.

Effects on the Injury Response Cycle

The healing properties of SWD are similar to those of other forms of heat application but tend to occur deeper within the tissues and are based on the treatment intensity (Table 4–11). During vigorous heating (dose 3), skin temperature in the treated area increases 4.3°F, and the intra-articular temperature of the knee increases 2.5°F.[8] Blood flow in the deeper tissues increases, and fibroblastic activity, collagen deposition, and new capillary growth are stimulated.[72] The number and quality of mature collagen bundles increase within the treated area, the result of increased *adenosine triphosphastase* activity, and the proportion of necrosed muscle fibers decreases.[73] Muscle spasm is reduced by the sedation of sensory and motor nerves. As with all heat applications, there is a local increase in cellular metabolic rate and in perspiration, which must be removed during the treatment.

Adenosine triphosphastase: An important source of energy for intracellular metabolism.

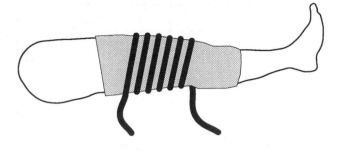

FIGURE 4–17 **Shortwave Diathermy Application via an Induction Cable.** The cable is wrapped around the body part with equal spacing along the length. Cables that are too close together concentrate the heat and may result in burns. Note the equal lengths running to and from the cable.

Setup and Application*

General Preparation

1. There must be **no** metal within the immediate treatment area (Table 4–12). The presence of metal will collect and concentrate the energy from the treatment in the same manner that an antenna collects radio waves.[74] Some manufacturers build metal-free tables for use with SWD.
2. For personal safety, the clinician should remove any rings, watches, bracelets, and so on.
3. Cover the area to be treated with a **dry** terry cloth towel to absorb perspiration. A portion of the treatment area must remain visible to check for burns during the treatment. Avoid any moisture buildup during the treatment because water tends to collect heat. The intensity must be turned to "zero" before drying the area.
4. Explain to the patient that mild warmth should be felt. Instruct the patient to inform you if any unusual sensations are experienced.

Condenser Method

Condenser Plate Setup

1. Adjust the plates so that they are parallel to the skin, 1 inch above the patient. On most units, it is essential that both plates be placed at an equal

TABLE 4–11 **Dosage Parameters Used with Pulsed Shortwave Diathermy**

Dose	Temperature Sensation	Indications	Pulse Width	Pulse Rate
NT	No detectable warmth	Acute trauma Acute inflammation Edema reduction	65 μsec	100–200 pps
1	Mild warmth	Subacute inflammation	100 μsec	800 pps
2	Moderate warmth	Pain syndromes Muscle spasm Chronic inflammation To increase blood flow	200 μsec	800 pps
3	Vigorous heating	Stretching collagen-rich tissues	400 μsec	800 pps

NT = Nonthermal

---

*Consult the user's manual of your particular modality.

TABLE 4–12   Precautions against Metal within the Field of Shortwave Diathermy

In the Environment	Near or on the Patient	In the Patient
Beds	Jewelry	Orthodontic braces
Treatment tables	Body piercings	Dental fillings
Chairs	Earrings	Implanted fixation devices
Wheelchairs	Watches	External fixation devices
Metal stools	Metal in pockets (keys, etc.)	Metal heart valves
CPM units	Belt buckles	Artificial joints
Splints	Zippers	Metal IUDs
Braces	Metal underwire bras	
Medical instruments	Hearing aids	
Electrical modalities		

CPM = continuous passive motion; IUDs = intrauterine devices.

distance above the tissue. This adjustment can be accomplished by using a spacer, such as a piece of wood. Place the spacer on the patient and lower the plate until the plate and the spacer touch. Remove the spacer and repeat for the other plate. The spacer must be removed before the treatment is started.

2. Consult the user's manual for the minimum and maximum distance allowed between the condenser plates.

Condenser Pad Setup

1. Cover the area to be treated with six layers of toweling.
2. Place the condenser pads on the toweling. If the pads are used on the same side of the body, place them as far apart as possible. If they are used on the opposite side of a body part (anterior or posterior, medial or lateral), avoid having the patient lie on the pad.
3. Secure the pads in place with sandbags or the like.

Induction Method

Cable Setup

1. Place six layers of toweling around the body part.
2. Using spacers, wrap the cable around the body part, leaving a minimum of 1 inch between the coils. The leads to and from the coil should be of equal length (see Fig. 4–17).
3. Secure the cable ends so that they do not touch each other, the patient, or the shortwave unit itself.

Coil Setup

1. Using spacers, form a coil of at least three circles approximately equal to the area being treated. There should be a minimum of 1 inch between the circles, and the leads should be of equal length. Use an insulator or 1 inch of padding to separate the end of the inner coil from the coil itself (see Fig. 4–17).

2. Insulate the skin with at least six layers of toweling.
3. Place the coil on the patient and lightly secure in place with sandbags.
4. Position the leads so they do not come into contact with each other, the patient, or the unit.

Drum Setup

1. Position the drum approximately 0.5 to 1 inch above the toweling. There is a direct relationship between the distance of the drum from the patient and the intensity of energy required for the treatment.

Application

1. Turn the unit on; allow it to warm up if necessary.
2. Some units must be tuned to allow for maximal energy transfer. If tuning is necessary, consult the user's manual and follow the manufacturer's instructions.
3. Instruct the patient not to move until the machine is shut off.
4. Increase the intensity until the athlete feels mild warmth.
5. If the electrodes must be moved or if it becomes necessary to dry the area, return the intensity to zero before making any adjustments.
6. Check the patient regularly. Observe the skin for signs of burns, and inquire as to any unusual sensations. Adjust as necessary.
7. After the treatment, return the intensity dial to "zero" and shut off the unit.

Duration of Treatment

At moderate intensities, treatments may be given for 20 to 30 minutes and may be repeated as needed for 2 weeks. When higher treatment temperatures are used, decrease the duration of treatment and apply on alternate days.

Precautions

- Many states require a physician's prescription for the application of SWD.
- Never allow the cables to touch each other. This may create a short circuit.
- The skin exposed to the treatment must always be covered by at least 0.5 inch of toweling.
- Do not allow perspiration to collect in the treatment field.
- Never allow the skin to come into direct contact with the heating unit or cables. Severe burns may result.
- Excessive amounts of adipose tissue overlying the treatment area can result in overheating the skin.
- Overheating of the patient's tissues may cause tissue damage without any immediate signs. Deep-tissue burning can cause destruction of muscular tissue or subcutaneous fat *necrosis*.
- A deep, aching sensation may be a symptom of overheating the tissues.
- It is difficult to heat only localized areas. Water pathways within the tissues dissipate heat formed in the treated area.

Necrosis: Cell death.

- The electromagnetic energy is not localized to the treatment area, radiating 2 to 3 feet from the source of continuous SWD and 2 feet from the source of pulsed diathermy.[75] Clinicians may be placed in the field of this scattering radiation, possibly overexposing them to diathermy. A distance of 3 feet from the source of the energy should be maintained to ensure the operator's safety.

Indications

- Joint inflammation (bursitis, tendinitis, synovitis). Use with caution as the deep heating may cause collagen destruction within the joint.
- Large areas, such as the paraspinal muscles, that cannot be effectively heated through other methods because of the size of the target tissues.
- Fibrositis.
- Myositis.
- Subacute and chronic inflammatory conditions in deep-tissue layers.
- *Osteoarthritis.*

Contraindications

- Ischemic areas: The increased metabolic rate increases the need for oxygen, causing further hypoxia.
- Peripheral vascular disease.
- Metal implants or metals such as jewelry: The metal collects and concentrates the energy, potentially causing burns.
- Perspiration and moist dressings: The water collects and concentrates the heat.
- Tendency to hemorrhage, including menstruation.
- Cancer.
- Fever.
- Sensory loss.
- Cardiac pacemakers.
- Pregnancy.
- Areas of particular sensitivity:
  - Epiphyseal plates in children
  - The genitals
  - Sites of infection
  - The abdomen with an implanted intrauterine device (IUD)
  - The eyes and face

Osteoarthritis: Degeneration of a joint's articular surface.

Chapter Quiz

1. Which of the following modalities has the greatest likelihood of frostbite?
   A. Ice immersion
   B. Reusable cold packs
   C. Ice massage
   D. Ice bag

2. Which of the following is a contraindication for the use of a paraffin bath?
   A. No range of motion
   B. Chronic conditions
   C. Pain
   D. Skin conditions

3. Which of the following modalities uses convection as the method of heat transfer?
   A. Ice bag
   B. Whirlpool
   C. Hot packs
   D. Infrared lamp

4. Which of the following is **not** a local effect of cold application?
   A. Decreased rate of cell metabolism
   B. Decreased muscle spindle activity
   C. Decreased nerve conduction velocity
   D. Decreased viscosity of fluids in the area

5. Which of the following modalities has the greatest depth of penetration into the tissues?
   A. Moist heat pack
   B. Hot whirlpool
   C. Infrared lamp
   D. Ice bag

6. Which of the following is **not** a local effect of heat application?
   A. Increased rate of cell metabolism
   B. Increased elasticity of soft tissue
   C. Increased muscle tone
   D. Decreased muscle spasm

7. How does the application of cold assist in reducing secondary hypoxic injury?

8. List the components and effects of intermediate treatment of an acute injury:

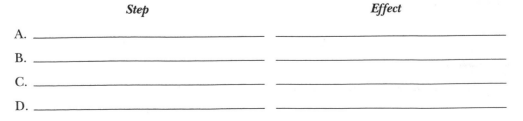

	Step	*Effect*
A.		
B.		
C.		
D.		

9. Why does the effect of cold application penetrate deeper and last longer than the effect of heat application?

10. Explain why the temperature of whirlpools must be altered as the surface area being treated increases.

11. List four physiological benefits associated with the use of an elastic compression wrap during ice pack treatments:

    A. _____

    B. _____

    C. _____

    D. _____

12. What are two possible detriments to the use of an elastic compression wrap during cold treatments?

    A. _____

    B. _____

CASE STUDY CONTINUATION

(The following discussion relates to Case Study 3, found on pages 104 through 109 of Chapter 3.)

The modalities presented in this chapter would benefit our patient throughout his rehabilitation program. Various forms of cold modalities can be used throughout the time frame indicated, and moist heat packs can be incorporated in the later stages of the program.

Ice Packs

Either crushed ice packs or reusable cold packs would be used during the early stages of this patient's program, administered in 20-minute treatments throughout the day. The patient would be placed in the supine position with his head and neck comfortably supported to decrease the amount of electromyographic activity in the trapezius. The cold application will decrease the amount of pain by increasing the pain threshold and by decreasing the rate of the nerve conduction velocity. Muscle spasm will be decreased secondary to reducing the muscle spindle's sensitivity to stretch. Acutely, this method of cold application will also decrease the metabolic activity in the treated area, thereby decreasing the amount of secondary hypoxic injury.

As the patient's treatment progresses, active and/or passive range of motion exercises (described later) would be performed after the removal of the pack. During the more advanced stages of the rehabilitation program, ice packs would be applied after the rehabilitation session to minimize the postexercise inflammatory response. Lastly, the patient would be instructed to use cold packs as a part of his home treatment program.

Ice Massage

Ice massage could be used in conjunction with stretching exercises. The patient would be in the seated position with the cervical spine flexed and laterally bent to the left to tolerance. Once the ice massage treatment has begun and the patient reports decreased pain, the trapezius could be further stretched until discomfort is once again reported. This process would be repeated for the 10- to 15-minute duration of the treatment.

This approach relies on ice massage numbing the area and decreasing the sensitivity of the local muscle spindles. This effect, combined with the passive stretching of the muscle, helps to decrease muscle spasm and to increase range of motion.

Moist Heat Packs

When the active inflammatory process subsides, moist heat can safely be applied before therapeutic exercise and other modalities. Similar to the application of cold packs, moist heat decreases the pain and spasm associated with the injury, but other benefits are realized as well. Moist heat promotes relaxation of the cervical musculature and increases tissue extensibility, increasing the effectiveness of the patient's range-of-motion program.

Concurrent Range-of-Motion Exercises

Range-of-motion exercises for side bending and rotation (30-second hold for five repetitions) are first begun with the patient in the supine position to decrease the effects of gravity. As the patient's pain and spasm begin to subside, these exercises can be progressed to being performed in an upright position.

REFERENCES

1. Bugaj, R: The cooling, analgesic, and rewarming effects of ice massage on localized skin. Phys Ther 55:11, 1975.
2. Ho, SS, et al: Comparison of various icing times in decreasing bone metabolism and blood flow in the knee. Am J Sports Med 23:74, 1995.
3. Knight, KL, Bryan, KS, and Halvorsen, JM: Circulatory changes in the forearm in 1, 5, 10 and 15°C water. Int J Sports Med 4:281, 1981.
4. Knight, KL: Circulatory effects of therapeutic cold applications. In Knight, KL (ed): Cryotherapy in Sport Injury Management. Human Kinetics, Champaign, IL, 1995, pp 107–125.
5. Weinberger, A and Lev, A: Temperature elevation of connective tissue by physical modalities. Critical Reviews in Physical and Rehabilitation Medicine 3:121, 1991.
6. Dahlstedt, L, Samuelson, P, and Dalen, N: Cryotherapy after cruciate knee surgery: Skin, subcutaneous and articular temperatures in 8 patients. Acta Orthop Scand 67:255, 1996.

7. Belitsky, RB, Odam, SJ, and Humbley-Kozey, C: Evaluation of the effectiveness of wet ice, dry ice, and cryogen packs in reducing skin temperature. Phys Ther 67:1080, 1987.
8. Bocobo, C, et al: The effect of ice on intraarticular temperature in the knee of the dog. Am J Phys Med Rehabil 70:181, 1991.
9. Oosterveld, FG, et al: The effect of local heat and cold therapy on the intraarticular and skin surface temperature of the knee. Arthritis Rheum 35:146, 1992.
10. Wilkerson, GB: Inflammation in connective tissue: Etiology and management. Athletic Training 20:299, 1985.
11. Grana, WA, Walton, WL, and Reider, B: Cold modalities. In Drez, D (ed): Therapeutic Modalities for Sports Injuries. Year Book Medical Publishers, Chicago, 1989, pp 25–32.
12. Lewis, T: Observations upon the reactions of the vessels of the human skin to cold. Heart 15:177, 1930.
13. Taber, C, et al: Measurement of reactive vasodilation during cold gel pack application to nontraumatized ankles. Phys Ther 72:294, 1992.
14. Weston, M, et al: Changes in local blood volume during cold gel pack application to traumatized ankles. J Orthop Sports Phys Ther 19:197, 1994.
15. Baker, RJ and Bell, GW: The effect of therapeutic modalities on blood flow in the human calf. J Orthop Sports Phys Ther 13:23, 1991.
16. Cote, DL, et al: Comparison of three treatment procedures for minimizing ankle sprain swelling. Phys Ther 68:1072, 1988.
17. Smith, TL, et al: New skeletal muscle model for the longitudinal study of alterations in microcirculation following contusion and cryotherapy. Microsurgery 14:487, 1993.
18. Halvorson, GA: Therapeutic heat and cold for athletic injuries. Physician and Sportsmedicine 18:87, 1990.
19. Ruiz, DH, et al: Cryotherapy and sequential exercise bouts following cryotherapy on concentric and eccentric strength in the quadriceps. Journal of Athletic Training 28:320, 1993.
20. Ferretti, G, Ishii, MC, and Cerretelli, P: Effects of temperature on the maximal instantaneous muscle power of humans. Eur J Appl Physiol 64:112, 1992.
21. Thompson, G, et al: Effect of cryotherapy on eccentric peak torque and endurance (abstract). Journal of Athletic Training 29:180, 1994.
22. Mattacola, CG and Perrin, DH: Effects of cold water application on isokinetic strength of the plantar flexors. Isokinetic Exercise Science 3:152, 1993.
23. Kimura, IF, Gulick, DT, and Thompson, GT: The effect of cryotherapy on eccentric plantar flexion peak torque and endurance. Journal of Athletic Training 32:124, 1997.
24. Ernst, E and Fialka V: Ice freezes pain? A review of the clinical effectiveness of analgesic cold therapy. J Pain Symptom Manage 9:56, 1994.
25. Whitney, SL: Physical agents: Heat and cold modalities. In Scully, RM and Barnes, MR (eds): Physical Therapy. JB Lippincott, Philadelphia, 1989, pp 844–875.
26. Brander, B, et al: Evaluation of the contribution to postoperative analgesia by local cooling of the wound. Anaesthesia 51:1021, 1996.
27. Knight, KL, et al: The effects of cold application on nerve conduction velocity and muscle force (abstract). Journal of Athletic Training 32:S5, 1997.
28. Griffin, JE and Karselis, TC: Physical Agents for Physical Therapists, ed 3. Charles C Thomas, Springfield IL, 1988.
29. Parker, TJ, Small, NC, and Davis, PG: Case report: Cold-induced nerve palsy. Athletic Training 18:76, 1983.
30. Green, GA, Zachazewski, JE, and Jordan, SE: A case conference: Peroneal nerve palsy induced by cryotherapy. Physician and Sportsmedicine 17:63, 1989.
31. Thieme, HA, et al: Cooling does not affect knee proprioception. Journal of Athletic Training 31:8, 1996.
32. Evans, TA, et al: Agility following the application of cold therapy. Journal of Athletic Training 31:232, 1995.
33. Arnheim, DD: Modern Principles of Athletic Training, ed 7. CV Mosby, St Louis, 1989.
34. Greenspan, JD, Taylor, DJ, and McGillis, SL: Body site variation of cool perception thresholds, with observations on paradoxical heat. Somatosens Mot Res 10:467, 1993.
35. Ingersoll, CD and Mangus, BC: Sensations of cold reexamined: A study using the McGill Pain Questionnaire. Athletic Training 26:240, 1991.
36. Streator, S, Ingersoll, CD, and Knight, KL: Sensory information can decrease cold-induced pain perception. Journal of Athletic Training 30:293, 1995.

37. Misasi, S, et al: The effect of a toe cap and bias on perceived pain during cold water immersion. Journal of Athletic Training 30:49, 1995.

38. Ingersoll, CD, Mangus, BC, and Wolf, S: Cold induced pain: Habituation to cold immersions (abstract). Athletic Training 25:126, 1990.

39. Myrer, JW, Measom, G, and Fellingham, GW: A comparison of subcutaneous and intramuscular temperature change between ice pack and cold whirlpool cryotherapy (abstract). Journal of Athletic Training 32:S5, 1997.

40. Myrer, JW, Draper, DO, and Durrant, E: Contrast therapy and intramuscular temperature in the human leg. Journal of Athletic Training 29:318, 1994.

41. Wilkerson, GB: Treatment of the inversion ankle sprain through synchronous application of focal compression and cold. Athletic Training 26:220, 1991.

42. Merrick, MA, et al: The effects of ice and compression wraps on intramuscular temperatures at various depths. Journal of Athletic Training 28:236, 1993.

43. Danielson, R, et al: Differences in skin surface temperature and pressure during the application of various cold and compression devices (abstract). Journal of Athletic Training 32:S34, 1997.

44. Perlau, R, Frank, C, and Fick, G: The effect of elastic bandages on human knee proprioception in the uninjured population. Am J Sports Med 23:251, 1995.

45. Lehman, JR, et al: Therapeutic heat and cold. Clin Orthop 99:207, 1974.

46. Cox, JS, et al: Heat modalities. In Drez, D (ed): Therapeutic Modalities for Sports Injuries. Year Book Medical Publishers, Chicago, 1989, pp 1–23.

47. Knight, KL and Londeree, BR: Comparison of blood flow in the ankle of uninjured subjects during application of heat, cold, and exercise. Med Sci Sports Exerc 12:76, 1980.

48. Swenson, C, Sward, L, and Karlsson, J: Cryotherapy in sports medicine. Scand J Med Sci Sports 6:193, 1996.

49. Benoit, TG, Martin, DE, and Perrin, DH: Hot and cold whirlpool treatments and knee joint laxity. Journal of Athletic Training 31:242, 1996.

50. Taylor, BF, Waring, VA, and Brashear, TA: The effects of therapeutic application of heat or cold followed by static stretch on hamstring muscle length. J Orthop Sports Phys Ther 21:283, 1995.

51. Curkovic, B, et al: The influence of heat and cold on the pain threshold in rheumatoid arthritis. Z Rheumatol 52:289, 1993.

52. Reed, BV: Wound healing and the use of thermal agents. In Michlovitz, SL (ed): Thermal Agents in Rehabilitation, ed 3. FA Davis, Philadelphia, 1990, pp 5–27.

53. Tsang, KW, et al: The effects of cryotherapy applied through various barriers. Journal of Sport Rehabilitation 6:345, 1997.

54. Healy, WL, et al: Cold compressive dressing after total knee arthroplasty. Clin Orthop 143, February, 1994.

55. Schroder, D and Passler, HH: Combination of cold and compression after knee surgery. A prospective randomized study. Knee Surg Sports Traumatol Arthrosc 2:158, 1994.

56. Levy, AS and Marmar, E: The role of cold compression dressings in the postoperative treatment of total knee arthroplasty. Clin Orthop 174, December, 1993.

57. Scheffler, NM, Sheitel, PL, and Lipton, MN: Use of Cryo/Cuff for the control of postoperative pain and edema. J Foot Ankle Surg 31:141, 1992.

58. Whitelaw, GP, et al: The use of the Cryo/Cuff versus ice and elastic wrap in the postoperative care of knee arthroscopy patients. Am J Knee Surg 8:28, 1995.

59. Barr, E, et al: Effect of different types of cold applications on surface and intramuscular temperature (abstract). Journal of Athletic Training 32:S33, 1997.

60. Nimchick, PSR and Knight, KL: Effects of wearing a toe cap or a sock on temperature and perceived pain during ice immersion. Athletic Training 18:144, 1983.

61. McCulloch, J and Boyd, VB: The effects of whirlpool and the dependent position on lower extremity volume. J Orthop Sport Phys Ther 16:169, 1992.

62. Newton, RA: Effects of vapocoolants on passive hip flexion in healthy subjects. Phys Ther 65:1034, 1985.

63. Downer, AH: Physical Therapy Procedures: Selected Techniques, ed 3. Charles C Thomas, Springfield, IL, 1981.

64. Press, E: The health hazards of saunas and spas and how to minimize them. Am J Public Health 81:1034, 1991.

65. Michlovitz, SL: Biophysical principles of heating and superficial heat agents. In Michlovitz, SL (ed): Thermal Agents in Rehabilitation, ed 2. FA Davis, Philadelphia, 1990, pp 88–108.

66. Smith, K, et al: The effect of silicate gel hot packs on human muscle temperature (abstract). Journal of Athletic Training 29:S33, 1994.

67. Tomaszewski, D, Dandorph, MJ, and Manning, J: A comparison of skin interface temperature response between the ProHeat® instant reusable hot pack and the standard hydrocollator steam pack. Journal of Athletic Training 27:355, 1992.

68. Cummings, J: Role of light in wound healing. In Kloth, LC, McCulloch, JM, and Feedar, JA (eds): Wound Healing: Alternatives in Management. FA Davis, Philadelphia, 1990, pp 287–301.

69. Kloth, LC and Ziskin, MC: Diathermy and pulsed electromagnetic fields. In Michlovitz, SL (ed): Thermal Agents in Rehabilitation, ed 3. FA Davis, Philadelphia, 1996, pp 213–284.

70. Castel, JC, et al: Rate of temperature decay in human muscle after treatments of pulsed short wave diathermy. Journal of Athletic Training 32:S34, 1997.

71. Draper, DO, et al: Temperature rise in human muscle during pulsed short wave diathermy: Does this modality parallel ultrasound? (abstract). Journal of Athletic Training 32:S35, 1997.

72. Brown, M and Baker, RD: Effect of pulsed shortwave diathermy on skeletal muscle injury in rabbits. Phys Ther 67:208, 1987.

73. Bansal, PS, Sobti, VK, and Roy, KS: Histomorphochemical effects of shortwave diathermy on healing of experimental muscular injury in dogs. Indian J Exp Biol 28:776, 1990.

74. Scott, DG and Wallbank, WA: Electrode burns during local hyperthermia. Br J Anaesth 70:370, 1993.

75. Martin, CJ, McCallum, HM, and Heaton, B: An evaluation of the radiofrequency exposure from therapeutic diathermy equipment in light of current recommendations. Clin Phys Physiol Meas 11:53, 1990.

76. De Coster, D, Bossuyt, M, and Fossion, E: The value of cryotherapy in the management of trigeminal neuralgia. Acta Stomatol Belg 90:87, 1993.

77. Bolster, MB, Maricq, HR, and Leff, RL: Office evaluation and treatment of Raynaud's phenomenon. Cleve Clin J Med 62:51, 1995.

78. Metzman, L, Gamble, JG, and Rinsky, LA: Effectiveness of ice packs in reducing skin temperatures under casts. Clin Orthop 330:217, 1996.

79. Urban, CD and Knight, KL: Insulating effects of elastic wraps used in ice, compression, and elevation. Presented at the Indiana Interagency Research Seminar, West Lafayette, IN, April, 1979.

80. Porter, MM and Porter, JW: Electrical safety in the training room. Athletic Training 16:263, 1981.

81. Therapeutic pools and tubs in health care facilities. In National Electric Code. National Fire Protection Association, Quincy, MA, 1996.

82. Ouellet-Hellstron, R and Stewart, WF: Miscarriages among female physical therapists who report using radio- and microwave-frequency electromagnetic radiation. Am J Epidemiol 138:775, 1993.

CHAPTER 5 | *Electrical Agents*

The purpose of this chapter is to describe the effects of passing an electrical current through the human body. Comprehension of the basic principles of electricity and familiarity with the terminology must occur before these effects can be fully understood. Various techniques, theories of application, and their effects on the injury response process are discussed in individual sections.

The effects of electricity on the body can be difficult to comprehend, and the thought of actually sending 500 V through a person's body is often intimidating to new students. Many application protocols seem to contradict the long-standing rules that we have been taught since early childhood. You have probably heard that "Electricity and water don't mix." In this chapter, it will become apparent that this is a natural and logical approach to electrotherapy and that electricity, when used properly and appropriately, is a safe and effective form of therapy. Just as important, you will also see that electrical stimulation is not a magical healing technique. It is an adjunct to traditional therapeutic techniques and rehabilitation exercises, and its use may not be appropriate in some instances.

The primary precautions and contraindications for the use of electrical stimulation lie in the placement of the electrodes. Current flow through the heart, *carotid sinus,* and pharynx must be avoided because it disrupts normal cardiovascular function. Electricity is not normally applied over sites of infection or cancer unless prescribed by a physician because of the unknown and unpredictable effects. The general contraindications to electrical stimulation are presented in Table 5–1. Contraindications particular to specific electrical stimulators are presented in their appropriate sections.

Because of the different treatment parameters that can be modified, each type of stimulation unit produces unique effects within the tissues and is capable

Carotid sinus: An enlargement of the carotid artery near the branch of the internal carotid artery, located distal to the inferior arch of the mandible. Baroreceptors at this site monitor and assist in the regulation of blood pressure.

TABLE 5–1   General Contraindications to Electrotherapy

Cardiac disability: Stimulation of the thorax or neck may result in disruption of normal respiratory or cardiac function.

Demand-type pacemakers: Electrical current flow may interfere with pacemaker's function.

Pregnancy: Stimulation of the abdominal, lumbar, or pelvic region may have an adverse effect on the developing fetus. Specific guidelines, however, have been developed to decrease pain for pregnant women, but these protocols must be closely monitored by a physician. Electrical stimulation has also been used during delivery, although the current may interfere with fetal monitoring machines.

Menstruation: Stimulation of the abdominal, lumbar, or pelvic region may increase hemorrhage.

Cancerous lesions: Electrical current may possibly result in a growth or spread of the tumor.

Sites of infections: Unless the treatment protocol is specifically designed to reduce infection.

Exposed metal implants: An example is a metal rod used for *external fixation* of fractures. Contact of a metal fixation rod to a grounded object can result in severe electric shock.

Areas of particular nerve sensitivity include:
- The carotid sinus
- The esophagus
- The larynx
- The pharynx
- On or around the eyes
- The upper thorax
- The temporal region

Severe obesity: Adipose tissue may provide insulation against effective stimulation.

Skin irritation from the gel, adhesive, or current flow in individuals who wear electrodes for extended periods. Altering the position of the electrodes reduces irritation.

TABLE 5–2   Therapeutic Uses of Electrical Currents

Controlling acute and chronic pain
Reducing edema
Reducing muscle spasm
Reducing joint contractures
Inhibiting muscle spasm
Minimizing disuse atrophy
Facilitating tissue healing
Facilitating muscle reeducation
Facilitating fracture healing
Strengthening muscle
Effecting orthotic substitution (Electrical stimulation can be used to force contractions of specific muscles during gait)

External fixation: A fracture-setting technique incorporating the use of metal rods that extend through the skin and are attached to a device outside the body.

of producing a wide range of therapeutic responses (Table 5–2). However, all therapeutic currents have certain characteristics that remain similar. This chapter is divided into three sections: The first introduces basic electrical principles, concepts, and terms; the second describes the effect that an electrical current has on the body; and the third describes the effects of various stimulation units.

FUNDAMENTALS OF ELECTRICITY

Electricity is the force created by an imbalance in the number of electrons at two points. This force, known as electromagnetic force, potential difference, or voltage, creates a situation in which electrons flow in an attempt to equalize the charges, creating an electrical current. In its simplest form, electrical current flows from the negative pole (**cathode**), an area of high electron concentration, to the positive pole (**anode**), an area of low electron concentration, taking the path of least resistance.

In addition to the presence of voltage, a complete circuit must be established for flow to occur. An uninterrupted circuit is a **closed circuit** when a complete loop is formed, allowing the current to flow to and from the source. An interrupted or incomplete path is referred to as an **open circuit.** When you walk into a room and flip a switch to turn on the light, you are closing a circuit that allows the electricity to flow from its source, through the light, and back to its source. Likewise, a closed circuit is created between your patient and an electrical stimulation device by attaching leads of opposite polarity to the body. The electrons flow from the generator, through the patient's body, and back to the generator.

ELECTRICAL STIMULATING CURRENTS

Electrical currents are classified as either **direct currents** (DC) or **alternating currents** (AC), depending on the course of flow. A third classification, **pulsed currents,** represents a current that has been modified to produce specific biophysical effects. The terms "alternating" and "direct" describe the uninterrupted flow of electrons, whereas "pulsed" indicates that the electron flow is periodically interrupted. Pulsed currents may flow in one direction, similarly to DC, or may have bidirectional movement, as in AC. However, pulsed currents are characterized by periods of no current flow.[1]

The primary properties of electrical flow are amplitude (intensity) and duration. The maximal distance to which the impulse rises above or below the baseline represents the amplitude of the wave. The isoelectric point sets the baseline where the electrical potential between the two poles is equal and no current flow occurs. The horizontal distance required to complete the shape represents the pulse duration. The term "pulse width" is often incorrectly substituted for pulse duration.[2] The total area within this waveform represents the amount of current the pulse contains.

Direct Currents

Direct currents are characterized by a continuous flow of electrons in one direction. The basic pattern of DC flow is the square wave and is recognized by continuous

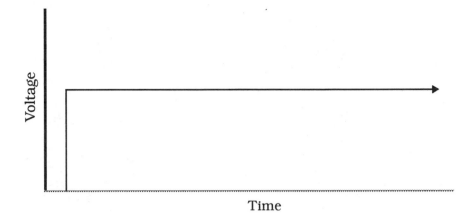

Time

FIGURE 5–1 **Direct Current.** Characterized by the constant flow of electrons in one direction, a direct current remains uninterrupted (does not return to the baseline) until the path is opened, thus stopping the flow of electrons.

current flow on only one side of the baseline as the electrons travel from the cathode to the anode (Fig. 5–1). Despite fluctuations in voltage or amperage, the current flow remains in one direction and stays on one side of the baseline. In medical applications, **the term "galvanic" is used to describe uninterrupted direct current.**

Perhaps the most common example of a DC is a flashlight. The battery possesses a positive pole, which lacks electrons, and a negative pole, which, because of chemical reactions, has an excess of electrons. Electrons leave the negative pole of the battery and flow through a wire to the bulb. After leaving the bulb, the electrons return to the positive pole of the battery (Fig. 5–2). When the number of electrons at the negative pole equals the number at the positive pole, no further potential for current flow exists. The battery is dead.

Alternating Currents

The direction and magnitude of the flow reverses with an AC, although the magnitude may not be equal in both directions. Unlike a DC, an AC circuit possesses no true positive or negative pole. Electrons, rather than constantly moving in one di-

FIGURE 5–2 **Example of a Direct Current.** Electrons exit the battery through the cathode (negative pole), flow through the wire and bulb, and return to the anode (positive pole).

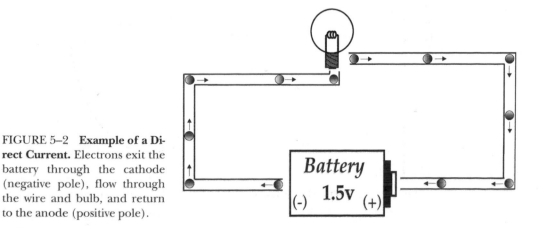

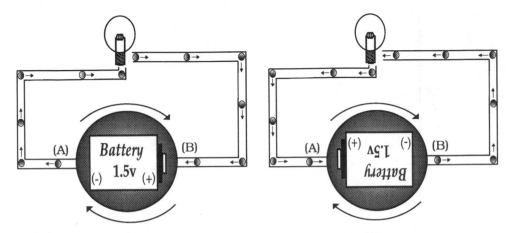

FIGURE 5–3 **Example of an Alternating Current.** Alternating currents possess no true positive or negative poles. In this type of current, electrons flow back and forth between poles (*A*) and (*B*).

rection, shuffle back and forth between the two electrodes as the electrodes take turns being the "positive" and "negative" poles. Household electricity uses AC.

Consider the flashlight example used to describe DC flow (see Fig. 5–2). If a battery were placed on a device that allowed it to rotate between the two wires, we could more or less duplicate an AC current.[3] Electrons would flow away from terminal (A) when the cathode is in line with it. When the anode aligns with terminal (A), electrons would flow toward it (Fig. 5–3). The basic pattern of an AC is the sine wave (Fig. 5–4).

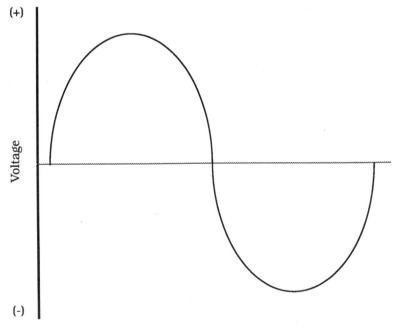

FIGURE 5–4 **The Sine Wave.** One cycle of an alternating current.

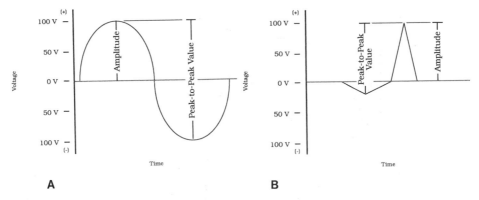

FIGURE 5–5 **Measures of Amplitude.** Peak amplitude and peak-to-peak values for (*A*) symmetrical and (*B*) asymmetrical pulses.

The **amplitude,** or "peak value," of an AC wave is determined by measuring the maximal distance to which the wave rises above or below the baseline. In the case of the pure sine wave shown in Figure 5–4, a peak value of 100 V appears on either side of the baseline. The peak value refers to the wave amplitude on only one side of the baseline without regard to its duration. The **peak-to-peak value** is measured from the peak on the positive side of the baseline to the peak on the negative side. In Figure 5–5A, the peak-to-peak value would be the absolute value of the difference between the two peaks, or 200 V. In an *asymmetrical* waveform, such as the faradic wave (Fig. 5–5B), the peak value is 100 V on the positive side of the baseline. The peak-to-peak value would be measured from the peak on the negative side (20 V) to the peak on the positive side (100 V), resulting in a peak-to-peak measure of 120 V.

The cycle duration of an AC is measured from the originating point on the baseline to its terminating point and represents the amount of time required to complete one full cycle. The number of times that the current reverses direction in 1 second is the current's number of cycles per second and is measured in **hertz** (Hz) (Fig. 5–6). An AC of 100 Hz would change its direction of flow 100 times during 1 second. A current of 1 megahertz (MHz) would change its direction 1 million times a second. Because ACs are measured in cycles per second, as the duration of the cycles increases, fewer cycles per second can occur. Although amplitude is often used to describe the magnitude of an electrical current, it does not take into account the actual amount of time that the current is flowing. Box 5–1 presents measures that take into consideration the cycle's duration.

Pulsed Currents

Pulsed currents are the unidirectional (**monophasic**) or bidirectional (**biphasic**) flow of electrons that are interrupted by discrete periods of noncurrent flow. Using the flashlight analogy from the DC section, turning the switch on and off,

---

Asymmetrical: Lacking symmetry (e.g., two halves are of unequal size and/or shape).

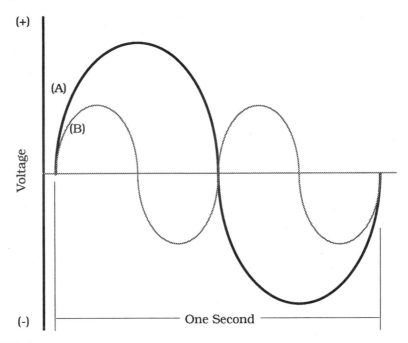

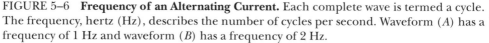

FIGURE 5–6 **Frequency of an Alternating Current.** Each complete wave is termed a cycle. The frequency, hertz (Hz), describes the number of cycles per second. Waveform (*A*) has a frequency of 1 Hz and waveform (*B*) has a frequency of 2 Hz.

causing the light to blink, is an example of a monophasic current. However, the pulses occur in a much more rapid progression.

The building block of pulsed currents is the **phase.** A phase is the individual section of a pulse that rises above or below the baseline for a measurable period of time. The number and type of phases then classify the type of pulse and, ultimately, the charge delivered by each phase is what affects the body's tissues.

BOX 5–1 Measures of a Current's Electrical Power

The **average current** of a wave is considered one-half of its complete cycle, taking into account the amount of time the current is flowing. To calculate the average value of a wave, the sine values of all angles up to 180° are added together and divided by the number of measurements. In the case of a perfect sine wave, this value is 0.637. This figure is then multiplied by the peak value to obtain the average value:

Average value = Mean of sines × Peak value
Average value = 0.637 × 100 V
Average value = 63.7 V

The **root-mean-square value** (RMS) takes into account both the amplitude and duration of the pulse. It describes the total amount of charge delivered by a single cycle and is useful when asymmetrical biphasic currents are used. This figure is important because it translates the power delivered by a biphasic current into the equivalent amount of power that would be needed by a direct current to produce the same amount of heat. In the case of a pure sine wave, the RMS value is calculated by multiplying the peak value by 0.707.

Monophasic Currents

one direction

Monophasic pulses have only one phase to a single pulse, and the current flow is unidirectional. Notice in Figure 5–7 that each pulse consists of only one component part, the phase. Despite the different shapes involved, there is only one phase, and it remains on one side of the baseline.

In this type of electrical current, amplitude is the maximal distance to which the wave rises above the baseline, and the duration is measured as the distance required to complete one full waveform (Fig. 5–8). The horizontal baseline is labeled as "time," so the distance a waveform travels represents the duration that the pulse is flowing. With monophasic currents, the terms "pulse," "phase," and "waveform" are synonymous.[4]

Biphasic Currents

Biphasic currents, such as those presented in Figure 5–9, consist of two phases, each occurring on opposite sides of the baseline. The lead phase of the pulse is the first area rising above or below the baseline, and the terminating phase occurs in the opposite direction. The pulse represented in Figure 5–10A is considered symmetrical because the two phases are equal in their magnitude and duration. In

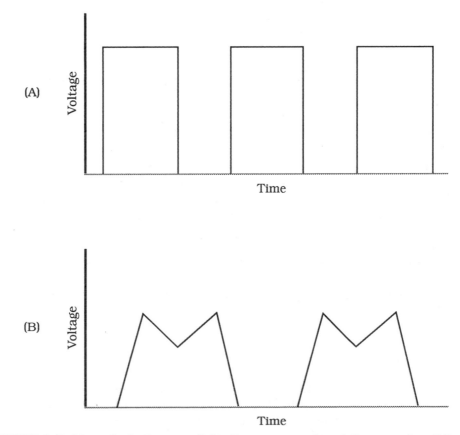

FIGURE 5–7 **Monophasic Currents.** Pulsatile current consists of discrete pulses. Like direct current, monophasic currents are characterized by the one-directional flow of electrons. (*A*) Square waves. (*B*) Twin-peaked monophasic.

(A)

(B)

(C)

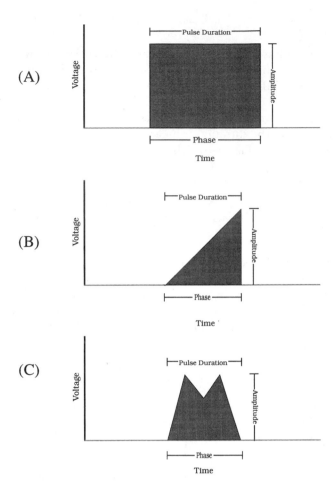

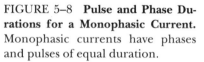

FIGURE 5–8 **Pulse and Phase Durations for a Monophasic Current.** Monophasic currents have phases and pulses of equal duration.

this case, each phase has equal, but opposite, electrical balance. Figures 5–10B and 5–10C represent asymmetrical pulses because each phase in the pulse has a different shape. When asymmetrical pulses are used, the characteristics of each phase should be considered separately. If the charges (area) of both phases are equal, the pulse is balanced; otherwise, it is unbalanced. Whereas the phases in a symmetrical pulse or balanced asymmetrical pulse cause the physiological effects of positive and negative current flow to cancel each other out, unbalanced asymmetrical pulses may lead to residual physiological changes based on the remaining net polarity. Symmetrical biphasic waveforms tend to be the most comfortable because they deliver relatively lower charges per phase.[5]

Pulse Attributes

The charge produced by an electrical generator is dependent on the duration and amplitude of the pulse. The relationship between intensity and duration of a single pulse determines the total charge delivered to the body. Increasing the amplitude and/or duration increases the total charge of the pulse.

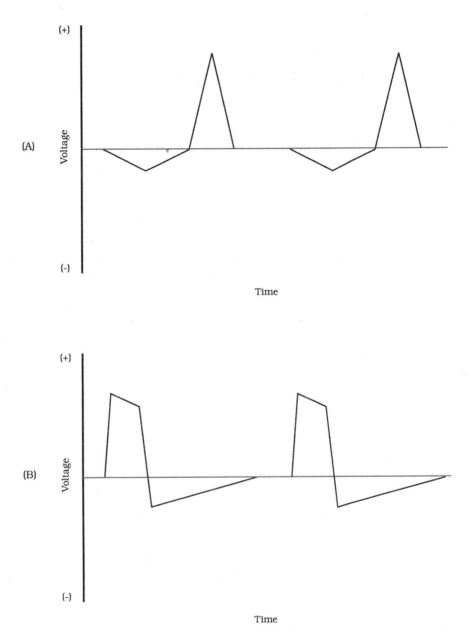

FIGURE 5–9 **Biphasic Currents.** An example of biphasic pulsed currents. (*A*) Original faradic waveform; (*B*) typical transcutaneous electrical nerve stimulation waveform.

Pulse and Phase Duration

As you will recall, the horizontal axis (or baseline) represents time. The distance that a pulse covers on the horizontal axis represents the **pulse duration:** the elapsed time from the beginning of the phase to the conclusion of the final phase, including the intrapulse interval.[1] The duration of a single pulse may be broken down into the time required for each component phase to complete its shape: the **phase duration** (see Figs. 5–8 and 5–10).

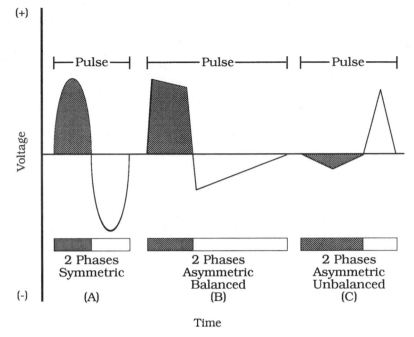

FIGURE 5–10 **Pulse and Phase Durations for a Biphasic Current.** Pulse and phase durations for (*A*) symmetrical biphasic, (*B*) balanced asymmetric biphasic, and (*C*) unbalanced asymmetric pulses.

In a monophasic current, the pulse duration and phase duration are equivalent terms. In biphasic currents, the pulse duration is the sum total of the two phase durations. Note that pulse durations cannot be measured for uninterrupted direct or alternating currents.

The phase duration is the most important factor in determining what type of tissues will be stimulated. If the phase duration is too short, the current will not be able to overcome the capacitive resistance of the nerve membrane and no action potential will be elicited. As the phase duration is increased, different tissues are depolarized by the electrical current (see Selective Stimulation of Nerves, page 202).

Interpulse Interval, Intrapulse Interval, and Pulse Period

Unlike a continuous current, a pulsatile current possesses periods when the current is not flowing. The duration of time between the conclusion of one pulse and the initiation of the next is the **interpulse interval.** A single pulse or phase may be interrupted by an **intrapulse interval;** however, the duration of the intrapulse interval cannot exceed the duration of the interpulse interval.[1] The intrapulse interval allows time for certain metabolic events, such as repolarization of cell membranes, whereas the interpulse interval provides time for mechanical and chemical recharging to occur. Jointly, the pulse duration and the pulse interval form the **pulse period,** the elapsed time between the initiation of one pulse and the start of the subsequent pulse (Fig. 5–11).

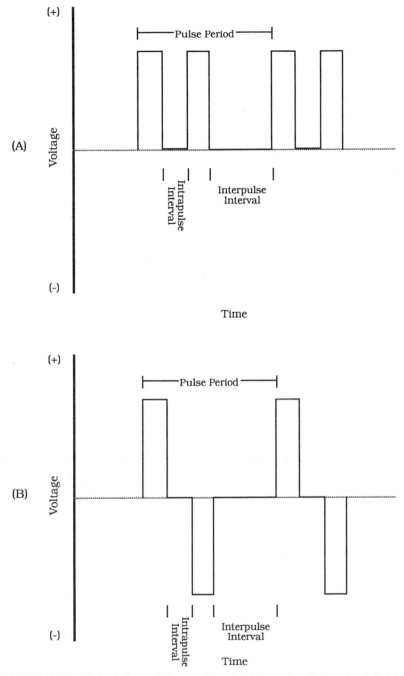

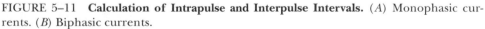

FIGURE 5–11 **Calculation of Intrapulse and Interpulse Intervals.** (*A*) Monophasic currents. (*B*) Biphasic currents.

By definition, uninterrupted currents (alternating and direct currents) do not possess pulses. Therefore, pulse duration and pulse periods do not exist for these types of currents.

Pulse Charge

A measurement of the number of electrons contained within a pulse, the charge of a pulse is expressed in **microcoulombs.** A *coulomb* is too large a unit to use when describing the charge produced by electrical stimulation units. Most electrotherapeutic modalities produce charges measured in microcoulombs (the charge produced by 10^{-6} electrons).

The pulse charge is a function of the amount of area within the waveform. Increasing or decreasing the amplitude or duration alters the charge of the pulse accordingly. The shape of the wave may also be altered to deliver more or less charge to the tissues per pulse.

Pulse Frequency

Any waveform repeated at regular intervals may be described in terms of its frequency or the number of events per second.[6] When a pulsed current is being used, the frequency is normally measured by the number of pulses per second (pps). The cycle frequency of an AC is measured by the number of cycles per second (cps) or Hertz (Hz) (see Fig. 5–6).

A confusing issue exists because the term "frequency" is used to describe base frequency of the electrical stimulator and also to describe the number of electrical pulses (or cycles) delivered to the tissues. Electrical stimulation units are grouped by their carrier frequency. **Low-frequency** currents, less than 1,000 cycles or pulses per second, are used for their biological effects; **medium-frequency** currents range from 1,000 to 100,000 cps; **high-frequency** currents, greater than 100,000 cps, are used for their heating effects, as seen with diathermy (see Chap. 4).

The number of electrical "bursts," either as individual pulses or, as in the case of alternating currents, as a series of cycles that cause depolarization of sensory and motor nerves, is also described in terms of their frequency (Table 5–3). To help alleviate this confusion within this text, the term "pulse frequency" is used to describe an adjustable output parameter. "Stimulation frequency" is used to denote

TABLE 5–3   **Pulse Frequency Ranges Commonly Used in Electrotherapy**

Descriptor	Pulses per Second (pps)	Neuromuscular Effects
Low	<10	Individual muscle contractions (twitch)
Medium	10–50	Summation of individual contractions resulting in increased muscle tone
High	>50	Tonic contraction

Coulomb: The amount of charge produced by 6.25×10^{18} electrons (negative charge) or protons (positive charge).

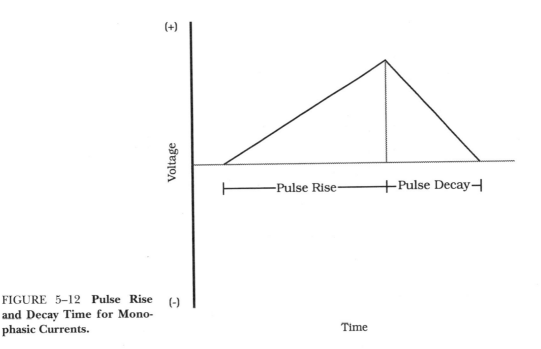

FIGURE 5–12 **Pulse Rise and Decay Time for Monophasic Currents.**

device-specific current frequencies. In each case, the actual numerical value of the frequency is the preferred nomenclature rather than "low," "medium," and "high."

An inverse relationship exists between the pulse frequency of an electrical current and the capacitive resistance offered by the tissues. A current having 10 pps would encounter greater tissue resistance than a current flowing at 1000 pps and would require an increased intensity to overcome the resistance.

Pulse Rise Time and Pulse Decay Time

Pulse rise is the amount of time needed for the pulse to reach its peak value and is usually measured in *nanoseconds* (almost immediate full pulse charge). Rapidly rising pulses cause nerve depolarization. If the rise is slow, the nerve accommodates to the stimulus and an action potential is not elicited. The counterpart of pulse rise time is the pulse decay time, the amount of time required for the pulse to go from its peak back to zero (Fig. 5–12).

Pulse Trains

Pulse trains may be considered individual patterns of waveforms, durations, and/or frequencies that are linked together. These linked patterns repeat at regular intervals (Fig. 5–13).

The gradual rise and/or fall in amplitude of a pulse train is the **amplitude ramp.** Ramping amplitude causes a gradual increase in the force of muscular contractions by the progressive recruitment of motor units. As the intensity of the ramp continues to rise, more motor units are recruited into the contraction. The patient appreciates a slow rise time because the stimulation is increased gradually

---

Nanosecond: One-billionth (10^{-9}) of a second.

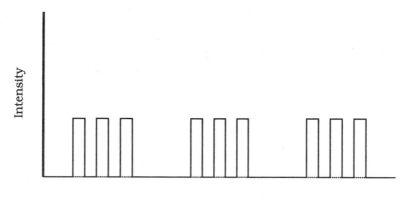

Time

FIGURE 5–13 **An Example of a Pulse Train.** A pattern of electrical pulses repeating at regular intervals.

and the "shock" of the current is reduced. When muscles are being stimulated, the gradual contraction produced by a slow rise time more closely resembles a voluntary muscle contraction. More and more fibers are recruited as the amplitude of the stimulus, or the phase duration, increases.[7]

MEASURES OF ELECTRICAL CURRENT FLOW

The strength of an electrical current is expressed in amperes and is related to the voltage of the current and the resistance it meets. This relationship, Ohm's law, is the fundamental principle governing electrical current flow (Box 5–2). The following sections describe the factors affecting the strength of an electrical current passing through the human body.

Electrical Charge

Electrical current results from the movement of electrons. The number of electrons required for electrical current flow is so great that it is impractical to count each one. Just as we may describe 12 objects as a dozen, or a dozen dozens as a gross, we may also describe a large number of electrons as a single unit. A **coulomb** is used to describe the charge produced by 6.25×10^{18} electrons (negative charge) or protons (positive charge) and is represented by the symbol "Q."

Coulomb's law describes the relationship between like and unlike electrical charges: Opposite charges attract and like charges repel. The strength of the attractive or repulsive forces may be amplified by increasing the magnitude of the charges or by decreasing the distance between the two objects.

Voltage

Voltage, also known as the electromotive force or **potential difference** between two poles, measures the tendency for current flow to occur. Electrons placed

BOX 5-2 Ohm's Law

Ohm's law describes the relationship between amperage, voltage, and resistance. Generally stated, **current (I) is directly proportional to voltage (V) and inversely proportional to resistance (R);** that is:

$$I = V/R$$

By using Ohm's law, or a derivation of it, the amperage, voltage, or resistance in a circuit can be calculated if two of the three variables are known. In a circuit where the potential is 120 V with 10 ohms of resistance, the amperage would be calculated as 120 V/10 ohms, or 12 A. Circuits having a very high voltage can still have a very small current flow if the resistance is high. For example, applying 1,000 V to a circuit with a resistance of 1,000,000 ohms would produce only 0.001 A. Likewise, low voltages can give rise to a very high current flow. Consider a 10-V circuit with 0.01 ohms of resistance. The resultant current would be 1,000 A.

To determine the effect that current (I) and resistance (R) have on voltage (V), we may transpose Ohm's law to give:

$$V = IR$$

For current to flow through a resistance, the voltage applied must be equal to or greater than the product of the amperage times the resistance. To produce a current of 12 A flowing through a circuit of 10 ohms, 120 V (12 A $\times$ 10 ohms) would be required.

The resistance (R) found in a circuit may be calculated by again transposing the formula so that we divide the voltage (V) by the resistance (I):

$$R = V/I$$

Therefore, if we are using a device that requires 120 V and 12 A, we can calculate the amount of resistance by dividing 120 V by 12 A to give 10 ohms.

You will notice that in all of our equations, current is equal to 10 A, voltage is equal to 120 V, and resistance is equal to 10 ohms. This illustrates the interrelationship between the variables. If we were to reduce the current to 5 A and increase the voltage to 200 V, the resistance would then be 40 ohms. In any case, the voltage applied to the circuit must be greater than the resistance, or no current will flow.

within a field strain themselves to move to the opposite pole, thus creating the potential for work to occur (Work = Force $\times$ Distance). The **volt** is the unit of potential difference and represents the amount of work required to move 1 coulomb of charge. The energy required to move this coulomb is termed a **Joule.** Traditionally, the symbol for voltage is "E," but recently the symbol "V" has come into vogue and is used to symbolize voltage in this text.

The flow of electrons is not a simple passage of particles through a medium. Rather, this flow consists of the passing of electrons between atoms in a manner similar to a bucket brigade. Picture a line of people passing buckets of water. In this analogy, the people represent atoms, and the buckets of water are electrons. The first person hands his or her bucket to the next person. This person then passes the bucket to the next person and the process repeats. The flow of electrons is quite similar; rather than a single electron passing through a wire, electrons are passed from atom to atom.

Current

Amperage describes the rate at which the electrical charge (measured in coulombs) flows. More specifically, 1 ampere (A) is the current when 1 coulomb passes a single point in 1 second. Conceptually, we may make the analogy to the number of people passing through a turnstile at any given time. If 1 coulomb passes a point in 1 second, the rate of flow is 1 A. If 2 coulombs pass a point in 1 second, the rate of flow is 2 A.

The symbol for current flow is "I." Most electrical modalities have current flow measured in milliamperes (mA), 1/1,000 of an ampere, or microamperes (μA), 1/1,000,000 of an ampere.

Resistance

All materials present some degree of opposition to the flow of electrical current. Those materials allowing current to pass with relative ease are labeled **conductors** and those that tend to oppose current flow **resistors.** A material's resistance to the movement of electrons is measured in **ohms.** One ohm is the amount of resistance needed to develop 0.24 calories of heat when 1 A of current is applied for 1 second. The symbol for resistance is "R," and for ohms, "Ω" (omega).

Conductance is a measure of the ease with which current is allowed to pass. Conductance is the mathematical reciprocal of resistance and is measured by the unit **mho**—"ohm" spelled backward.

The type, length, and cross-sectional area of the material and the temperature of the circuit determine the amount of resistance offered to the flow of electrons (Table 5–4). These four elements together determine the total resistance to current flow. As we have already discussed, the potential difference at each end of the circuit must be great enough to overcome the resistance, or no current will flow.

Impedance

In an AC, two additional properties, *inductance* and *capacitance,* act to resist the flow of an AC. Collectively known as **impedance,** this form of resistance is also measured in ohms, but uses the symbol "Z."

Inductance is the ability of a material to store electrical energy by means of an **electromagnetic field** and is measured by the *henry.* Variation in the magnitude and direction of electrical current creates a *flux* that induces voltage. Inductors tend to oppose electrical current flow. A transformer used to convert household

---

Inductance: The degree that a varying current can induce voltage, expressed in henries (H).

Capacitance: The frequency-dependent ability to store a charge. The symbol for capacitance is C and is expressed in farads (F).

Henry: A measure of inductance (H). One henry induces an electromagnetic force of 1 V when the current changes at a rate of 1 A per second.

Flux: A residual electromagnetic field created by two unlike charges.

TABLE 5–4 Factors Determining the Resistance of an Electrical Circuit

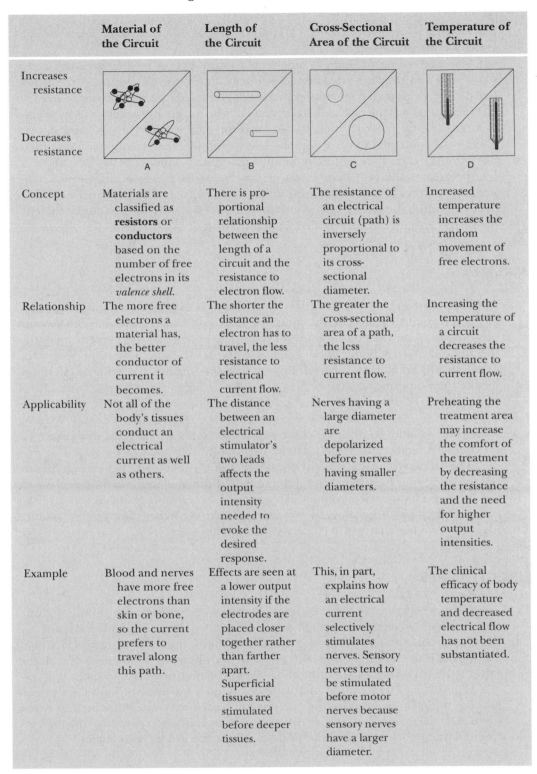

	Material of the Circuit	Length of the Circuit	Cross-Sectional Area of the Circuit	Temperature of the Circuit
Increases resistance / Decreases resistance	A	B	C	D
Concept	Materials are classified as **resistors** or **conductors** based on the number of free electrons in its *valence shell.*	There is proportional relationship between the length of a circuit and the resistance to electron flow.	The resistance of an electrical circuit (path) is inversely proportional to its cross-sectional diameter.	Increased temperature increases the random movement of free electrons.
Relationship	The more free electrons a material has, the better conductor of current it becomes.	The shorter the distance an electron has to travel, the less resistance to electrical current flow.	The greater the cross-sectional area of a path, the less resistance to current flow.	Increasing the temperature of a circuit decreases the resistance to current flow.
Applicability	Not all of the body's tissues conduct an electrical current as well as others.	The distance between an electrical stimulator's two leads affects the output intensity needed to evoke the desired response.	Nerves having a large diameter are depolarized before nerves having smaller diameters.	Preheating the treatment area may increase the comfort of the treatment by decreasing the resistance and the need for higher output intensities.
Example	Blood and nerves have more free electrons than skin or bone, so the current prefers to travel along this path.	Effects are seen at a lower output intensity if the electrodes are placed closer together rather than farther apart. Superficial tissues are stimulated before deeper tissues.	This, in part, explains how an electrical current selectively stimulates nerves. Sensory nerves tend to be stimulated before motor nerves because sensory nerves have a larger diameter.	The clinical efficacy of body temperature and decreased electrical flow has not been substantiated.

Valence shell: An imaginary shell in which the electrons responsible for chemical reactivity orbit around the nucleus of an atom.

current into a lower-voltage DC is an example of an inductor. Inductance is negligible in biological systems.[1]

Capacitance is the ability of a material to store energy by means of an electrostatic field and provides frequency-dependent opposition to electric current flow. Created by an insulator separating two conductors, charges may be stored even after the applied voltage has been discontinued. The output of capacitors is measured in farads (F), microfarads, (μF, 10^{-6} F), or picofarads (pF, 10^{-10} F). A farad stores a charge of 1 coulomb when 1 V is applied. As we will see when frequency is discussed, the lower the capacitance of a circuit, the higher the frequency of an AC it allows.[8]

Because many cell membranes act as capacitors by separating positive and negative charges between the inside and outside of the cell, capacitance is a factor in determining the effects of current flow on the body. Higher-frequency currents meet less capacitive skin resistance than lower-frequency currents.

Wattage

The relationship between voltage and amperage is expressed in units of wattage (P) and is used to designate the **power** of a current. Power describes the amount of work being performed in a unit of time. The voltage of the current measures the amount of work being done; amperage defines the time unit. One watt is the power produced by 1 A of current flowing with the force of 1 V. With this in mind, we can then describe wattage as:

$$P = VI$$

Using the variables from Box 5–2, we can calculate the power used by a device requiring 12 A from a 120-V source to be 1440 W.

The change in wattage of an electrical circuit reflects the net change in amperage and/or voltage. If either amperage or voltage is increased or decreased, the wattage changes accordingly. However, if one variable is increased and the other decreased, the wattage increases or decreases depending on the relative magnitude of the changes in voltage and amperage.

CIRCUIT TYPES

An electrical current introduced into a conductive medium may flow along one set route (**series circuit**), through many different pathways (**parallel circuit**), or through a combination of each. Consider an old-fashioned string of Christmas tree lights. If the string is wired as a series circuit, when one bulb burns out, all the other lights go out as well because the current has no other path to take.

In a string of lights wired in a parallel circuit, a burned-out bulb does not affect the other lights because the current still has other routes by which to reach them. Electricity operates under different constraints when traveling through series and parallel circuits, and each type of circuit has unique properties.

Series Circuit

Electrons in a series circuit have only **one pathway available for travel.** Connecting a wire between the two poles of a battery forms a simple series circuit. In more

BOX 5-3   Calculation of Ohm's Law in Series and Parallel Circuits

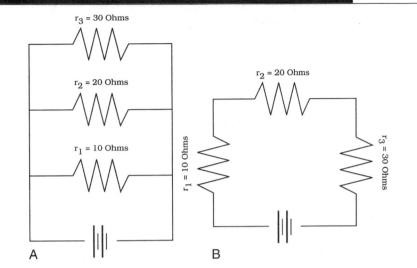

In a Series Circuit:

If we know that a potential of 120 V is applied to a circuit with 60 ohms of resistance, the amperage can be calculated by using Ohm's law. Using the values from Figure *A* above, the equation for calculating the current flow through the series of resistors is:

$$I = V/R_t$$
$$I = 120 \text{ V}/60 \text{ ohms}$$
$$I = 2 \text{ A}$$

If each of three resistors has a different resistance (say 10 ohms, 20 ohms, and 30 ohms), the voltage will fluctuate between resistors. By applying a derivation of Ohm's law, $V = IR$, the voltage across each resistor may be calculated as:

$V_1 = Ir_1$	$V_2 = Ir_2$	$V_3 = Ir_3$
$V_1 = 2 \text{ A} \times 10 \text{ ohms}$	$V_2 = 2 \text{ A} \times 20 \text{ ohms}$	$V_3 = 2 \text{ A} \times 30 \text{ ohms}$
$V_1 = 20 \text{ V}$	$V_2 = 40 \text{ V}$	$V_3 = 60 \text{ V}$

By adding $V_1 + V_2 + V_3$, you can see that the sum of the potential across the individual resistors equals the total power applied to the circuit. The current (amperage) remains the same throughout a series circuit. The voltage and the resistance vary.

In a Parallel Circuit:

To calculate the total resistance for a parallel circuit, we must keep in mind that the flow in each pathway is inversely proportional to its resistance. Because voltage is constant, this value may be canceled out and the mathematical reciprocal (1/n) of the resistance may be used (Fig. *B* above).

$$I = V/R_t$$
$$I = 120 \text{ V}/5.56 \text{ ohms}$$
$$I = 21.6 \text{ A}$$

complex series circuits, resistors are aligned "end to end" so that the current leaving one resistor will enter the next. In a series circuit, **the current remains the same** in all components along the circuit **and the total resistance is equal to the sum of the individual resistors.** Box 5–3 presents the calculations of Ohm's law within a series and parallel circuit.

BOX 5–3 **Continued**

The amount of current flowing across each resistor (and path) is calculated by:

$i_1 = v/r_1$	$i_2 = v/r_2$	$i_3 = v/r_3$
$i_1 = 120\ V/10\ ohms$	$i_2 = 120\ V/20\ ohms$	$i_3 = 120\ V/30\ ohms$
$i_1 = 12\ A$	$i_2 = 6\ A$	$i_3 = 4\ A$

where:

i_n = Amperage across resistor n
v = Voltage applied to the circuit
r_n = Resistance in ohms

Unlike series circuits, the parallel circuits have the same voltage across each path. The amperage and resistance differ from path to path. Therefore, if the voltage across one path can be calculated, the voltage for the entire circuit is known.

Parallel Circuit

Electrons in a parallel circuit are provided with alternative pathways for travel, and electrons tend to take the path of least resistance. Paths within the parallel circuit may then branch into other parallel or series circuits, but in either case, **each path has its own amperage and the voltage remains constant.** The flow in each of these pathways is inversely proportional to the resistance provided. This is quite similar to checking out of a grocery store. When we are finished shopping, we tend to get in the line with the fastest clerk rather than the slowest. In any given time frame, more people will check out through the fastest clerk, and fewer through the slowest. Refer to Box 5–3 for the calculations of Ohm's law within a parallel circuit.

TABLE 5–5 **Electrical Terms**

Amperage (I):	The rate at which an electrical current flows. One ampere is equal to the rate of flow of 1 coulomb per second. It is analogous to the rate of flow of water through a pipe. $I = V/R$.
Charge:	See Coulomb.
Coulomb (Q):	The basic unit of charge is the coulomb, the net positive or negative electrical charge produced by 6.25×10^{18} electrons or protons.
Coulomb's law:	Like charges repel and unlike (opposite) charges attract each other.
Joule (J):	Basic unit of work in the International System of Units. Representing the work done by moving 1 coulomb, 1 J equals 0.74 foot-pounds of work. The conversion equation is: $J = QV$.
Ohms (Ω):	Unit of electrical resistance (R). $R = V/I$.
Ohm's law:	Current is directly proportional to voltage and inversely proportional to resistance. $I = V/R$.
Voltage (V):	The potential for electron flow to occur. Analogous to the height of a waterfall, it indicates how much energy is available in the system. The greater the height of a waterfall, the more energy it can impart to a mill below. $V = I/R$.
Watts (W):	Unit of electrical power (P). May be calculated from the relation Watts = Volts × Amperage ($P = VI$). Watts measure the ability to perform work.

To review: An electrical current is the flow of electrons through a medium. Electron flow is measured in coulombs per second, and the voltage of the current is based on the potential difference for flow to occur. The rate of electron flow, the amperage, represents how many coulombs are being moved past a single point in 1 second. The movement of the current is always met with some degree of resistance, measured in ohms. Ohm's law describes the relationship between amperage, voltage, and resistance. The total power delivered by the current is wattage, calculated by multiplying the amperage times the voltage. Table 5–5 lists common electrical terms, their definitions, and equations describing basic laws of electricity.

Electrical circuits are classified as being series or parallel. Within a series circuit, the electrons have only one path to take. The amperage remains constant, but the voltage fluctuates. Within a parallel circuit, the electrons have the option of taking more than one route, but the path of least resistance is preferred. In a parallel circuit, the amperage is varied among the paths, but the voltage remains constant.

CHARACTERISTICS OF ELECTRICAL GENERATORS

Electrical modalities may be driven by either standard household current (120-V AC) or by batteries (1.5-V to 9-V DC). Before this current is delivered to the body, it must be modified to the desired stimulation parameters.

In a simplified view, the current passes through one or more transformers to change it to the desired type (AC to DC, or DC to AC) and another to control the output current. A device, generically known as a generator, shapes the current (waveform) used by the modality. Other components within the generator control the characteristics of the electrical pulses.

Each element of the waveform has an effect on the tissues' reaction to the current flow. The following sections discuss each generator characteristic and relate how each affects the treatment.

Current Attributes

The manner in which the stimulating current is applied to the body affects its ability to depolarize excitable tissue. The actual intensity of the current, the amount of current per unit of body area, and the duty cycle influence the effect that the treatment has on human tissues.

Average Current

Average current describes the absolute value of current per unit of time. The physiochemical and thermal changes in the tissues are based on the average current.[9] Average current is meaningful only for monophasic currents and unbalanced biphasic currents. Because the net charge for balanced biphasic and alternating currents is zero, the root-mean-square value should be used for these currents (see Box 5–1).

By increasing the number of pulses per second or by increasing the pulse duration, the average current is increased and so is the perception of the stimulus. There is much more current per unit of time in high-frequency generators than with other types. Long pulse durations combined with a high average current result in an increased sensation of pain.

The average current found in most electrical stimulation units is measured in milliamperes. This measure is not meaningful for a balanced symmetrical current because the phase charges for this type of current are equal and for the average current are zero.

Current Density

The physiological effects derived from electrical stimulation are related to the current density and the amount of current per unit area. The current density is inversely proportional to the size of the electrode. For example, if you are passing 300 V through an electrode of 10 square inches, the resulting current density would be 30 V per square inch. If the electrode's surface area is reduced by half, 300 V are then passing through an electrode of 5 square inches, with a current density of 60 V per square inch. If the electrode's surface area is again reduced, to a size of 1 square inch, the result is a current density of 300 V per square inch.

As the current density increases, so does the perception of the stimulus. If the stimulus was comfortable to the patient in our first example, it would be much more uncomfortable in the last example because the same amount of current is being delivered by one-tenth of the initial surface area.

Duty Cycle

The ratio of the amount of time the current is flowing (ON) to the amount of time without current (OFF) is known as the duty cycle. Expressed as a percentage, duty cycles are calculated by dividing the time the current is flowing by the total cycle time (the time the current is flowing plus the time it is not). For example, to calculate the duty cycle of a generator producing 10 seconds of stimulation, followed by 10 seconds without current flow, the following equation would be used:

$$\text{Duty cycle (percentage)} = \frac{\text{Time current is ON}}{\text{Total cycle time}} \times 100$$

$$= \frac{10 \text{ seconds (ON)}}{10 \text{ seconds (ON)} + 10 \text{ seconds (OFF)}} \times 100$$

$$= \frac{10 \text{ seconds}}{20 \text{ seconds (Total cycle time)}} \times 100$$

$$= 0.5 \times 100$$
$$= 50 \text{ percent duty cycle}$$

This relationship may also be expressed as a ratio. Using the parameters from the previous examples:

$$\text{Duty cycle (ratio)} = 10:20$$
$$= 1:2$$

Duty cycles play a role in neuromuscular stimulation by preventing muscle fatigue. Muscular stimulation is started with a 25 percent duty cycle and is progressively increased as the condition improves.[10]

The Body Circuit

The human body is a mass of tissues and fluids, each having varying ability to conduct an electrical current. A tissue's ability to conduct electricity is directly related to its water content. As the percentage of the water in tissue increases, its ability to transmit electricity increases.

Tissues are classified as being either **excitable** or **nonexcitable** (Box 5–4). Excitable tissues are directly influenced by the current parameters of intensity, pulse duration, and pulse frequency. Nonexcitable tissues do not respond directly to current flow but may be influenced by the electrical fields caused by the current.

The outer layer of the skin has a low water content, making it a poor electrical conductor. Bone, tendons, fascia, and adipose tissue are also poor conductors of electrical currents because of their low water content (20 percent to 30 percent). Muscle, nerve, and blood have a high water content (70 percent to 75 percent) and are good conductors of electrical currents. The cell membrane produces the greatest resistance to current flow. The internal organs, especially the heart, have a low resistance to electrical current flow (Box 5–5).

The current enters the body through a series circuit. Because the composition and texture of skin are relatively consistent, there is only one path for the flow to take. Once the current enters the tissues, it may take many different paths, forming a parallel circuit, with the current preferring to follow the path of least resistance, such as those formed by muscle, nerves, effusion, and blood.

The passage of current through living tissues produces varying biophysical effects, including physiochemical effects and physiological reactions. Thermal

---

BOX 5–4   Excitable Tissues

Excitable Tissues	Nonexcitable Tissues
Nerve fibers	Bone
Muscle fibers	Cartilage
Blood cells	Tendons
Cell membranes	Ligaments

When an excitable tissue (nerve, muscle, etc.) remains undisturbed, its resting potential stays constant. The resulting potential acts as a stored energy source to be used in the transmission of impulses; the energy is stored as separated electrical charges on either side (inside and outside) of the cell membrane. In this sense, the membrane serves as a capacitor. The amount of depolarization required to bring these tissues to threshold is about the same for each.

A decrease (depolarization) or increase (hyperpolarization) in the cell membrane's electrical charge is required before an action potential can take place. Any stimulus, be it electrical, mechanical, chemical, thermal, or hormonal, at a sufficient magnitude, can cause a depolarization by changing the permeability of the cell, resulting in an action potential. A membrane requires approximately 0.5 msec to recover its excitability after an action potential. This "down time" after the action potential is the absolute refractory period. If a second impulse at the same intensity occurs within this period, the membrane will not discharge. After the absolute refractory period, there is a relative refractory period, during which another depolarization can occur if the magnitude of the stimulus is increased (see Box 1–2).

BOX 5–5 **The Path of Least Resistance**

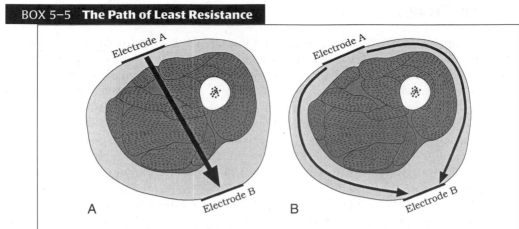

We tend to visualize an electrical current flowing in a straight line from one electrode to another, and in some cases this is correct. Recall, however, that electrons follow the path of least resistance and that the amperage and voltage must be sufficient to overcome the total resistance imposed by the circuit.

Consider a situation in which electrodes are placed on the anterior and posterior surfaces of the thigh. We may think that the current will flow directly through the tissues from one electrode to another as presented in *A* above. Most therapeutic treatment dosages lack the electrical power, voltage, and amperage required to overcome the sum of the resistance formed by the cross-section of the tissues. In most cases, the current travels around the periphery by conducting through superficial blood vessels and nerves (*B* above). The deeper tissues are affected by stimulation of superficial nerves.

Transthoracic and transcranial stimulation is often contraindicated, but not necessarily out of fear of sending a current through the heart or brain. Appropriately placed electrodes can affect the functions of these organs secondary to stimulation of superficial nerves. Many stimulation techniques, such as those for temporomandibular joint dysfunction and auriculotherapy, involve application of electricity to the head. However, at these intensities the current stays within the tissues that are immediately subcutaneous.

Caution should always be exercised when applying an electrical current anywhere on the upper torso, neck, or head.

changes could potentially occur within the tissues, but at therapeutic doses the effect is negligible.[9]

Electrodes

The site where the electrodes touch the skin serves as a point of conversion between the flow of electrons used by the generator and the flow of ions within the body's tissues.[6] To form a closed circuit between the generator and the body's tissues, at least one electrode from each of the generator's output leads must be in contact with the skin. Properly prepared and placed electrodes increase the efficiency of the electrical current while allowing for improved patient comfort (Table 5–6).

The electrodes themselves may be metal, carbon-impregnated silicone rubber, or a metallic meshed cloth. In most cases, a **medium** is required to reduce the

TABLE 5–6 Methods of Reducing Skin-Electrode Resistance

Moisten electrodes with water or conductive gel (sponge or rubber electrodes).
Remove dirt, oil, or flaky skin by washing with soap and water, alcohol, or acetone.
Warm area with a moist heat pack.
Gently scrub area with fine emery paper.
Remove excess hair.
Saturate sponges with commercial saline solution rather than tap water.
Use silver electrodes.

resistance between the skin and the electrode and provide even current distribution. Metal electrodes commonly use moistened sponges for this purpose. Carbon-rubber electrodes may also use moist sponges, gauze, or a conducting gel. To conduct the current, sponges and gauze must be thoroughly saturated (but not soaked) with water. Although tap water is commonly used for this purpose, the quality and mineral content of water in many areas may needlessly increase electrical resistance. Usually this is not a problem, but patients who are sensitive to electrical currents may experience more comfort if the sponge is saturated with a commercially available saline solution.

Conducting gels are salt-free coupling agents designed to minimize skin-electrode resistance and are used with carbon rubber or metal electrodes. Their chemical properties allow long-term use with little breakdown associated with current flow or evaporation, and because of the gel's high water content and low mineral content, skin irritation and allergic reactions are minimized. Before placing the electrode on the patient's skin, a liberal amount of the gel should be spread over the entire area of the conducting surface. Once the electrode has been positioned on the skin, it should be slightly rotated and slid to ensure even distribution of the medium.

Nonadhesive electrodes used during short-term treatments are generally held in place by elastic straps. In the case of long-term treatments, the electrodes are either self-adhesive or they must be secured through the use of adhesive patches. Gel, rather than water, should be used for this type of treatment. Generally these types of electrodes and their adhesives are very durable and water-resistant.

The type of electrode and the conductive medium used can affect the efficiency and comfort of electrical stimulation. Of the standard electrode types, carbon-rubber electrodes deliver the most current at the lowest skin impedance, about 200 ohms, allowing for a more comfortable stimulation. Silver electrodes (most commonly used with iontophoresis, microcurrent stimulators, and electrodiagnostic units) provide about 20 ohms of resistance, so less energy is required to pass the current through them.[11,12] However, silver electrodes are quite expensive. Self-adhesive electrodes have been shown to produce the most discomfort during the treatment, with an increased burning sensation occurring under the electrode's metal connector.[12]

Electrode Size

The size of the electrode inversely affects the density of the current; as the size of the electrode decreases, the **current density** increases. Consider, for example, a current passing through two electrodes, one having a surface area of 10 square

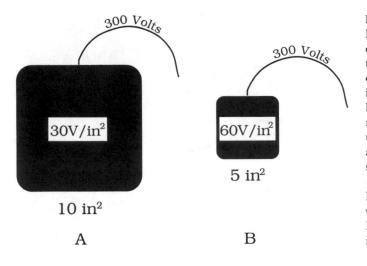

FIGURE 5–14 **Current Density.** Electrodes must transmit the entire voltage flowing through the circuit. In this case the large electrode (*A*) has 300 volts flowing through it. Electrode (*B*) is half the size of (*A*), yet 300 volts must pass through it as well. In this example, Electrode (*A*) has a current density of 30 volts per square inch (in^2) and Electrode (*B*) has 60 volts per square inch. In this example the stimulation would be more intense under Electrode (*B*) because of the increased current density.

inches and the other 5 square inches. The smaller electrode (5 square inches) would have twice as much current passing through it per square inch than the larger one (Fig. 5–14).

The electrode's contact with the skin also influences the stimulation parameters, comfort, and muscular tension associated with electrical stimulation.[13] As the electrode surface area increases, there is a greater current flow at any given voltage.[1]

Smaller electrodes require less current to stimulate tissues than larger electrodes because of the high current density. By manipulating the relative sizes of the electrodes, various physiological responses may be elicited. The size of an electrode to be used is determined by the size of the body area being treated and/or the other electrodes being used. A "small" electrode used on the quadriceps could easily be a "large" electrode when it is used on the forearm. In addition, as we will see in the next section, the size of an electrode is relative to the other electrode(s) being used.

There is a positive correlation between the maximal isometric torque produced during electrical stimulation and the size of the electrodes.[12] The resistance to current flow (impedance) offered by the skin is reduced as the size of the electrode increases. Larger electrodes produce stronger contractions without causing pain, but the stimulation of the tissues is less specific because the current is spread over a larger area.[4,13]

Electrode Placement

The treatment site, current intensity, and type of excitable tissue being stimulated are determined by a combination of electrode size and their relative location on the body. Certain areas of the skin are more conducive to electrical stimulation than other areas. These sites, collectively referred to as **stimulation points,** represent **motor points, trigger points,** and **acupuncture points** (Box 5–6).

The proximity of electrodes to one another determines which tissues are stimulated, the depth of the stimulation, and the number of parallel circuits that are formed. When electrodes are placed close together, the current flows superficially, with a relatively small number of parallel paths developed. As the distance

---

BOX 5–6 Stimulation Points

Certain areas of the skin conduct electricity better than other areas. These locations, collectively known as stimulation points, represent areas that require less current to produce muscle contractions, sensation, or pain. Many therapeutic techniques are designed to specifically stimulate one or more of these stimulation points. The proximity of these areas to each other results in a single electrode stimulating all three points.

Motor Points

Each muscle has one or more skin surface areas that are hypersensitive to electrical current flow. These points, known as **motor points,** are discrete areas above the location where motor nerves and blood vessels enter the muscle mass. Because of their low electrical resistance, stimulation of these points elicits a stronger contraction at lower intensities than the surrounding tissues. Motor points associated with an injured area show an increased sensitivity to current flow and palpation.

Although there is a degree of consistency in the location of motor points, there is some variation between individuals and, depending on the pathology involved, can vary within the same person over time. Appendix C presents commonly accepted motor points and is presented for reference purposes. These points must be located on each athlete by finding the point at which the strongest contraction results from the lowest intensity of stimulation.

Trigger Points

Trigger points are pathological, localized areas of pain that are hypersensitive to stimulation. Stimulation of these areas "triggers" radiating or referred pain. Unlike motor points, trigger points may be found not only in muscle but also in other soft tissues, such as ligament, tendon, and fascia (see Appendix A).

Acupuncture Points

Acupuncture points are specific sites on the skin possessing a decreased electrical skin resistance and increased electrical conductivity. These points are connected by meridians through which blood and energy flow.[95,96,143] Superficial master points, consisting of 12 main channels, 8 secondary channels, and a network of subchannels, connect areas of the skin to deeper channels and allow systemic regulation of many body functions. These master points are especially effective in alleviating pain along the entire meridian. Although acupuncture has been successfully used for many centuries, its theoretical basis has never been fully substantiated.

---

between electrodes is increased, the current is allowed to reach deeper into the tissues. If the distance between the two electrodes is too great, such a large number of parallel circuits is formed that the specificity of the stimulation decreases (Fig. 5–15).

The orientation of the electrodes in relation to the body part must also be taken into consideration. Muscle fibers are four times more conductive when the current flows with the direction of the fibers than when it flows across them.[6]

Although each electrical circuit must have two leads from the generator, more than one electrode can be connected to a single lead. Through bifurcation, two or more electrodes can originate from a single lead. It is not uncommon for both leads to possess two electrodes each, or for one lead to have two electrodes and the other lead to have only one. The relationship between the total current density of one electrode (or set of electrodes) to the other electrode determines the electrode configuration, which may be classified as **bipolar** or **monopolar.**

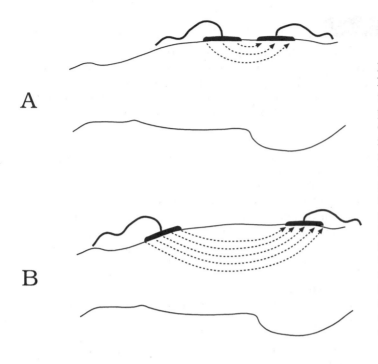

A

B

FIGURE 5–15 **Electrode Proximity.** (*A*) When electrodes are placed in close proximity to each other, the current flow forms relatively few parallel paths and does not penetrate as deeply into the tissues. (*B*) As the distance between the electrodes is increased, the number of parallel paths increases and the current tends to flow more deeply within the tissues. However, along with this the focus of the stimulation becomes less defined because the current meets more resistance and more parallel pathways are formed.

Bipolar Technique

Bipolar application involves the use of electrodes of equal or near-equal size (Fig. 5–16). Both electrodes are located in the target treatment area. Because the current densities are equal, an equal amount of stimulation should occur under each electrode or set of electrodes. Other factors may affect the quality and equality of stimulation under each electrode. If electrode "A" is placed over a motor point or other hypersensitive stimulation point (see Box 5–6) and electrode "B" is not, the effects of the treatment will be weighted toward electrode "A." This scenario would be appropriate if a single point, such as a trigger point, were being targeted during the treatment. In this case, a monopolar configuration would be preferable because a single, well-localized area is being targeted. However, if the treatment goal is to elicit a muscle contraction, electrodes "A" and "B" both should be placed over motor points within the same muscle or muscle group.

Monopolar Technique

Monopolar application involves the use of two classifications of electrodes: (1) an **active electrode** placed where the treatment effect occurs and (2) a **dispersive electrode** used to complete the circuit. The active electrode is placed on or near the body part to be treated, and the dispersive electrode is fastened to the body at a distant location (Fig. 5–17). The high current density focuses the effect of the treatment under the smaller electrodes. As the distance between the active and dispersive electrodes increases, more parallel electrical paths are formed, resulting in less specific stimulation of deep motor nerves.[4]

The surface area of the dispersive electrode is significantly larger than that of the active electrodes. Because of the relatively low current density, little or no stimulation should occur under the dispersive electrode. If sensation is experi-

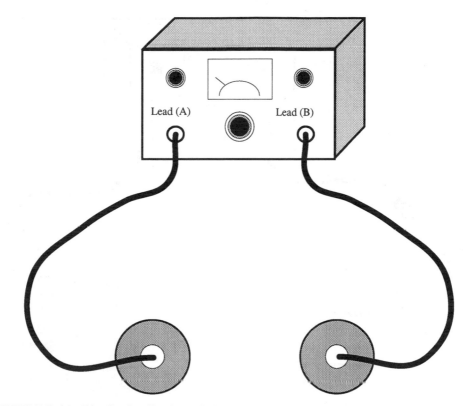

FIGURE 5–16 **Bipolar Application of Electrical Stimulation.** The surface area of the electrodes originating from each lead is equal. This creates an equal current density, and the effects of the stimulation occur equally under each electrode. Each lead may be split to accommodate two electrodes. As long as the electrodes are of equal size and the resulting current density is equal, the application is classified as bipolar.

enced under this electrode, reapply the dispersive electrode to a different site, rewet it, or use a larger electrode. Sensation under the dispersive electrode does not negate the effects of the treatment, but it is unnecessary. Motor nerve stimulation under this electrode indicates that the current densities of the electrodes are too similar. In this case, a larger dispersive electrode or a smaller active electrode should be used.

Quadripolar Technique

Quadripolar application involves the use of two sets of electrodes, each originating from its own *channel;* it may be considered the concurrent application of two bipolar circuits. The current from each of the two channels may intersect and intensify and localize the treatment effects as is found with interferential stimulation. Other quadripolar configurations include parallel placements, as are found in certain transcutaneous electrical nerve stimulation techniques, or agonist-

Channel (electrical): An electrical circuit consisting of two poles that operate independently of other circuits.

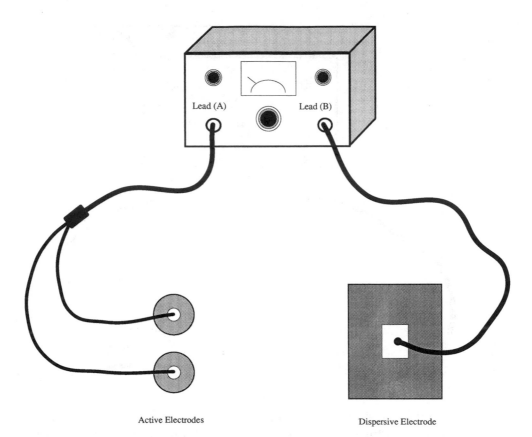

Active Electrodes   Dispersive Electrode

FIGURE 5–17   **Monopolar Application of Electrical Stimulation.** The total area of the active electrode is significantly less than the area of the dispersive electrode. The imbalance in current density focuses the stimulation to the area under the active electrodes.

antagonist placements used in neuromuscular electrical stimulation techniques (Fig. 5–18).

Movement of Electrical Currents Through the Body

Most forms of electrical stimulation are applied transcutaneously. The exceptions are certain bone growth generators that may have electrodes surgically implanted in the muscle or bone. When a current is passed through the skin, it has the potential to upset the resting potential of peripheral axons. Under the cathode, a depolarization of the nerve occurs, whereas stimulation under the anode results in a hyperpolarization of the nerve (see Box 5–4 and Box 1–2).[14] **Rheobase** is the term used to describe the minimum amount of voltage, under the negative pole, required to produce a stimulated response when the phase duration is unlimited (e.g., a direct current is used).

Once a therapeutic electrical current enters the body, the movement of ions replaces the flow of electrons (Box 5–7). As described by Coulomb's law, ions move away from the pole having the same charge and migrate toward the pole having the opposite charge. When an AC or pulsed biphasic current is used, the ions move back and forth between the electrodes based on the number of cycles

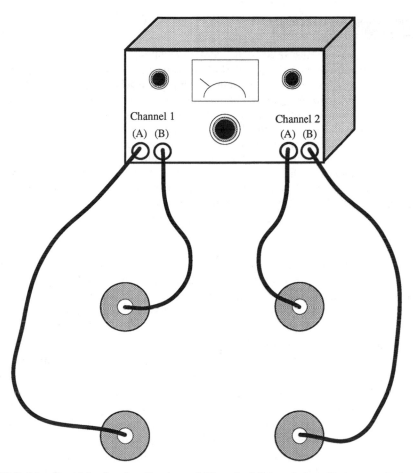

FIGURE 5–18 **Quadripolar Application of Electrical Stimulation.** Two sets of electrodes operating with two independent channels.

per second, as shown in Figure 5–3. When a DC or pulsed monophasic current is used, this migration is in one direction only.

Medical Galvanism

Galvanic stimulation involves the application of a low-voltage direct current to the body, with a known polarity under each electrode. By controlling the polarity of the electrodes, certain involuntary cellular and biochemical responses may be elicited. True galvanism requires an uninterrupted direct current to achieve a net galvanic change under the electrodes. The *pH* of tissues under the cathode becomes basic, whereas acidic changes are noted under the anode. Galvanic stimulation is the only type of current that elicits a muscle contraction from denervated muscle, but the phase duration is so long that C fibers are also stimulated, making the contraction painful.

---

pH: (potential of hydrogen) A measure of acidity or alkalinity (bases). A neutral solution has a pH of 7. Acids have a pH of less than 7; bases greater than 7.

BOX 5–7   Ionic changes

In its normal state, an atom has a number of electrons equal to the number of protons. Because the charges of the electrons (negative) and protons (positive) are equal, the atom has a zero (neutral) charge. Atoms that no longer have a zero net charge are known as ions. When an atom loses one or more electrons, it becomes a positive ion (cation) because the number of protons is greater than the number of electrons. Likewise, atoms that gain electrons become negatively charged ions (anions) because the number of electrons is greater than the number of protons.

Ions behave differently from their neutrally charged relatives. Because they possess an electrical charge, they are subject to electromagnetic and electro-osmotic influences. When placed in the path of a direct current, positively charged ions migrate toward the negative pole and vice versa.

Through an **electro-osmotic** process, ions are attracted to the pole possessing the opposite charge and repelled from the pole having the same charge. Positively charged sodium ions (Na^+) move toward the cathode, where they gain an electron and form an uncharged sodium atom. Through the reaction of sodium with water, proteins are liquefied, causing a general softening of the tissues in the area and a decrease in nerve irritability.[15] Physiological events under the anode are essentially opposite those occurring at the cathode. Here, tissues harden because chemical mediators force a coagulation of protein.

These effects are not as pronounced when monophasic, biphasic, or alternating currents are used. The short pulse duration and long interpulse interval reduce the chemical effects of pulsed currents.[16] Symmetrical or balanced asymmetrical biphasic currents or ACs result in no galvanic changes because both phases have an equal but opposite charge. An unbalanced asymmetrical current can result in residual chemical changes if the duration of the current is sufficient.

Selective Stimulation of Nerves

During the application of electrical stimulation, different nerve types are stimulated in an orderly, predictable manner. A nerve's response to electrical stimulation is based on three factors: (1) the relative diameter of the nerve, (2) the depth of the nerve in relation to the electrode, and (3) the duration of the pulse. During electrical stimulation, sensory nerves are stimulated first, followed by motor nerves, and then pain fibers. Only after these structures have been depolarized (or if these nerves are incapable of depolarizing) can the electrical current directly affect muscle fibers.

The amplitude necessary to stimulate a nerve is inversely proportional to the nerve's diameter. Nerves with larger diameters are stimulated to threshold before nerves with smaller diameters. Because the larger cross-sectional area of the nerve provides less capacitive membrane resistance, less current is required (Box 5–8).

Superficial sensory nerves receive a greater amount of stimulation than do the more deeply placed motor nerves. To activate a more deeply situated motor nerve, the current must first pass through the more superficial sensory nerves. Pain fibers are more superficial than motor nerves, but they also tend to have a smaller diameter. Their resistance to current flow is so great that motor nerves reach threshold first, allowing muscle contractions to be elicited before pain is

---

BOX 5–8   The Law of Dubois Reymond

Causing a nerve to depolarize is a relatively easy task; simply apply enough voltage with sufficient amperage and depolarization is bound to occur. However, this type of stimulation is rarely therapeutic or selective.

According to the Law of Dubois Reymond, the variation in current density, rather than the absolute current density, causes the depolarization of nerves or muscle tissue.[144] Variations in current density overcome the cell membrane's resistance at a lower intensity than at unchanging densities. To depolarize excitable tissues in an orderly and sequential manner, the following criteria must be met:[145]

- The current must be of sufficient intensity to cause depolarization of the cell membrane.
- The rate of rise of the leading edge of the pulse must be rapid enough to prevent accommodation.
- The duration of the current must be long enough in one direction that the nerve has the time to depolarize and repolarize.

---

felt. However, superficial pain fibers may be stimulated before the deeper motor nerves. Surface stimulation of the skin always results in the activation of sensory receptors before motor or pain nerves.[17]

Short pulse durations allow the greatest range in stimulation intensity for excitation of the three nerve types. There is a great range among the currents required to stimulate sensory nerves, motor nerves, and pain fibers. As the phase duration is increased, two events occur. First, less amperage is required to stimulate each nerve type. Second, the interval between each nerve level is decreased. Figure 5–19 depicts a typical strength-duration curve that describes the relationship between phase duration and the threshold of excitation of the nerve types indicated. Theoretically, if the phase duration were continued out along the baseline, there would be a point at which each type of nerve would be stimulated almost simultaneously and at a very low intensity.

Stimulation Levels

Many stimulation techniques describe the intensity of the current applied with reference to the type of nerve stimulated. **Subsensory-level** stimulation occurs within the output interval between the point at which the output intensity (be it voltage or amperage) rises from zero to the point at which the patient first receives a discrete electrical sensation. **Sensory-level** stimulation describes an output that stimulates only sensory nerves. This level is found by increasing the output to the point at which a slight muscle twitch is seen and then decreasing the output intensity by approximately 10 percent. **Motor-level** stimulation describes an intensity that produces a visible muscle contraction without causing pain. **Noxious-level** stimulation is current applied at an intensity that stimulates pain fibers.

Central and Peripheral Nervous System Interference

When a stimulus sufficient to cause depolarization of a cell membrane remains unchanged, the resting potential of the membrane returns to its prestimulus level. This process, **accommodation,** occurs when the rate of discharge of the nerve's ac-

In neural activation the amplitude and phase duration are usually inversely related.

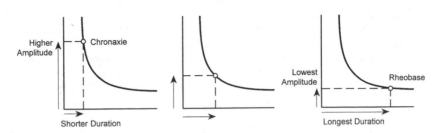

The optimal excitation of the nerve occurs between its rheobase and chronaxie (or simply where the nerve bends) as plotted on the strength - duration curve.

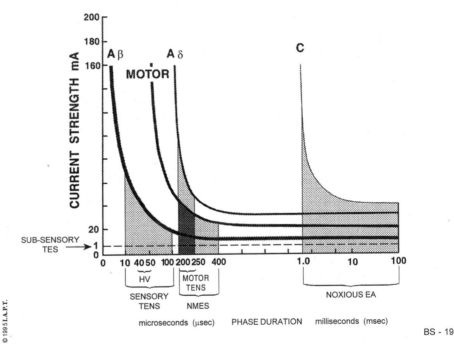

FIGURE 5–19   **Strength-Duration Curve.** Because of the capacitive resistance formed by the walls of cell membranes, short pulse or phase durations are more selective in the nerve fibers stimulated than pulses having a longer duration. Shorter-duration currents require increasing amounts of current to stimulate the same type of nerve fiber than currents having a longer duration. (Courtesy of IAPT. Used with permission.)

tion potential decreases while the depolarization stimulus, in this case an electrical current, remains unchanged. Cells undergoing accommodation require a more intense stimulus to reach the threshold of depolarization (Fig. 5–20).

The threshold for the initiation of an action potential varies according to the stimulation applied. Slowly rising pulses require a greater amount of depolarization to initiate an action potential. Nervous tissue accommodates very quickly; thus, an abrupt pulse rise is needed. Muscle fibers accommodate more slowly than nerve fibers, so a gradual pulse rise may be used.[9] This parameter is typically preset by the generator and is not changeable.

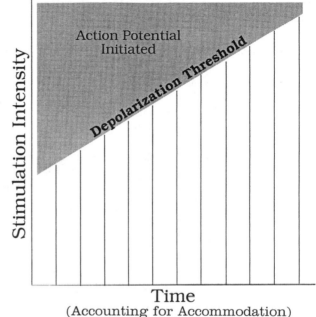

FIGURE 5–20 **Changes in Depolarization Threshold during Accommodation.** When excitable tissues are exposed to an unchanging stimulus, the cell membrane adapts to the stimuli, requiring an increased level of stimulation to trigger an action potential. This figure illustrates how the level of stimulation, over time, would have to be increased to cause depolarization of the cell membrane. The onset of accommodation can be combatted when using electrical stimulation by adjusting the output parameters such as intensity, frequency, and duration at random intervals. These modulation parameters are built into many electrical stimulators.

The central nervous system (CNS) may also play a role in decreasing the long-term sensory stimulation associated with electrical stimulation.[18] Through the process of **habituation,** the CNS filters out a continuous, nonmeaningful stimulus. This can be seen in everyday life: You sit down to study in the kitchen. Your roommates have gone out for the evening, so the house is quiet except for the humming of the refrigerator. After you begin studying, the sound of the refrigerator gets pushed further and further into the background of your consciousness. Eventually, you no longer realize that the sound is there. This stimulus stays in the background until the refrigerator stops humming. At this point, you are struck by the silence of the room.

The concepts of accommodation and habituation can be demonstrated in applying an electrical modality. Increase the intensity of an electrical modality to the point at which the patient expresses slight displeasure in the comfort of the stimulus. Allow the person to experience the current flow for about 5 minutes, and then ask if the intensity can be increased. More times than not, the patient will say "Yes." This ability to increase the intensity represents accommodation of the involved nerves.

Many electrotherapeutic modalities have modulation parameters to combat the effects of accommodation. The generator randomly alters the intensity, frequency, and/or duration of the pulses to prevent the body from receiving a constant, unchanging stimulus.

ELECTRICAL STIMULATION GOALS AND TECHNIQUES

This section presents common goals of electrical stimulation and techniques on how to achieve them. The section on clinical application in this chapter relates these goals to the different types of electrical stimulation units commonly used in the treatment of orthopedic and minor neurological conditions.

TABLE 5-7   Comparison of Physiologically versus Electrically Induced Muscle Contractions

Physiologically Induced Contractions	Electrically Induced Contractions
• Small-diameter, slow-twitch muscle fibers are recruited first. • Contractions and recruitment are asynchronous to decrease muscle fatigue. • Golgi tendon organs protect muscles from too much force production.	• Large-diameter, fast-twitch muscle fibers are recruited first. • Contractions and recruitment are synchronous, based on the number of pulses per second. • Golgi tendon organs cannot override the developing tension within the musculotendinous unit.

Muscle Contractions

Virtually any type of electrotherapeutic modality can elicit a contraction in normal, healthy muscle, if applied at a sufficient intensity, by causing a depolarization of the motor nerve's membrane. When the magnitude of the stimulation is sufficient, an action potential is initiated, sending a signal to the motor unit that results in contraction of the muscle. These contractions may be used to retard the effects of atrophy, reeducate muscle, reduce edema, or augment the force-generating capacity of healthy muscle. Electrical stimulation has been demonstrated to be as effective as voluntary muscle contraction in strengthening the quadriceps when used during the first 4 weeks after anterior cruciate ligament (ACL) surgery. On a 1-year follow-up of patients, no significant strength differences were found between these two treatment protocols.[19] It should be noted, however, that both groups of patients resumed identical rehabilitation regimens after the 4-week test period.

Electrical stimulation of innervated muscle activates the motor nerve rather than the muscle fibers directly. Because the capacitance of motor nerves is less than that of muscular tissue, the current overcomes the resistance of the nerve first (Table 5-7). For this reason, every effort should be made to place the electrodes over the muscle's motor points (see Appendix C).

The motor nerves are recruited into the contraction based on their size and proximity to the electrode. Large-diameter motor neurons are recruited before smaller ones, and nerves in proximity to the electrode respond before those more distant.

Motor nerves that have been denervated for less than 3 weeks are still capable of depolarization and can be selectively recruited through the use of a short pulse duration that has a slowly rising waveform. In this case, motor nerves can continue to produce a muscle contraction via electrical stimulation until *wallerian degeneration* sets in.[9]

When a muscle is denervated, communication with the muscle fibers can no longer occur through the motor nerve, so the fibers must be directly stimulated to evoke a contraction. Denervated muscle reacts to stimulation from a galvanic current or a monophasic current having a long phase duration, but not from ACs or pulsed

---

Wallerian degeneration: Gradual physiological breakdown of a nerve axon that has been severed from its body.

currents having a short duration. This reaction is because the current flows for a longer time in one direction when using a DC, allowing depolarization of the muscle fiber membranes to occur. In cases in which the patient has suffered a spinal cord injury but the peripheral nerves are still intact, such as an *upper motor neuron lesion,* muscle contractions can still be obtained through the use of nongalvanic stimulation.[9]

Pulse Amplitude

As the intensity of the stimulus increases, so does the strength of the contraction. The force of the muscle contraction is linearly correlated to the amount of current introduced into the tissues.[20,21] The depth of penetration of the current increases as the peak current increases, thus recruiting more nerve fibers. Pain fibers are of relatively small diameter when compared with motor nerve fibers and are normally only stimulated at higher intensities and with longer phase durations, allowing for muscle recruitment without a disproportional amount of discomfort. However, the pain associated with the intensity of the stimulation often prevents maximum contractions from being achieved.

Cold treatments are often used for their anesthetic effects. Researchers have attempted to determine if the application of cold treatments prior to neuromuscular electrical stimulation would, by decreasing the discomfort associated with the stimulation, allow an increase in the torque produced by involuntary muscle contractions. Research on this subject has produced mixed results.[22,23] The pain experienced during high-amplitude electrical stimulation is caused not only by stimulation of the cutaneous pain receptors but also by the nociceptors located deep within the muscle.[24] Although these studies neither support nor refute the efficacy of cold application before electrically induced muscle contractions, this technique could be beneficial for individuals who have increased sensory discomfort during electrical current application.

Pulse Frequency

When the stimulation is applied at a pulse rate of less than 15 pps (or in the case of AC, Hz), there are distinguishable muscle contractions for each pulse. At this pulse rate there is sufficient time for the mechanical process required for the muscle fibers to return to their original length before the next pulse begins. Each of these individual contractions is referred to as a **twitch** contraction.

Because of **summation,** individual contractions become less and less distinguishable between 15 and 25 pulses per second. In this case, the pulses occur in such rapid succession that the muscle fibers do not have the time to return to their original position before the next pulse begins (Fig. 5–21). As the pulse frequency increases, the amount of summation increases as a result of the greater overlap in the mechanical process of muscle contraction.[9]

Summation continues until the muscle reaches the stage of *tetany.* At this point, the muscle enters a *tonic contraction.* Increasing the frequency of the stimu-

---

Upper motor neuron lesion: A spinal cord lesion resulting in paralysis, loss of voluntary movement, spasticity, sensory loss, and pathological reflexes.

Tetany: Total contraction of a muscle achieved through the recruitment and contraction of all motor units.

Tonic contraction: Prolonged contraction of a muscle.

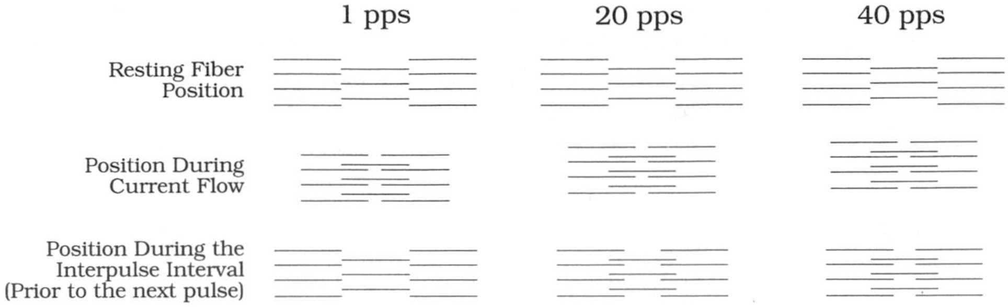

FIGURE 5–21 **Muscle Fiber's Reaction to Pulse Frequency.** The tone of a muscle undergoing electrically induced contractions varies with the pulse frequency. At less than approximately 15 pps, the muscle fibers have the time to return to their original starting position. As the pulse frequency increases, the duration of the interpulse interval decreases, prohibiting the muscle fibers from returning to their original starting position before the next pulse.

lation will do little to further smooth the muscle tone. It will, however, promote muscle fatigue if used for a sufficient duration. The exact number of pulses per second required to reach tetany varies between muscle groups. Postural muscles have been found to reach tetany before nonpostural muscles.[8]

A strong tetanic contraction is required to delay atrophy or enhance strength. Low pulse frequency stimulation (20 pps) reduces fatigue, but the muscle develops 45 percent less force than it could at higher frequencies.[2] Very high pulse frequencies have been shown to make it possible to produce tetany with greater comfort than lower frequencies.[25] Medium-frequency biphasic currents selectively fatigue type II muscle fibers, resulting in decreased torque production as the treatment progresses.[26] This effect may be counteracted by increasing the amount of rest between treatment cycles or decreasing the pulse frequency during treatment.

Phase Duration

Recall that pulsed currents are built from phases. Monophasic currents consist of one phase, whereas biphasic pulses consist of two phases (the prefixes "mono" and "bi" are easy memory aids for this). When monophasic currents are being discussed, the terms "phase duration" and "pulse duration" may be used interchangeably.

To recruit only motor nerves, a moderate phase duration should be used.[9] When attempting to recruit the muscle fiber directly, a slowly rising pulse is recommended. Short phase durations require greater amplitude to evoke an action potential than phases of longer durations. Phase durations of less than 1 millisecond (msec) will not be able to stimulate denervated muscle, regardless of the current's amplitude.[7,8] The optimal phase duration for elicitation of maximal muscle contractions has been shown to be in the range of 300 to 500 microseconds (μsec).[27]

Strength Augmentation

The following effects are based on the output parameters described under Muscle Contractions in this chapter. Also, the reader should keep in mind that electrically induced muscle contractions are less desirable than voluntary contractions and should supplement, but not substitute for, voluntary contractions when attempting to increase the overall strength of a muscle.

Strength gains realized through the use of electrical stimulation are attributed to two factors.[28] First, strength gains are a response to placement of an increased functional load on the muscle. For strength gains to occur via electrical stimulation, the functional load placed on the muscle must equal a significant proportion of the torque produced by the maximal voluntary isometric contraction (MVIC). You may recognize this factor as being, in part, the basis of the *overload principle*. To produce overload, the muscle must exceed the minimum electrically evoked torque (EET) production threshold, the point at which the contraction produces measurable and meaningful tension on the muscle. As the strength of the muscle increases, the EET increases as well.[29]

The increased functional load produced by electrical stimulation is supplemented by the increased recruitment of **type II muscle fibers,** the second factor in strength augmentation. When muscles are voluntarily contracted, **smaller type I motor nerves** are recruited before the type II fibers. Because electrical current depolarizes larger-diameter nerves first, type II fibers are brought into the contraction sooner and fatigue first.[26,30,31] The two elements of type II fiber recruitment and increased functional load work together so that muscle strengthening through electrical stimulation may occur at levels producing 30 percent of the tension found in the MVIC.[2,28]

As previously mentioned, electrical stimulation is not a replacement for voluntary muscle contractions, but an adjunct technique. Although effective in increasing isometric muscle strength, electrical stimulation is less effective in increasing quadriceps torque than the use of biofeedback (see Chap. 7).[32] Strength gains obtained by electrical stimulation follow the same parameters of specificity as any other form of exercise; that is, isometric training improves only isometric strength, and that improvement does not carry over to isotonic or isokinetic strength.[33]

Several concerns must be taken into consideration when attempting to increase muscle strength through electrical stimulation. If the duty cycle of the stimulation is too great, an unacceptable level of fatigue may occur in the muscle because of increased use of the *phosphocreatine system*. Also, the protective function of Golgi tendon organs is overridden during electrical stimulation. Precautions must be taken to damper the terminal ends of the patient's range of motion. For these reasons, the patient should always be given a safety switch that, when depressed, shuts off the stimulation unit in the event that the stimulation and/or muscle tension becomes too intense.

Pain Control

Electrical currents are used to reduce the amount of pain experienced by either assisting in the healing process or affecting the transmission and perception of pain. Lessening the mechanical pressure placed on nerve endings or decreasing

---

Overload principle: For strength gains to occur, the body must be subjected to more stress than it is accustomed to. This is accomplished by increasing the load, frequency, or duration of the exercise.

Phosphocreatine system: A compound that is important in muscle metabolism.

TABLE 5–8 **Electrical Parameters Used in Pain Control Approaches**

Approach	Target Nerves	Phase Duration	Pulse Frequency	Intensity
Sensory level	A-beta	<100 μsec	60–100 pps	Submotor
Motor level	Motor nerves	150–250 μsec	2–4 pps	Strong contraction
Noxious level	A-delta C fibers	1 msec	Variable	As painful as can be tolerated

the degree of muscle spasm or edema eliminates the mechanical and chemical events that stimulate pain transmission. In specific pain control approaches, electrical stimulation may simply "mask" the pain or encourage the body to release its pain-controlling substances, endogenous opiates. Refer to Levels Theory of Pain Control in Chapter 2 for more information regarding the neurophysiological approaches to pain control.

High-pulse-frequency, short-duration, sensory-level currents are thought to activate the gate mechanism of pain modulation. In this case, the stimulation of sensory nerves closes the gate to the transmission of pain. Low-pulse-frequency, long-duration, high-intensity stimulation and noxious-level stimulation are thought to stimulate the release of the body's natural opiates—β-endorphin from the pituitary gland and enkephalins from the spinal cord (Table 5–8).

In the initial phases of pain control, electrotherapeutic treatments stimulate the dorsal horn of the spinal cord. Activation of type I, II, III, and IV neurons may cause the dorsal horn to transmit less noxious information to the supraspinal levels.[34] Decreased nerve conduction of small, pain-carrying nerves reduces the amount and rate of noxious impulses transmitted up the spinal cord. In large motor nerves, decreased nerve conduction decreases the amount of pain-producing muscle spasm in the treated area.[35] Peripheral stimulation could relieve chronic pain if applied to the site of pain or to an area serviced by the involved peripheral nerve.

As mentioned in Chapter 2, the placebo effect of electrotherapeutic modalities cannot be overlooked. Many studies exploring the effects of electrical current flow (and other modalities and medications as well) on pain perception report that patients receiving sham treatments described a decrease in the amount of pain experienced, supporting the theory that cognitive processes are involved in pain modulation.[36–41]

Wound Healing

The use of a low-intensity DC may reduce the time needed for superficial wound healing 1.5 to 2.5 times that needed for wounds not receiving such treatment.[42] Depending on the polarity of the electrode, certain inflammatory mediators, including neutrophils, macrophages, epidermal cells, and fibroblasts, are attracted or repelled from the area.[43,44] This form of electrical current encourages hydration, increases the number of growth factor receptors, increases the rate of collagen formation,[45] stimulates the growth of fibroblasts and granulation tissues,[46] and reduces the number of mast cells in the injured area.[47] Last, leukocytes migrate toward the anode, resulting in increased blood clotting in the area.[43]

Evidence exists that confirms the usefulness of electrical stimulation in the resolution of open superficial wounds.[43,48,49] Explanations for the effectiveness of tissue repair include increased circulation, increased blood clot formation, antibacterial effects, influences on migration of cells, and the presence of an "injury potential" in damaged tissues. When tissues are damaged, an electrical potential is created between the healthy and damaged tissues.[50,51] This injury potential is theorized to electrically control tissue repair. Most of the evidence supporting the use of electrical stimulation in wound healing in humans has involved chronic conditions, with the majority of the cases being *dermal ulcers*.

Using animal models, DCs have also shown efficacy in promoting healing of the medial collateral ligament. Traumatized ligaments treated with electrical stimulation demonstrated an increased rupture force, increased amount of energy absorption, and decreased stiffness and laxity compared with nonstimulated ligaments.[52] When applied to healing tendons, DC appeared to suppress the proliferation of adhesion-causing cells compared to treated tendons.[53]

Control and Reduction of Edema

After orthopedic trauma, surgery, certain diseases, and burns, electrical stimulation is often used to control or reduce the amount of edema in the involved area. **Sensory-level stimulation** attempts to stop the formation of edema by preventing the fluids, plasma proteins, and other solids from escaping into surrounding tissues. If edema has already formed, **motor-level stimulation** attempts to assist the venous and lymphatic system in returning the edematous substances back to the torso, where they can be filtered and removed from the body.

Sensory-Level Stimulation for Edema Control

In acute trauma, electrical stimulation applied to, or directly around, the injury site has been found to limit the volume of edema formed in laboratory animals. This method of application is termed sensory-level because the intensity of the stimulation is kept below the motor threshold level. The central concept of this theory is to limit the formation of edema rather than to remove existing edema. In fact, attempting these techniques when swelling has already formed may actually inhibit edema reduction.

One proposed mechanism for this response is a reduction in capillary pressure and capillary permeability, which discourages plasma proteins from entering the extracellular tissues.[54] Another potential mechanism used to explain this form of edema control theorizes that a pulsed, monophasic current produces a vascular spasm and prevents fluids from leaking out of the vessels.[55]

The theoretical and applied approach to sensory-level edema control is described in the High-Voltage Pulsed Stimulation section of this chapter.

Dermal ulcer: A slow-healing or nonhealing break in the skin.

Motor-Level Stimulation for Edema Reduction

The role of the motor-level response in reducing edema formation is less controversial and has demonstrated more clinical efficacy than the sensory-level approach. In this mode, muscular contractions encourage venous and lymphatic return by squeezing the vessels, moving the fluids proximally, and "milking" the fluids out of the area. Many types of electrical stimulation devices can be employed to produce an involuntary muscle contraction that forces the fluids out of the area. This technique is also referred to as "muscle milking" or the "muscle pump."

Electrodes are arranged on the involved extremity so that they follow the course of the primary vein exiting the swollen area. A low pulse frequency, usually 1 pps, is used to allow enough time for the contents of the venous and lymphatic system to move between muscle contractions. Another technique is to increase the number of pulses per second so that a tonic contraction is achieved. A 50 percent duty cycle is then used to obtain the desired off-and-on contractions.

The output intensity is adjusted so that the contraction is within the patient's tolerance, and contraindicated joint movement is avoided. Although electrically induced muscle contractions do increase the rate of venous return, the volume of flow is less than that which occurs with voluntary contractions. If the individual is capable of producing strong contractions, this method should be preferred over electrically induced contractions.

As would be expected from what we know of the venous and lymphatic return mechanisms (see Chap. 1), the efficiency of this technique is improved when the limb is elevated so that gravity may assist in the fluid flow. In addition, the use of an elastic wrap or tubular compressive stockings applied to the extremity assists in edema reduction.

Fracture Healing

Electrical currents have traditionally been used to assist in the healing of *nonunion fractures,* although the effectiveness of this technique on acute fractures is now again being investigated. Normally, fractures heal through the process of *osteogenesis.* If the fracture fails to heal properly, further repair must occur through endochondral bone formation, the process by which the soft-tissue callus transforms itself into bone.[56] Historically, nonunion fractures required the surgical grafting of bone into the fracture site to assist the healing process.

The use of electrical stimulation to aid in the healing of bone is based on the theory that bone cannot differentiate between the body's innate charges needed for normal bone remodeling (see Wolff's Law in Chap. 1) and those derived from outside sources, such as electrical generators. The natural source of these intrinsic stresses are piezoelectric charges caused by the deformation of the bone's col-

---

Nonunion fracture: A fracture that fails to heal spontaneously within a normal time frame.

Osteogenesis: Healing of fracture sites through the formation of callus, followed by the deposition of collagen and bone salts.

lagen matrix.[57] These piezoelectric charges require an intermittent stress to be delivered to the bone. Static or constant stresses do not produce an electric charge.

Collectively known as bone-growth generators, these units attempt to produce electromagnetic fields that mimic the normal electrical signals produced by bone or activate the bone's piezoelectric properties. Each approach encourages the deposition of calcium through increased osteoblastic activity, regardless of the technique used to introduce the current. Generally, those generators applied transcutaneously use ACs, whereas those having electrodes implanted in the body use direct currents.[58] The cathode is placed near the fracture site when the electrodes are implanted into the tissues because new bone callus is electropositive.[59] Implanted electrodes are then surgically removed once successful healing has been obtained.

Generators with external electrodes are similar to diathermy units (see Chap. 4) in that their electrodes produce strong electromagnetic fields. These fields then create electric currents at the fracture site.

The usefulness of bone-growth generators is still debatable.[56,58,60] Evidence exists that electrical bone-growth generators may actually delay fracture healing, with stress fractures perhaps being the most negatively impacted.[61] This negative effect may be, at least in part, a result of the fact that many generators use a current "orders of magnitude" more powerful than that required for healing.[57]

After a long hiatus, the effectiveness of electrical bone-growth generators in assisting the healing of acute fractures is again being investigated. Implantation of electrodes into acutely fractured bones and the subsequent introduction of a direct current to the healing structure have shown an increased bending rigidity and bone mineral density in animal models.[61]

The prescription of bone-growth generators is the physician's domain, and it is most likely their use will be prescribed only in extraordinary circumstances. These units appear to be most effective only in certain nonunion fractures and require long-term treatments (6 months or more). As it appears that the currently proposed protocol for treating acute fractures involves implanting electrodes into the damaged bone, the risks and time delays of the associated surgery may limit use of this device to cases in which the patient is at risk for a nonunion or *malunion fracture*. However, clinicians should be familiar with the functions, benefits, and limitations of this device. As this technology grows and the efficacy of this modality is established, its possibilities for use in the treatment of acute fractures increase.

SUMMARY

Therapeutic currents are classified as being either alternating, direct, or pulsed. Alternating and direct currents are characterized by an uninterrupted flow of electrons. In pulsed currents, the flow of electrons is intermittently paused. A pulsed current may be monophasic, having a unidirectional current flow, or biphasic, having a bidirectional flow of electrons.

When a therapeutic electrical current is introduced into the body, the flow of electrons causes the movement of ions. This current enters the body through a set

---

Malunion fracture: The faulty or incorrect healing of bone.

of electrodes that forms a closed circuit between the generator and the patient. Within the tissues, physiological effects are related to current parameters such as amplitude, duration, and frequency. Depending on the mix of these variables, responses such as neuromuscular stimulation, pain control, control and reduction of edema, and wound healing are evoked.

MULTIMODALITIES

The development of microprocessors, improved circuitry, and better battery supplies has led to an evolution in the design and function of electrical stimulators. Until recently, each type of electrical stimulating current described in this chapter required its own specific generator. Today, a single **multimodality** is capable of producing a multitude of currents and may include other therapeutic agents, such as ultrasound (Fig. 5–22). These devices use a computer chip to produce the various types of waveforms discussed in this chapter.

The user simply selects the type of output desired, usually described by the type of current, and selects a preprogrammed treatment regimen (e.g., motor-

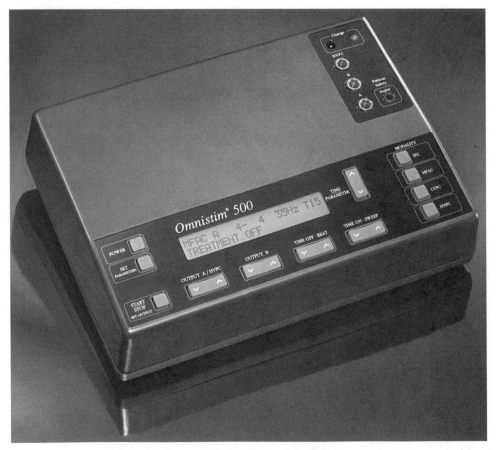

FIGURE 5–22 **An Electrical Stimulation "Multimodality."** These generators are capable of producing alternating, direct, monophasic, and biphasic currents. (The Omnistim 500, courtesy of PTI, Topeka, KS.)

level edema reduction, sensory-level pain control). Because of the differences among multimodalities, their use is not described in this text.

CLINICAL APPLICATION OF ELECTRICAL MODALITIES

This part of the chapter describes the theory, effects, and application of various forms of electrical stimulation. Although each stimulation method is presented as a distinct modality, as described in the previous section, many generators are capable of producing a wide range of electrical characteristics.

Many states require that electrical stimulation devices be applied only under a physician's order. Clinicians and students should be aware of state laws governing their profession's use of these devices as well as the policies and procedures for use at their institution. Likewise, an appropriately credentialed individual should supervise use of these devices. This supervision is even more essential during the learning process.

Basic Guidelines for the Setup and Application of Electrotherapy

An outline of the process used in preparing the generator, electrodes, and the patient for electrotherapy follows. The steps involved in using the generator are later detailed for each stimulation approach.

Preparation of the Generator

1. If a portable or battery-operated unit is being used, make sure the batteries are fully charged. If a clinical model is being used, make sure it is properly plugged into a grounded wall socket. If the treatment involves water immersion, the unit **must** be plugged into a ground-fault interrupter circuit. Avoid the use of extension cords.
2. Make sure the electrode leads are not tangled. The leads should be inspected regularly for frays, broken insulation, and loose connections. Frayed leads should be repaired or replaced before they are used.
3. Ensure that all dials are in their zero (OFF) position.

Preparation of the Electrodes

1. Clean the electrodes to remove any residual gels or skin oils. Rubber electrodes should be cleaned with alcohol, and gel-based, self-adhesive electrodes should be cleaned with soap and water.
2. Carbon-impregnated rubber electrodes should be used only with a wet medium, such as a sponge. Gels should not be used unless specifically recommended by the manufacturer.
3. If conductive sponges are used, moisten them with water. If sponges are not required, apply an even coat of conductive gel to the electrodes.
4. Connect the leads to the unit and to the electrodes.
5. In all cases, read and follow the manufacturer's recommendations for the electrodes being used.

Preparation of the Patient

1. Ensure that the patient has no contraindications to the treatment about to be performed.
2. Determine the electrode placement technique to be used.
3. The points to be stimulated should be cleansed with alcohol to remove any body oils, lotions, dirt, and grime. Keep in mind that body hair increases resistance to electrical current flow. When possible, place the pad over areas of low hair density.
4. If a monopolar technique is being used, attach the dispersive electrode to a large body mass, such as the thigh or lower back. If the lower back is selected for the site of the dispersive electrode, place the electrode so that it lies on one side of the spinal column and not across it. The indentation formed by the erector muscles causes incomplete contact with the dispersive electrode and may result in sensation under this electrode. Avoid placing the dispersive electrode over the abdomen or torso.
5. If the electrodes are not self-adhesive, use rubber and Velcro straps, elastic wraps, or sandbags to secure the electrodes in place.
6. If this is the patient's first exposure to electrical stimulation, explain the sensations to be expected (e.g., "tingly sensation" or "muscle twitch"). Be aware that some individuals are very apprehensive about electrotherapeutic treatments. The patient should be advised against any unnecessary movements because this may break the circuit between the electrodes.

Termination of the Treatment

1. Many units automatically stop the current flow when the treatment time has expired. If this is not the case with your unit, or if the treatment is being terminated prematurely, gradually decrease the INTENSITY and/or depress the STOP button.
2. Remove the electrodes from the body, and wipe away any residual water or gel.
3. Check the treatment area for burns, skin irritation, or discoloration.
4. An interview should be conducted immediately on the conclusion of the treatment to ascertain the effectiveness of the parameters used. The results should be noted in the medical or treatment file. Future modifications of the treatment protocol should be indicated.

High-Voltage Pulsed Stimulation

High-voltage pulsed stimulation (HVPS) is the application of a monophasic current to the body, with a known polarity under each set of electrodes (Fig. 5–23). This technique is often incorrectly referred to as high-voltage galvanic stimulation, but this is bad nomenclature (Box 5–9). HVPS is a versatile form of electrical stimulation and has a wide variety of uses, including muscle reeducation, nerve stimulation, reduction of edema, and pain control.

A typical high-voltage generator produces a twin-peaked waveform (see Fig. 5–7) or a train of two single pulses with a phase duration of 5 to 260 microseconds (μsec). The average current does not normally exceed 1.5 mA, or a pulse charge

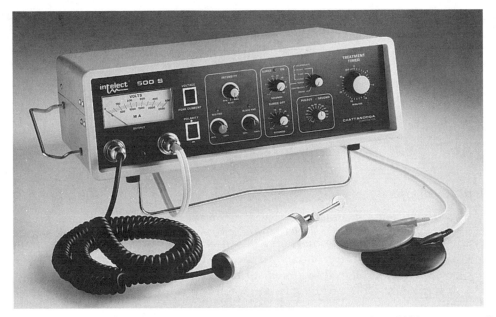

FIGURE 5–23 **A High-Voltage Pulsed Stimulation Unit.** (The Intelect 500S, courtesy of the Chattanooga Group, Hixon, TN. Used with permission.)

of 4 microcoulombs (Table 5–9). Because of the low pulse charge, voltages of greater than 150 V are required to stimulate motor and sensory nerves.[2] The relatively low phase duration allows for the activation of sensory and motor nerves without stimulating pain fibers.

The interpulse interval is much longer than the pulse duration. Consider a current consisting of pulses having a duration 140 μsec and a frequency of 125 pps. In 1 second, the current is actually "flowing" for 0.0175 seconds; during 1 minute, the current is flowing for only 1.05 seconds. Because of the short amount of time the current is flowing, there is time for dissipation of the residual ions attracted to the body area. As a result, the amount of physiochemical reaction beneath the electrodes is limited and no skin pH changes occur under the cathode.[62] The fact that galvanic changes do not seem to occur within the tissues indicates that many of the effects attributed to polarity during HVPS may possibly be a result of some other mechanism.

BOX 5–9 What's in a Name? (Part I)

The term "high-voltage pulsed galvanic stimulation" is an oxymoron similar to "jumbo shrimp" or a "perfectly straight crooked line." The contradiction arises from the use of the terms "pulsed" and "galvanic" in describing the flow of the same current. As you will recall from the discussion on direct current flow, galvanic refers to "a continuous, waveless, unidirectional current."[66] Therefore, a galvanic current cannot be pulsed. The confusion stems from the constant use of this term in the literature and in manufacturers' descriptions.

TABLE 5–9 **Typical Current Parameters Used by High-Voltage Pulsed Stimulation Units**

Parameter	Range
Total current flow	1.5 mA
Pulse frequency	1–256 pps
Pulse duration	5–100 μsec
Phase duration	20–45 μsec

Biophysical Effects

Neuromuscular Stimulation

The short phase duration found on most HVPS generators allows a moderately high-intensity muscle contraction with relatively little discomfort. Unlike muscle contractions produced by other electrical modalities, the pulse frequency seems to have little effect on the maximum tension produced in a muscle being stimulated by HVPS. Although HVPS has been reported to produce torque nearing that obtained through a maximal voluntary contraction, pulse frequencies above 30 pps appear to have little effect on increasing the strength of the contraction.[63,64]

Generation of these contractile forces has not been shown to translate into increased muscular strength. The short-term benefits derived from HVPS neuromuscular stimulation are unclear, with study results ranging from significant increases in isometric strength to significant decreases in strength relative to a nonexercising control group.[65]

The most important role for HVPS in neuromuscular stimulation is to "teach," or reeducate, a muscle how to contract after periods of immobilization or transient denervation. Other types of currents, such as biphasic or alternating, that employ the use of a duty cycle (as found on neuromuscular stimulators) should be used when strength augmentation is desired. An example of the parameters used for producing muscle contractions is presented in Table 5–10. These parameters are modified to meet the goals of the specific treatment regimen being implemented.

TABLE 5–10 **Neuromuscular Stimulation Using High-Voltage Pulsed Stimulation Units**

Parameter	Setting
Intensity	Strong, comfortable contractions.
Pulse frequency	Low for individual muscle contractions (<15 pps).
	Moderate for tonic contractions (35–50 pps).
Polarity	Positive or negative.
Alternating rate	Alternating.
Electrode placement	Bipolar: Proximal and distal to the muscle (or muscle group) to be stimulated.
	This method offers the most direct method of stimulating specific areas.
	Monopolar: Over motor points or muscle belly.

TABLE 5–11 **Pain Control Using High-Voltage Pulsed Stimulation via the Gate Control Mechanism**

Parameter	Setting
Intensity	Sensory level
Pulse frequency	60–100 pps
Phase duration	<100 μsec
Mode	Continuous
Electrode placement	Directly over the painful site

Pain Control

High-voltage pulsed stimulation may be used as an adjunct treatment in controlling acute and chronic pain through both sensory-level (gate control) and motor-level (opiate release) stimulation. The gate control mechanism of pain modulation can be activated through the application of sensory-level currents at 100 to 150 pps (Table 5–11). Because of the relative lack of portability of some high-voltage generators, HVPS is not always the modality of choice for treatments that require long-term stimulation.

High-voltage pulsed stimulation can also be used to stimulate the release of opiates. Although the phase duration associated with HVPS does not easily activate A-beta fibers, the high output intensity (voltage) can stimulate these fibers (Table 5–12). A monopolar electrode configuration should be used, with the active electrodes being only as large as the area being stimulated. External hand-held probe electrodes are often used for this method of application (Fig. 5–24). Pain reduction can also be obtained through the brief-intense stimulation protocol (Table 5–13).

The use of the positive polarity for acute pain and of negative polarity for chronic pain has been recommended.[66] Acute pain is associated with an acid reaction that **may** be repelled by the effects of the positive polarity. In the case of chronic pain, the negative pole is used for its reputed liquefying and vasodilative properties.

In practicality, long-term pain relief derived from HVPS application most probably stems from the other biophysical effects described in the following sec-

TABLE 5–12 **Pain Control Using High-Voltage Pulsed Stimulation via the Opiate Release Mechanism**

Parameter	Setting
Intensity	Motor level
Pulse rate	2–4 pps
Phase duration	150–250 μsec
Mode	Continuous
Electrode placement	Directly over painful site, distal to the spinal nerve root origin, trigger points, or acupuncture points

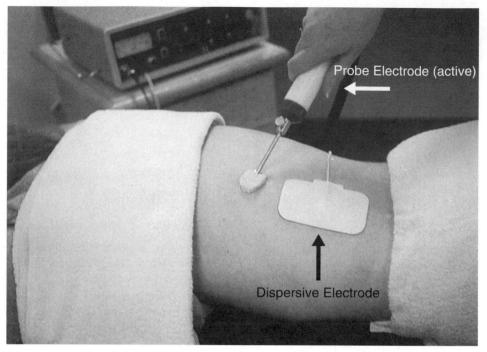

FIGURE 5–24 **Use of an Electrode Probe with High-Voltage Pulsed Stimulation.** This form of electrical stimulation is used to target stimulation points. Because of the current density under the probe, this type of stimulation is monopolar.

tions. Reduction of edema, decreased muscle spasm, muscle reeducation, and increased blood flow assist in decreasing the mechanical and chemical factors triggering the nociceptors. These factors are usually not sufficient, however, to decrease pain caused by *delayed-onset muscle soreness.*[67,68]

Control and Reduction of Edema

Sensory-level HVPS has typically been used to limit the formation of acute edema after trauma. Motor-level stimulation is used to reduce the amount of swelling that has formed in the traumatized tissues during the subacute or chronic stages of inflammation.

TABLE 5–13 **Pain Control Using High-Voltage Stimulation via the Brief-Intense Protocol**

Parameter	Setting
Intensity	Noxious
Pulse rate	>120 pps
Phase duration	300–1000 μsec
Mode	Probe (15–60 sec at each site)
Probe placement	Gridding technique, stimulating hypersensitive areas working distal from the painful area to proximal to it

Delayed-onset muscle soreness: Residual muscle soreness, caused secondary to damage of the muscle cells, which appears within 24 hours after heavy muscular activity, particularly with eccentric muscle actions.

Sensory-Level Edema Control

In acute injuries in which the application of HVPS is intended to prevent or limit the amount of swelling, the time of intervention after the onset of the injury, the pulse frequency used, and the construction of the treatment sessions are critical in obtaining positive treatment outcomes. The permeability of the local microvessels must be decreased before the major swelling occurs. If the stimulation is applied too late in the injury response process, decreased vascular permeability may inhibit reabsorption of the edematous proteins and fluids back into the venous and lymphatic system, virtually trapping them within the extracellular tissues and inhibiting edema reduction.[69]

The sensory-level application of HVPS in limiting the formation of edema has been extensively tested in animal models. Cathodal stimulation applied at 10 percent below the motor threshold with a frequency of 120 pps and delivered to the traumatized tissues via immersion appears to be effective in limiting the formation of post-traumatic edema.[55] When applied immediately after trauma, this protocol, delivered in four 30-minute treatments interspersed with 60-minute rest periods, suppressed edema formation for 17 hours, whereas a single 30-minute treatment curbed edema formation for 4 hours.

The pulse frequency also influences the effectiveness of sensory-level edema control. A low pulse frequency (e.g., 1 pps) does not significantly limit edema formation.[70–72] A single 30-minute treatment administered once daily does not significantly curb long-term edema formation.[54,70,73–75]

For sensory-level edema control to be effective, the treatment must be initiated as soon as possible after injury, preferably within 6 hours.[55] To preserve the benefits associated with the recommended treatment protocol, care must be taken to limit edema formation between treatment sessions and treatment bouts (Table 5–14). The injured limb should be elevated and/or a compression wrap applied to discourage fluids from leaking into the interstitial space while encouraging venous and lymphatic return.

Blood clot formation was once thought to be enhanced under the positive electrode, and the use of anodal stimulation to control acute edema has been suggested. However, this treatment approach has not been substantiated.[55,66]

Motor-Level Edema Reduction

Chapter 1 of this text described how muscle contractions assist in venous and lymphatic return by manually forcing the contents of these vessels out of the extremity. Motor-level edema reduction attempts to replicate this effect by eliciting the required muscle contractions. This technique is used during the subacute or chronic stage of injury because the force of muscle contraction and/or the associated joint motion may either limit the effectiveness of this technique or may be contraindicated.

To increase the milking effect, a low pulse frequency (e.g., 1 pps) and a strong, comfortable muscle contraction within the patient's tolerance should be used. The electrodes should be placed over the motor points of the major muscle groups through which the vessels course, following the path from the swollen area proximally to the torso (Table 5–15).

Elevating the limb, allowing gravity to assist in the venous return process, enhances the effectiveness of this treatment. As with all edema reduction techniques, the patient should be given home-care instruction to keep the limb elevated and wrapped between treatment sessions.

TABLE 5–14   Sensory-Level Control of Edema Formation Using High-Voltage Pulsed Stimulation

Parameter	Setting
Intensity	Sensory level.
Pulse duration	Maximum duration allowed by the generator.
Pulse frequency	120 pps.
Polarity	Negative electrodes are placed over the injured tissues.
Mode	Continuous.
Electrode placement	The immersion method should be used when possible, or the active electrodes should be grouped over and around the target tissues.
Treatment duration	Four 30-minute treatments, each followed by 60-minute rest periods **or** Four 30-minute treatments, each followed by 30-minute rest periods.
Comments	This treatment approach should be initiated as soon as possible after the onset of the trauma. The treated body part should be wrapped and elevated between sessions. This treatment regimen should be discontinued or not initiated if gross swelling forms.

Blood Flow

Although it is not clear if HVPS significantly increases local blood flow, any influence would be dependent on the output intensity and pulse frequency. Motor-level stimulation increases metabolism of the affected tissues, increasing their need for oxygen. This demand is apparently met by increasing the amount of blood delivered to the area. The number of pulses per second may also influence the increase in blood flow, although this relationship is less understood.

Isometric contractions producing muscular tension between 10 percent and 30 percent of the maximal voluntary contraction produce a slight increase in local

TABLE 5–15   Motor-Level Reduction of Edema Using High-Voltage Pulsed Stimulation via the Muscle-Milking Technique

Parameter	Setting
Intensity	Strong, yet comfortable muscle contraction. Avoid joint movement that may be contraindicated.
Pulse frequency	Low.
Polarity	Positive or negative.
Mode	Alternating.
Electrode placement	Bipolar: Proximal and distal ends of the major muscle (or muscle group) proximal to the edematous area. Monopolar: Active electrodes follow the course of the venous return system.

blood flow, but at a level significantly less than that associated with voluntary contractions.[76] Increasing the output intensity is positively correlated with increased blood flow.[77] However, strong muscle contractions, joint motion, and the associated stresses placed on the involved tissues are often contraindicated.

Pulse frequencies of 10, 20, and 50 pps significantly increased blood flow, although these conclusions have not been obtained by all researchers.[78] Pulse frequencies of 2 and 128 pps have also produced a significant increase in blood flow, but no significant increase has been demonstrated at 32 pps.[77] Various forms of monophasic pulses have not been shown to significantly increase or decrease blood flow relative to other forms of monophasic pulses.[78]

If increasing blood flow is the aim of the treatment, clinicians should probably look first toward other modalities. Ideally, voluntary muscle contractions or therapeutic exercise should be used to meet this goal, providing that the patient is able. If not, the use of moist heat or 3-MHz ultrasound (for superficial blood flow) or 1-MHz ultrasound (deep blood flow) should be considered.

Wound Healing

The use of HVPS to facilitate wound healing probably stems from the success seen with the application of low-intensity DCs. The use of HVPS is similar in that each electrode serves as either the positive or negative pole. The possible shortcoming of this technique may be that the pulses are of insufficient duration to cause responses equal to that of a low-intensity DC.

Evidence does exist that HVPS, depending on the polarity of the treatment electrode, attracts leukocytes, epidermal cells, and fibroblasts[44] and increases *collagenase* levels in the treated area.[79] High-voltage pulsed current has also been shown to inhibit the growth of certain bacteria in infected wounds.[80]

Because most of the biophysical effects of electricity on wound healing are polarity-specific, the application protocol should reflect the desired outcomes of the treatment. To account for the effects of polarity during the treatment of cutaneous wounds, the application of 20 minutes of negative polarity followed by 40 minutes of positive polarity stimulation has been recommended.[81]

Electrode Placement

High-voltage pulsed stimulation may be applied using either a monopolar or bipolar technique. Monopolar application is used when the focus of the treatment is over a wide area, such as in the control and reduction of edema, sensory-level pain control, and point stimulation. Bipolar techniques are most often used when attempting to evoke a contraction from a specific muscle or in motor-level pain control.

Instrumentation

Power: When this switch is in its ON position, the current is allowed to flow to the internal components of the generator.

Reset: This safety feature ensures that the voltage is reduced to zero before each new treatment is started.

Collagenase: A substance that causes collagen to break down.

Timer: This control sets the duration of the treatment and subsequently displays the remaining time. On some units, the TIMER serves as the master power switch.

Start-stop: When this button is depressed to start the treatment, the circuit is closed, allowing the current to flow to the patient's tissues. When it is depressed again, the circuit is opened, interrupting the current flow.

Intensity (voltage): This knob adjusts the amplitude of the pulse from zero (OFF) to the maximal value of the unit. The applied output is displayed on the OUTPUT meter.

Pulse (phase) duration: This control selects the duration of each pulse or pair of pulses. Short pulses selectively stimulate sensory nerves, medium-duration pulses stimulate motor nerves, and long pulses activate pain fibers. This parameter may not be available on all units.

Pulse rate: This parameter controls the number of pulses (or pulse trains) per second. Low numbers of pulses per second stimulate endorphin release for pain control, moderate levels produce tetanic contractions, and the upper levels are useful in activating the gate mechanism of pain control.

Pulse multiplier: This switch multiplies the number of pulses per second by a selectable value. For example, if the pulse rate is set at 12 pps and the pulse multiplier is set at 10, the resultant output would be 120 pps.

Polarity: This switch determines the polarity (positive or negative) of the ACTIVE electrode(s). Depending on the manufacturer of the product, the polarity may be changed during the course of the treatment without first decreasing the voltage. Other units require that the voltage be reduced before changing polarity.

Mode: When this switch is set to CONTINUOUS, the current is always flowing to each of the active electrodes. Switching to the ALTERNATING modes causes the current to be routed to only one set of active electrodes at a time. Many units also have a PROBE selection that activates the hand-held electrode.

Alternating rate: This switch sets the amount of time the current is routed to each active electrode. For example, selecting an electrode alternating rate of 2.5 seconds routes the current to one set of electrodes for 2.5 seconds, then the other set for the same amount of time. On many units, this function is meaningful only when the MODE is set to ALTERNATING and two sets of active electrodes are attached to the "ACTIVE" electrode jack.

Alternating the electrodes is useful for reciprocal stimulation of agonist-antagonist muscle groups. Another use is to stimulate different muscle groups to produce a milking action to reduce edema.

Balance: During the course of a treatment, the greater sensation may be experienced under one set of active electrodes than the other. This situation may be corrected through the BALANCE adjustment dial. When this dial is in its midposition, an equal amount of current is routed to both sets of electrodes. If this dial is moved in one direction, toward the "B" electrodes for example, a greater amount of current flows to the "B" electrodes and less to the "A" electrodes.

The imbalance in stimulation under the electrodes can be the result of many factors. These may include improper preparation of the electrodes, the location of the electrodes, and loose connections between the electrodes and the generator or between the electrodes and the patient's body. If adjusting the BALANCE dial does not equalize the sensation, discontinue the treatment, reapply the electrodes, and start again.

Setup and Application

Initiation of the Treatment

1. *Turn the unit on:* Activate the POWER switch.
2. *Reset output parameters:* Fully reduce the INTENSITY control and depress the RESET button.
3. *Select output parameters:* Based on the goal of the treatment, adjust the POLARITY, DURATION (width), FREQUENCY, and electrode ALTERNATING rates.
4. *Set treatment duration:* Indicate the duration of the treatment by adjusting the TIMER.
5. *Begin treatment:* Press the START button to close the circuit between the generator and the patient's tissues.
6. *Increase intensity:* Slowly increase the INTENSITY control until the appropriate current level is obtained.
7. *Adjust electrode balance:* If necessary or applicable, adjust the BALANCE control to maximize comfort.

Alternate Methods of Application

Water Immersion

High-voltage pulsed stimulation may be combined with water immersion to treat irregularly shaped areas, such as the hand or foot (Fig. 5–25). The water touching the skin serves as the active electrode. With this in mind, the dispersive electrode should be as large as possible to keep the focus of the electrical stimulation on the part being treated.

The active electrodes are placed in the tub with the insulated (rubber-coated) side facing toward the body part. Intense stimulation would occur if the patient were to contact one of the electrodes. The dispersive electrode is placed on the closest large body mass. When treating the foot and/or ankle, the thigh is a logical site. The application of the current is similar to that in all other forms of HVPS. It is important to instruct the person not to remove the treated body part from the water; if the intensity of the treatment is too strong, a greater proportion of the body part should be immersed (see Current Density).

Treatment of acute injuries with water immersion also raises the same concerns about edema management as ice immersion. Because the limb is placed in a gravity-dependent position, the hydrostatic pressure within the capillaries is increased and the formation of edema is encouraged rather than discouraged. After treatment, the treated limb should be wrapped and elevated to encourage venous return.

Probe

A probe (tap key) can be used to specifically stimulate trigger points or other localized areas. The probe serves as a very small active electrode in a monopolar configuration that results in a very high current density being placed on a limited group of tissues. A dispersive electrode is required to complete the circuit. A typical probe consists of a handle with a metal tip that is designed to hold a conductive medium.

The handle contains an INTENSITY control knob and an INTERRUPT button. The probe is activated by setting the electrode alternating switch to PROBE

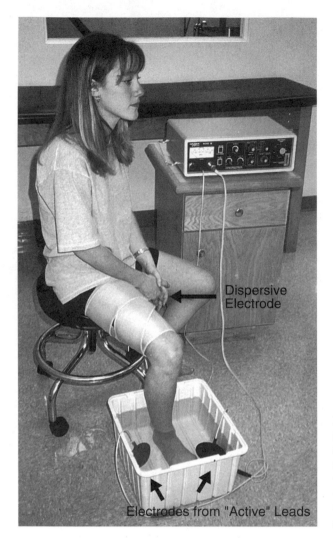

Dispersive
Electrode

Electrodes from "Active" Leads

FIGURE 5–25 **High-Voltage Pulsed Stimulation Delivered via Water Immersion.** In this form of electrical stimulation, water serves to conduct the current from the electrodes to the body. This setup is useful when treating a large, irregularly shaped area.

or by plugging the probe into a separate jack on the generator. In either case, the INTENSITY adjustment on the probe overrides the adjustment on the generator. This allows the operator to remotely adjust the intensity of the treatment. The INTERRUPT button allows the operator to open and close the circuit. When the button is depressed, the circuit is closed and the patient's tissues are stimulated.

Duration of Treatment

The standard duration of HVPS treatments is 15 to 30 minutes, and the treatments may be repeated as many times a day as needed.

Precautions

- Stimulation of muscles can cause unwanted tension to be placed on the muscle fibers, the tendons, or the bony insertion.
- Muscle fatigue can arise if an insufficient duty cycle is used.

- Improper use can cause electrode burns or irritation.
- Intense or prolonged stimulation may result in muscle spasm and/or muscle soreness.

Indications

- Reeducation of peripheral nerves
- Delay of denervation and disuse atrophy by stimulating muscle contractions
- Reduction of post-traumatic edema
- Maintenance of range of motion
  - Reduction of muscle spasm
  - Inhibition of spasticity
  - Reeducation of partially denervated muscle
  - Facilitation of voluntary motor function
- Increase in local blood circulation

Contraindications

The contraindications to the use of this device are described in Table 5–1.

Transcutaneous Electrical Nerve Stimulation

Although all electrical modalities described in this chapter deliver their current transcutaneously, the term "transcutaneous electrical nerve stimulation" (TENS) has evolved to describe a specific electrotherapeutic approach to pain control. It describes the process of altering the perception of pain through the use of an electrical current (Box 5–10). Depending on the parameters used during treatment, electrical stimulation may reduce pain through activation of the gate control mechanism or centrally through the release of endogenous opiates.

The use of TENS in the treatment of pain is a spin-off of the work conducted by Melzack and Wall (cited in Roeser et al.[82]) during their gate control pain modulation experiments (see Chapter 2). Anecdotal claims of permanent relief from

---

BOX 5–10   What's in a Name? (Part II)

Transcutaneous electrical nerve stimulation, or TENS, is the term used to describe an electrotherapeutic modality used in pain control. In reality, each of the electrical modalities described in this chapter could be termed TENS. Transcutaneous means "through the skin," and "nerve stimulation" implies that the current has sufficient intensity to cause the depolarization of sensory, motor, or pain nerves. Therefore, whenever electrodes are attached to the body, an electrical current is passed through them, and the patient reports a tingling sensation, TENS is being performed.

The names given to electrotherapeutic modalities most probably arise from, and are most certainly reinforced by, marketing of the product. As multimodalities become more prevalent, names such as "TENS" and "HVPS" will most likely be replaced by more accurate descriptors of the current being used (e.g., low-voltage biphasic, high-voltage monophasic).

TABLE 5–16 **Electrical Parameters Used in Transcutaneous Electrical Nerve Stimulation**

Parameter	Range
Intensity	0–100 mA
Pulse frequency	1–150 pps
Pulse duration	10–500 μsec

chronic pain after a single, brief TENS treatment—although possibly true—are an exaggeration and oversimplification of the practical effects and application of TENS. It has been found effective in the management of acute or chronic musculoskeletal pain but has little effect on reducing *visceral* or *psychogenic* pain.

The effectiveness of TENS treatment is as varied as its application techniques. The outcome of TENS treatment is dependent on the nature of the pain, the individual's pain threshold, electrode placement, the intensity of the stimulation, and the electrical characteristics of the stimulus[83] (Table 5–16). Traditionally, TENS units incorporate an asymmetrical biphasic pulsed current (see Fig. 5–9B). However, some manufacturers use variants of this pulsed current including a symmetrical biphasic or monophasic waveform. When this treatment is given for extended periods, the waveform should be designed so that there is no net physiochemical effect on tissues.

Biophysical Effects

Despite the fact that a TENS unit can cause muscle contractions, the primary, if not the only, use of TENS is to control pain. TENS decreases the patient's perception of pain by decreasing the conductivity and transmission of noxious impulses from the small pain fibers to the CNS. By affecting the large motor fibers, TENS may interfere with the normal guarding pattern of the muscle (muscle spasm), further reducing painful stimuli.[35,84] The pulse rate and pulse duration, combined with the current intensity, activate responses at different pain-modulating levels (Table 5–17). The determination of the exact parameters to use on any given patient is as much of an art as it is a science. The combination of output parameters is more important in obtaining the desired outcome than any single parameter.[84]

The pain reduction associated with TENS application occurs primarily through modulation of the body's nervous system. Neither sensory-level nor moderate motor-level TENS application significantly increases blood flow in the treated area. Indeed, evidence supports the concept that TENS application may activate the preganglionic and postganglionic neurons and actually cause a mild vasoconstriction.[85] Most prolonged TENS applications can modulate the activity of dorsal horn neurons secondary to stimulation of peripheral nerves and chemical stimulation of visceral organs primarily by the release of endogenous opiates.[34] Last, pain relief obtained through the various forms of TENS application may be

---

Visceral: Pertaining to organs enclosed by the abdominal cavity.
Psychogenic: Pain of mental rather than physical origin.

TABLE 5–17 Protocol for Various Methods of Transcutaneous Electrical Nerve Stimulation Application

Parameter	High TENS	Low TENS	Brief-Intense TENS
Intensity	Sensory	Motor	Noxious
Pulse frequency	60–100 pps	2–4 pps	Variable
Pulse duration	60–100 μsec	150–250 μsec	300–1000 μsec
Mode	Modulated rate	Modulated burst	Modulated amplitude
Treatment duration	As needed	30 min	15–30 min
Onset of relief	<10 min	20–40 min	<15 min
Duration of relief	Minutes to hours	Hours	<30 min

Source: Adapted from Bechtel and Fan,[94] p 41.

obtained through psychological factors either exclusively from, or in addition to, the neurophysiological effects.[86,87]

Clinicians should note that there is sufficient evidence to indicate that moderate levels of caffeine (200 mg, approximately equal to two or three cups of coffee) can decrease the effectiveness of TENS.[88] Caffeine competes with adenosine, a primary mediator of TENS-induced pain reduction, for its receptor sites. As caffeine binds to these sites, adenosine is prohibited from filling its receptors, causing a decreased effectiveness in TENS pain reduction.

Note that, although the following techniques decrease the individual's **perception** of pain, the treatment has little effect on the underlying pathology. This modality should be used in conjunction with other therapies that attempt to treat the source of the pain.

High-Frequency TENS (Sensory Level)

Conventional TENS treatment, applied with a high pulse frequency (60 to 100 pps), short pulse duration (less than 100 μsec), and sensory-level intensity activates the pain-modulating gate at the spinal cord level. Painful impulses are transmitted along slow-transmitting, unmyelinated, small-diameter nerves, whereas nonpainful sensory information travels at a faster rate along neurons of larger diameter.

Because of the short phase duration and high pulse frequency used with conventional TENS, large-diameter sensory nerve A-delta fibers are selectively stimulated.[89] Activation of A-delta nerve fibers causes presynaptic inhibition of A-beta and C fibers within the substantia gelatinosa, blocking transmission of painful impulses to the T cells. In other words, the gate is closed to pain transmission and opened to the transmission of sensory information. This method of TENS application is also referred to as **high TENS,** based on the high pulse rate used.

High-frequency, low-intensity stimulation to *somatic receptive fields* decreases the activity of spontaneously firing nerves, decreases the activity in noxiously evoked dorsal horn neurons, and decreases neural activity compared with the low-frequency TENS, high-intensity TENS protocol, which is described in the follow-

---

Somatic receptive field: Area that is used to apply a stimulus obtaining the optimum response.

ing section.[34] In addition, patients who are seeking pain reduction subjectively prefer the high-TENS protocol.[90]

Accommodation and habituation are concerns when high TENS is used for an extended period. If the stimulation parameters are kept constant, the nervous system may adapt to the unchanging stimulus. Most TENS generators have current modulation parameters designed to diminish these effects. The generator should be adjusted so that the output is modulated to decrease accommodation, with burst and frequency modulation being the most preferred by patients.[91,92] Even so, the current intensity is normally increased during the course of the treatment.

High TENS is effective in the treatment of acute soft tissue injury, but care must be taken to avoid unwanted muscle contractions. Other indications for high TENS include treatment of pain associated with musculoskeletal disorders, postoperative pain, inflammatory conditions, and myofascial pain.

Low-Frequency TENS (Motor Level)

Low-frequency TENS (**low TENS**) is applied with a low pulse frequency (2 to 4 pps), long phase duration (150 to 250 μsec), and motor-level intensity, in treatment bouts lasting a minimum of 45 minutes. These stimulation parameters activate small-diameter nociceptors and motor fibers. Pain relief obtained through this method is thought to occur by the release of β-endorphin, which results in narcoticlike pain reduction.[93]

Low-frequency, high-intensity TENS stimulates the pituitary gland to release chemicals that trigger the production of pain-reducing β-endorphins. During the treatment, the pituitary gland releases ACTH and β-lipotropin into the bloodstream. Once present, these two mediators trigger the release of β-endorphin that binds to the receptor sites of A-beta and C fibers, blocking the transmission of pain.

Actual relief of pain may not be experienced for some time after the treatment has been completed, but the effects last much longer than with high TENS.[16,94,95] Suggested uses for low TENS include the treatment of chronic pain, pain caused by damage to deep tissues, myofascial pain, and pain caused by muscle spasm. Because this method of TENS application involves muscle contractions, care must be taken to avoid any joint movement that may be contraindicated. Studies have indicated little difference between the degree of pain reduction obtained from high and low TENS treatments.[83,96]

Brief-Intense TENS (Noxious Level)

This method of TENS application is delivered at a high pulse frequency (greater than 100 pps), long pulse duration (300 to 1000 μsec), and motor-level intensity in treatment bouts lasting a few seconds to a few minutes. Pain relief is achieved by activating mechanisms in the brain stem that dampen or amplify pain impulses. Although this application protocol is sometimes referred to as **noxious-level TENS,** true noxious-level stimulation is not actually obtained because the limited phase duration found on TENS generators is too short to activate C fibers.

Pain relief is obtained in this TENS protocol by the formation of a negative feedback loop within the central nervous system. The intense stimulation activates ascending neural mechanisms that, on reaching the brain, make the person conscious of the pain caused by the stimulation. During the impulse's passage through the midbrain, a "short circuit" occurs, stimulating the release of endogenous opiates in the raphe nuclei. A descending pain suppression system is activated that loops efferent impulses down the spinal cord.[86] Here, the opiates inhibit the release of substance P, a neurotransmitter of noxious impulses, thus blocking the transmission of pain.[97]

A high level of analgesia is achieved through this application protocol, but the effects are more transitory than those derived from high and low TENS. Because of the short duration of pain relief, this technique is recommended for pain reduction before rehabilitation exercises.[95]

Other Biophysical Effects of TENS

Range of motion, muscle strength, and the reduction of delayed-onset muscle soreness may be improved secondary to pain reduction, although these benefits have not been fully substantiated. The use of low TENS may be more effective at improving range of motion than high-TENS protocol.[97,98] During the early stages of rehabilitation, patients using TENS have demonstrated the ability to reduce the need for pain medication and a more rapid return to active exercise relative to patients not using TENS.[38]

Electrode Placement

The placement of TENS electrodes for optimal treatment is not an exact science and many times is derived through trial and error. The determination of electrode placement is made easier if a set of logical constructs is followed. Placement techniques may be described by the electrodes' location relative to the painful area. Methods include direct placement, contiguous placement, placement at stimulation points, dermatome placement, and placement at the level of the involved spinal nerve root.

High TENS is most commonly employed with direct, contiguous, dermatome, or nerve root–level electrode placement. Low-TENS and brief-intense TENS treatments target the stimulation points. This is not an absolute formula, as the parameters can be mixed and matched to obtain the best treatment results.

Most TENS units use four electrodes, two originating from each of two channels used. However, some units may have as few as two electrodes or as many as eight (two electrodes originating from each of four channels). When two or more channels are used, electrode placement is further defined by one channel's electrode placement relative to the other possible placements (Fig. 5–26).

The effects of TENS can be maximized if the nerve(s) involved in the transmission of pain can be identified and stimulated. For example, the reduction of pain associated with an injured thumb is facilitated if the radial nerve, or portions of its path, is stimulated, rather than the median or ulnar nerve.

Direct Placement

The electrodes are placed on the skin directly over or around the painful site and are arranged so that each channel runs parallel to the midline of the body part.

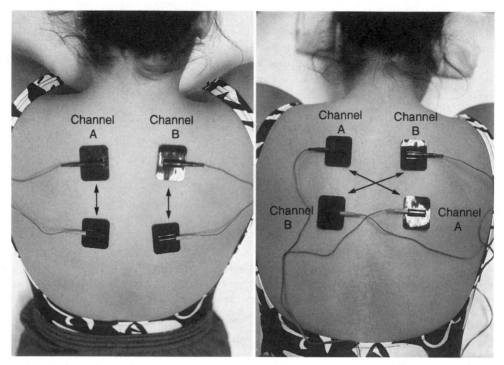

FIGURE 5–26   **Parallel and Crossing Electrode Placements.**

The electrodes are then connected so that the channels flow parallel to each other and the midline of the body.

Contiguous Placement

In conditions such as postoperative incisions, lacerations, and other circumstances that contraindicate direct electrode placement on the site of pain, contiguous placement can be used where the electrodes are located in the immediate vicinity of the painful site. The currents from each channel may run parallel to each other or cross at the center of the painful site.

Stimulation Point Placement

Areas such as motor, trigger, and acupuncture points may be targeted for TENS treatments (see Box 5–6). These points are very sensitive to stimulation and in many instances are located in proximity to each other. Because of the close location of these areas, a single TENS electrode may stimulate all three points at once.

Dermatome Placement

In cases in which pain is distributed across one or more dermatomes, placing electrodes along the affected and the contralateral dermatome can achieve pain reduction. One technique involves placing one electrode at the corresponding spinal cord nerve root and the other at the distal end of the dermatome.

Spinal Cord–Level Placement

This method stimulates the spinal cord nerve root associated with the pain. The electrode should be placed parallel to the spinal column between the transverse processes. Both dermatome and spinal cord–level placement are unexacting methods of TENS treatment. These forms of application should be used only when the surface area of the afflicted area is inaccessible (e.g., with casts or non-removable immobilization devices).

Contralateral Placement

This technique involves placing the electrodes on the opposite side of the body approximating the location from which the pain is arising on the injured side. This method is based on the theory of bilateral transfer in which the sensory impulses from one side of the body would become "confused" with the noxious impulses arising from the other side when the nerve tracts cross in the spinal cord.

Instrumentation

Intensity: On most units there is one intensity dial for each channel. Although the intensity of each channel is controlled individually, the other current parameters (pulse duration and pulse frequency) regulate the activity in all channels.

Pulse duration: Usually labeled "PULSE WIDTH" on the unit, this adjustment should be set according to the treatment method being used.

Pulse frequency: Also labeled "PULSE RATE," this adjustment sets the number of pulses per second used during the treatment.

Mode: Modes are used to alter the current in an attempt to reduce the amount of accommodation that occurs. The various modes that are commonly selectable are:

Constant: Current flow occurs at a constant amplitude, rate, and pulse duration. This mode is best described as unmodulated, to avoid confusion with uninterrupted current. This mode is used when the treatment is not required for an extended length of time and accommodation is not a concern.

Burst: In the burst mode, pulse frequencies are interrupted at regular intervals. Bursts allow "OFF" time from stimulation and assist in reducing muscle fatigue in low-TENS treatments.

Modulated rate: This setting alters, at a preset percentage, the frequency at which the stimulus is delivered. For example, if the pulse rate were adjusted to 100 pps, the unit would alternate the rate between 90 and 110 pps. Modulating the frequency has been found effective in the treatment of chronic musculoskeletal pain.[95]

Modulated amplitude: The pulse amplitude is increased and decreased by a preset percentage. Modulating the amplitude has been shown to provide short-term analgesia in the area.

Multiple modulation: Intensity, frequency, and pulse duration are alternately modulated in such a way that there is delivery of a steady amount of current to the body, but the body has a varying sensory perception of the treatment. This mode decreases the effects of accommodation during prolonged TENS application.

Setup and Application

Initiation of the Treatment

1. *Adjust output parameters:* Depending on the method of TENS application to be used (see Table 5–17), set the pulse duration (WIDTH) and pulse frequency (RATE) dials to the midrange of the parameters to be used.

2. *Select the electrodes:* High TENS should be applied with larger electrodes, whereas low-TENS and brief-intense TENS should use progressively smaller electrodes.

3. *Set the output mode:* Select the appropriate MODE for the method and duration of the TENS application.

4. *Make sure the unit is off:* Make sure that the output intensity is reset to zero, and turn the unit on. Note that many TENS units have the power switch built into the intensity knob(s). In this case, the intensity level of zero is equal to "OFF."

5. *Increase the output intensity (channel 1):* Slowly turn up the INTENSITY of channel 1. If this treatment involves sensory-level stimulation, continue increasing the intensity until a slight muscle contraction is visible, then reduce the intensity by approximately 10 percent. (The patient should be monitored for comfort while the intensity is being increased.)

6. *Increase the output intensity (channel 2):* If more than one channel is being used, increase the intensity of the remaining channels.

7. *Balance the channels:* Adjust the intensity of the channels so that an equal amount of stimulation occurs under each set of electrodes.

8. *Fine-tune the output:* When "fine-tuning" the treatment parameters, most manufacturers recommend first adjusting the intensity, then the pulse duration, and finally the pulse frequency.

9. *Provide home-care instructions:* If the patient is being sent home or to class while wearing this unit, instruction should be provided on how to adjust the intensity. If indicated, instructions should also be provided on how to disconnect the unit before taking a shower or retiring for the night, and during recharging.

Alternate Forms of Application

Point Stimulators

Devices such as the Neuroprobe (Medical Research Lab, Inc., 1 Armour Court, Lake Bluff, IL) are modified TENS devices designed to locate and stimulate trigger and acupuncture points by measuring the amount of resistance provided by the skin. Neuroprobes and galvanic stimulators are the only types of current that directly cause activation of C fibers.

Auriculotherapy

Auriculotherapy describes TENS stimulation of acupuncture points on the ear.[37,99] This method of application is based on the premise that an injured or diseased body reflects pain or tenderness to specific points on the ear. These points, arranged in the form of an inverted fetus, are said to represent the point at which all the acupuncture channels meet and respond to stimulation by decreasing the perception of pain in the corresponding area of the body (Fig. 5–27). Although not supported by much research, this form of electrostimulation has been found effective in reducing pain caused by musculoskeletal trauma.[99]

Duration and Frequency of Treatment

Conventional high-frequency TENS may be used as needed, but caution should be used when applied while the patient is sleeping. The use of a TENS device dur-

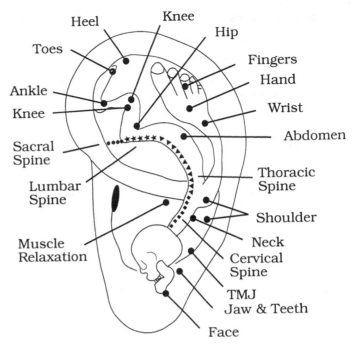

FIGURE 5–27 **Auriculotherapy Points.** These acupuncture points are arranged on each ear, roughly in the shape of an inverted fetus. Stimulation of these points reportedly decreases pain in the corresponding body area. Note that there are both French and Chinese mappings of these points.

ing athletic competition has been attempted; however, because of the potential of TENS to mask pain, its use should be discouraged. An alternate approach would be to keep the electrodes affixed to the athlete and apply stimulation while the athlete is on the bench.

Low-frequency TENS may be given as needed in treatment bouts not exceeding 30 minutes. Brief-intense–type TENS application should be performed only once a day, in treatment bouts not exceeding 30 minutes.

Precautions

- Transcutaneous electrical nerve stimulation is a symptomatic treatment that can mask underlying pain and other conditions.
- Improper use can result in electrode burns or skin irritation.
- Intense or prolonged stimulation may result in muscle spasm and/or muscle soreness.
- Intake of 200 mg or more of caffeine may reduce the effectiveness of TENS.[88]
- Narcotics use decreases the effectiveness of TENS.

Indications

- Control of chronic pain
- Management of postsurgical pain
- Reduction of post-traumatic acute pain

Contraindications

In addition to the contraindications described in Table 5–1, TENS is contraindicated in:

- Pain of central origin
- Pain of unknown origin

Interferential Stimulation

Interferential stimulation (IFS) units generate two ACs on two separate channels. One channel produces a constant high-frequency sine wave (4000 to 5000 Hz), and the other channel produces a sine wave with a variable frequency. As theorized, these independent channels combine to produce an interference wave possessing a frequency of 1 to 100 Hz. The medium-frequency carrier currents penetrate the tissues with very little resistance, whereas the resulting interference currents are in a range that allows effective stimulation of biological tissues (Fig. 5–28).

To realize the combined effects of two separate waveforms, we must first understand the effect that one series of waves has on the other. When two waves are in perfect phase—that is, the wavelengths are equal and the phases cross the baseline at the same point—the amplitude of the combined wave is equal to the sum

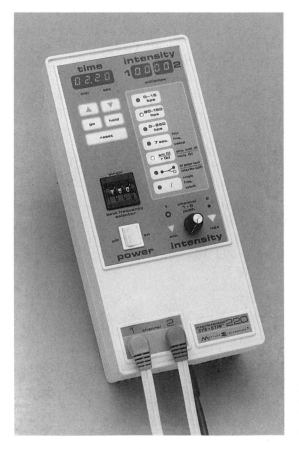

FIGURE 5–28 **An Interferential Stimulator.** (The Sys*Stim 220, courtesy of Mettler Electronics Corporation, Inc., Anaheim, CA.)

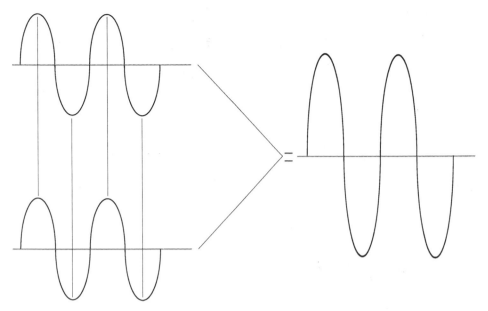

FIGURE 5–29   **Constructive Interference.** Two waves in perfect phase collide to form one single, larger wave.

of its two parts. This effect is termed **constructive interference** because the two waveforms build a larger single wave (Fig. 5–29).

The opposite effect occurs in **destructive interference.** In this case, two wave-forms are perfectly out of phase. The positive peak of the first waveform occurs at the same point on the horizontal baseline as the negative peak of the second wave. When these two waves meet, the amplitudes cancel each other out, resulting in a wave intensity of zero (Fig. 5–30).

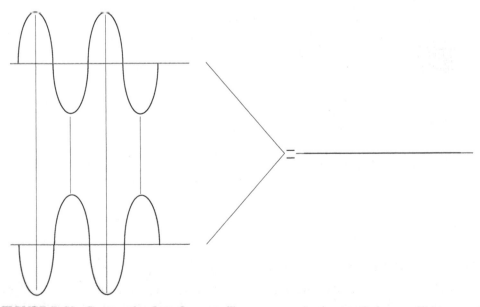

FIGURE 5–30   **Destructive Interference.** Two waves perfectly out of phase collide, cancel each other out, and produce no wave.

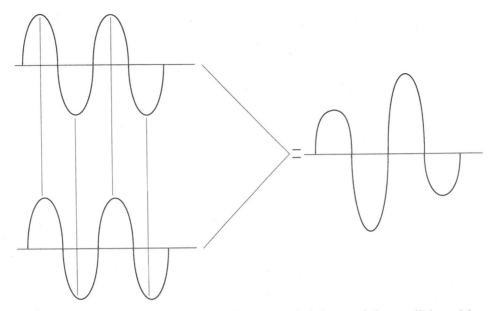

FIGURE 5–31 **Continuous Interference.** Two waves slightly out of phase collide and form a single wave with progressively increasing and then decreasing amplitude.

Interferential generators combine constructive and destructive interference patterns to form a **continuous interference** pattern. This occurs when two circuits have slightly different frequencies (±1 Hz). The resultant waveform is one that drifts between constructive and destructive interference patterns (Fig. 5–31). These circuits may be superimposed in the tissues (quadripolar technique) or within the generator itself (bipolar technique). Superimposing the circuits within the generator itself allows for precise mixing of the waves.[100]

The rate at which the resultant waveform changes is known as the **beat pattern,** the difference in frequency between the two circuits. One channel has a fixed frequency in the range of 5000 Hz, and the frequency of the second channel is variable. By selecting a beat frequency of 1 Hz, the second channel produces a current with a frequency of 5001 Hz, whereas selecting a beat frequency of 100 Hz increases the frequency of the second channel to 5100 Hz. The beat produced by IFS elicits responses similar to the waveforms produced by TENS units, but is capable of delivering a greater total current to the tissues (70 to 100 mA).[101] Refer to Table 5–18 for other electrical parameters.

Capacitive skin resistance is inversely proportional to the frequency of the current. An AC of 50 Hz encounters approximately 3000 ohms of resistance per 100 cm^2 of skin. Increasing the frequency to 4000 Hz reduces capacitive skin resistance to approximately 40 ohms.[14] Consequently, IFS encounters less skin resistance than other low-frequency forms of stimulation. Inside the tissues, the interference between the two waves reduces the frequency to a level that has biological effects on the tissues.

Biophysical Effects

Interferential stimulation has been used to control pain and elicit muscle contractions to increase venous return. A variation of IFS, with a superimposed duty cycle, is used to reeducate muscle and to increase muscular strength.

TABLE 5–18 Electrical Parameters Used in Interferential Stimulators

Parameter	Range
Intensity	1–100 mA
Carrier frequency	2500–5000 Hz
Beat frequency	0–299 Hz
Sweep frequency	10–500 μsec

Pain Control

Mechanisms of pain control are similar to those found with TENS. High beat frequencies, about 100 Hz, when accompanied by sensory-level stimulation, activate the spinal gate, inhibiting the transmission of noxious impulses (Table 5–19). Low beat frequencies of 2 to 10 Hz, when combined with motor-level intensities, initiate the release of opiates and result in a narcoticlike pain reduction (Table 5–20). Stimulation of acupuncture points with a frequency of 2 Hz or 100 Hz results in pain mediation at specific receptor sites, whereas a 30-Hz frequency affects the widest range of receptors, but the pain reduction tends to occur to a lesser degree.[102]

Neuromuscular Stimulation

Medium beat frequencies of approximately 15 Hz may be used to reduce edema. Venous and lymphatic return can be increased by way of muscle contractions. The IFS does not appear to significantly increase blood flow in the injured area.[103]

Time-modulated Alternating Current

After the 1972 Summer Olympics, much attention was given to an electrical strength training regimen used by Russian athletes. A Soviet physician, Dr. Yakov Kots, reported that athletes training under this technique demonstrated a 30 percent to 40 percent strength improvement over those training with isometric exercise alone. Other reported benefits of this technique included increased muscular endurance and changes in the velocity of muscular contractions. These results, owing in part to Dr. Kots's failure to specify the parameters used by these athletes, have never been duplicated in the United States.[2,20,22,23,26,28,104,105] This method of application has gained the name "Russian stimulation" based on its country of origin.

Classical Russian stimulation involves the use of a 2500-Hz carrier sine wave with burst modulation (Table 5–21). The theory behind Russian stimulation, as

TABLE 5–19 Pain Control via Gate Control Using Interferential Stimulation

Parameter	Setting
Intensity	Sensory level
Electrode configuration	Quadripolar
Beat frequency	High
Sweep frequency	Long duration, ramped change

TABLE 5–20 **Pain Control via Opiate Release Using Interferential Stimulation**

Parameter	Setting
Intensity	Strong, yet comfortable muscle contraction
Electrode configuration	Quadripolar
Beat frequency	Low
Sweep frequency	Long duration, abrupt shift

with IFS, is that the higher frequencies would decrease the amount of capacitive skin resistance and allow more current to reach the motor nerve at lower intensities.[2] Although the strength-gain benefits have not been duplicated, this form of electrical stimulation is an excellent method to decrease muscular atrophy.

Although sometimes found as dedicated units, IFS units are often capable of modulating bursts, providing for Russian-type stimulation.

Reduction of Edema

Chronic post-traumatic edema can be reduced by the use of IFS.[105] This effect is attributable to milking of the venous and lymphatic return systems through electrically evoked muscle contractions. Care must be taken to avoid unwanted joint motion that could produce further injury of the involved structures.

Electrode Placement

Quadripolar Technique

The four electrodes are positioned around the painful area so that each channel runs perpendicular to the other and the current crosses at the midpoint (Fig. 5–32). The interference effects branch off at 45° angles from the center of the treatment, in the shape of a four-leaf clover. Tissues within this area receive the maximal treatment effect. When the electrodes are properly positioned, the stimulation should be felt only between the electrodes, not under the electrodes.[14]

Referring to Figure 5–32, notice that the interference effect covers only about half of the area between the electrodes. If the patient has a very discrete area of pain, the interference pattern should be able to encompass the appropriate tissues. However, in cases in which the pain is diffuse, maximal pain reduction may not occur. This problem can be reduced through rotating the interference effect area. By slightly unbalancing the currents, the interference pattern "ro-

TABLE 5–21 **Electrical Parameters Used in Time-Modulated Alternating Current Stimulation**

Parameter	Setting
Intensity	To tolerance
Carrier frequency	2500 Hz
Beat frequency	1–100 Hz

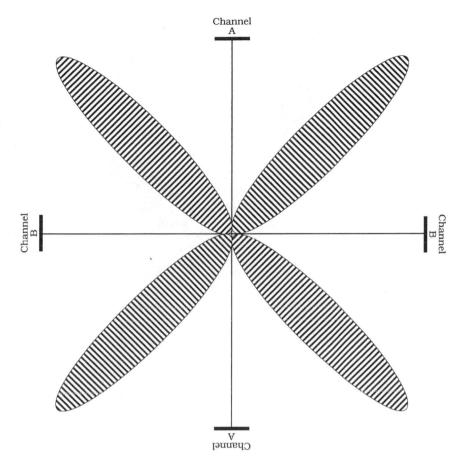

FIGURE 5–32 **Interference Pattern.** Maximal benefit from interferential stimulation occurs at 45° angles from the intersection of the channels.

tates" or "scans" 45° back and forth between the electrodes, resulting in treatment of a larger area (Fig. 5–33).

Bipolar Electrode Placement

When IFS is applied using a bipolar technique, the mixing of the two channels occurs within the generator rather than in the tissues. Two channels are used within the generator, with a single output channel applied to the tissues. Although bipolar IFS does not penetrate the tissues as deeply as quadripolar application, a more precise mixing occurs.

When muscle contractions are the goal of the treatment session, either through IFS or Russian stimulation, bipolar electrode placements are used. When the effects are targeted for one specific muscle or muscle group, only one channel is used. Four electrodes are incorporated into a dual channel, agonist-antagonist treatment regimen.

Instrumentation

Power: When this switch is in its ON position, the current is allowed to flow to the internal components of the generator.

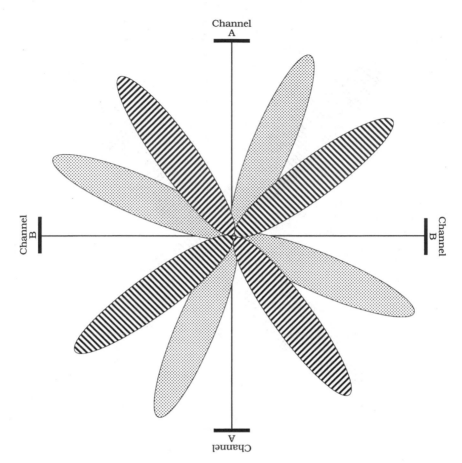

FIGURE 5–33 **Dynamic Interference Vectoring.** The normal vector pattern is rotated throughout the treatment to stimulate a broader tissue area.

Reset: This safety feature ensures that the intensity is reduced to zero before the treatment is started.

Timer: This control sets the duration of the treatment and subsequently displays the remaining time. On some units, the TIMER serves as the master power switch.

Start-stop: This switch is used to initiate and terminate the treatment.

Intensity: This control adjusts the amplitude of the pulse and is displayed in milliamperes (mA). When quadripolar stimulation is being used, the intensity control regulates both channels simultaneously.

Mode: This switch allows the user to choose between true interferential therapy and bipolar stimulation. The interferential mode allows the current to stimulate deep tissue. In the bipolar mode, only one channel is used, and the resultant current flow stimulates relatively subcutaneous nerves.

Russian stimulation: This mode changes the output from amplitude-modulated to burst-modulated for evoking strong muscle contractions. This technique may use one or both channels. This is an option on many IFS units, and other units provide Russian stimulation as well.

Beat frequency: The "beat" is the result of the fixed rate of the carrier wave and the variable rate of the second channel.

On-off control: When Russian-type stimulation has been selected from the MODE control, this adjusts the duty cycle by determining the amount of time the current is ON versus OFF.

Balance: This dial allows the user to control the balance of electrical current under each set of electrodes and to equalize the sensory stimulation. It may only be meaningful during quadripolar stimulation.

Setup and Application

Initiation of the Treatment

1. *Vacuum electrodes:* If the unit uses electrodes that are secured by means of a vacuum, refer to the operator's manual for instructions on their use.
2. *Turn on the unit:* Turn on the unit by activating the POWER switch.
3. *Reset parameters:* Fully reduce the INTENSITY control and depress the RESET button.
4. *Select application mode:* Determine the MODE of application: quadripolar, bipolar, or Russian stimulation.
5. *Adjust beat frequency:* Select the appropriate BEAT frequencies based on the goals of the treatment.
6. *Adjust sweep frequency:* Use the appropriate SWEEP frequency for this treatment protocol.
7. *Adjust treatment duration:* Set the duration of the treatment by adjusting the TIMER.
8. *Begin treatment:* Press the START button to close the circuit between the generator and the patient's tissues.
9. *Increase output intensity:* Slowly increase the INTENSITY control until the appropriate current level is obtained.
10. *Adjust balance:* If necessary, adjust the BALANCE control to obtain maximal treatment comfort.

Duration of Treatment

Interferential stimulation may be applied once or twice daily in treatment bouts normally ranging from 15 to 30 minutes. Burst-modulated stimulation is normally applied three times a week in 30-minute bouts.

Precautions

- Improper use can result in electrode burns or skin irritation.
- Intense or prolonged stimulation may result in muscle spasm and/or muscle soreness.

Indications

- Acute pain
- Chronic pain
- Muscle spasm

Contraindications

In addition to the contraindications presented in Table 5–1, the use of INF is contraindicated in:

- Pain of central origin
- Pain of unknown origin

Neuromuscular Electrical Stimulation

Neuromuscular electrical stimulation (NMES) is used for muscle reeducation, reduction of spasticity, delay of atrophy, and muscle strengthening (Fig. 5–34). The use of electrical stimulation reverses the order in which muscle fibers are recruited into the contraction. During voluntary muscle contractions, small-diameter type I motor nerves are the first to contract. Because of their construction, type I fibers do not generate much force but are able to sustain the contraction for a prolonged period. Electrical stimulation causes large-diameter type II motor nerves to evoke a contraction before the type I fibers. Because type II fibers are capable of producing more force, the strength of the contraction is increased.

This reversal of the order of motor nerve recruitment is a result of the relative sizes of the nerves and their depths below the surface of the skin. Electrical stimulation first causes a depolarization of large-diameter nerves because their cross-sectional area provides less resistance to current flow. In addition, type II motor nerves, being more superficial, receive greater stimulation than the deeper type I nerves.

The amount of torque produced is directly related to the amount of current introduced into the muscle.[20] The strength of the contraction can be further altered through manipulation of the electrode placement. Generators for NMES use a wide range of waveforms, but the majority of the units currently on the mar-

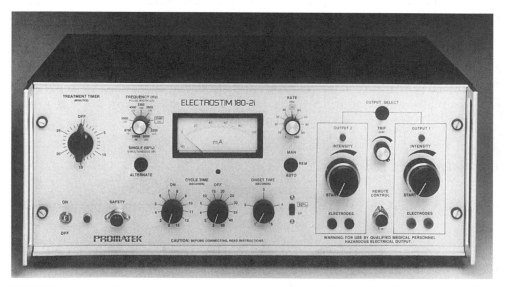

FIGURE 5–34 A Neuromuscular Electrical Stimulation Unit. (The Electrostim 180-2, courtesy of Promatek Medical Systems, Inc., Joliet, IL.)

TABLE 5–22 Electrical Parameters Used in Neuromuscular Electrical Stimulation

Parameter	Setting
Peak amperage	To tolerance
Pulse duration	50–300 μsec
Pulse frequency	1–200 pps
Pulse charge	≤10 mQ

mQ = microcoulombs; pps = pulses per second; μsec = microseconds.

ket use a biphasic wave. A review of the literature indicates that no one waveform is universally comfortable but that perceived comfort is based on individual preference. Symmetrical pulses tend to be less painful over a large muscle mass because there is an equal amount of stimulation under both electrodes.[27]

Neuromuscular stimulation is a frequency-dependent modality. The current must be strong enough to overcome the capacitive resistance of the tissues before the motor nerves can be stimulated. The capacitive tissue resistance is inversely proportional to the frequency of the current. Therefore, the relatively low frequencies used by NMES generators must produce a greater current to overcome this resistance. Commonly used electrical parameters in NMES generators are presented in Table 5–22.

Biophysical Effects

Neuromuscular Stimulation

Because of the large amplitude and long pulse duration, NMES provides stronger stimulation than other forms of electrical stimulation. The increased pulse duration and amperage, however, tend to result in decreased comfort. Increasing the duration of the pulses results in increased stimulation of pain nerve fibers. When the aim of the treatment session is to increase muscular strength, the output of the treatment should be as high as the patient will allow; if the aim is muscle reeducation, a mild tonic contraction for "cueing" is all that is required.[2]

The efficacy of NMES in improving isometric muscle strength has been substantiated in the literature. The improvement in strength occurs as a result of increasing the functional stress placed on the muscle and as a result of the reversal of motor nerve recruitment.[28] NMES has been shown to elicit a contraction that produces torque equal to 90 percent of the maximal voluntary contraction.[21]

Patients who are reeducating muscle through NMES have the potential for significantly increasing strength more than those who are not exercising. It has been demonstrated that groups using NMES applied with a 60 percent duty cycle displayed a significant increase in strength over an isometrically trained group.[106,107] After ACL reconstruction, high-intensity NMES may increase the strength of the involved quadriceps muscle to 70 percent, compared with 57 percent for voluntary contractions and 51 percent for low-intensity NMES.[108]

TABLE 5–23 **Effects Associated with Neuromuscular Electrical Stimulation**

Electrically induced isometric quadriceps contractions can significantly increase strength in certain joint positions.
- Knee joint positions ranged from 30°–90° of flexion.
- The amount of hip flexion can influence the strength of the contractions, possibly secondary to providing the muscle group with a mechanical advantage.
- Strength gains summarized ranged from 7%–48%.

Electrical stimulation can increase isokinetic strength at certain speeds.
- No significant strength increases have been reported at speeds greater than 120° per second.
- Speeds of 65° per second showed the most substantial increases.

No **statistically significant** strength increases have been demonstrated to occur between strength gains obtained via ES, voluntary contractions, and a combination of ES and voluntary contractions.
- Most of the literature reviewed indicated greater strength gains in voluntary contractions than in electrically induced contractions.
- Although the differences in strength gains obtained from voluntary contractions compared with those obtained from ES were not statistically significant, the results may be **clinically significant.** Strength increases obtained from ES were on average 10% greater than those derived from voluntary contractions.

Source: Adapted from Selkowitz.[111]

Muscular contractions obtained through NMES have been shown to increase peripheral blood flow to the extremity being stimulated. This occurs as a result of the increased metabolic rate associated with the contractions. During treatment, blood flow increases during the first minute, whereas it reaches a steady state for the remainder of the treatment.[109] This response is independent of the stimulation intensity. Sympathetic changes in blood flow may also occur in the opposite side of the body.[110]

Table 5–23 presents several different types of benefits and effects reported to be associated with NMES and various protocols.

Reduction of Edema

In reducing edema, NMES is similar to other forms of electrotherapy. The protocol described for motor-level reduction of edema using HVPS can be used with this device. Venous and lymphatic return are enhanced through the milking of these vessels by muscle contractions. Because the aim of this method is to produce individual muscle contractions, a low (1 to 10 pps) pulse frequency or a 50 percent duty cycle is used. The intensity of the current should produce a visible contraction but should not cause unwanted movement of the joint. As with other methods of edema reduction, the benefits of this treatment are enhanced if the limb is placed in a non-gravity-dependent position.

Electrode Placement

Bipolar electrode placement is commonly employed in NMES treatments. The electrodes are placed over the proximal and distal ends of the muscle or muscle group. Because large electrodes lie over several muscles and/or motor points, a more generalized contraction is obtained. The use of small electrodes may elicit a more specific contraction through direct stimulation of the muscle's motor point. As the electrodes are brought closer together, the effect of the stimulation becomes more superficial, and the relative intensity of the contraction decreases.

Quadripolar application requires the use of two separate channels. This method of application is commonly used when stimulating agonist-antagonist muscle groups.

A monopolar technique may be employed through the use of one small and one large electrode or through the use of a hand-held applicator. This method of electrode placement is useful when a specific muscle, or a small muscle group, is the target of the treatment.

The size of the electrodes should be only as large as is required to stimulate the desired tissues. Electrodes that are too small result in a very high current density, whereas electrodes that are larger than needed may stimulate unwanted nerves.

Instrumentation

Power: When this switch is in its ON position, the current is allowed to flow to the internal components of the generator.

Reset: This safety feature ensures that the output is reduced to zero before the treatment is started.

Timer: This control sets the duration of the treatment and subsequently displays the remaining time.

Intensity: This knob adjusts the amplitude of the pulses.

Pulse rate: This parameter determines the type of muscle contraction to be elicited. Depending on the muscle, or muscle group, being stimulated, a pulse rate of less than 15 pps causes a distinct contraction for each impulse. Between 15 and 25 pps, the muscle begins to contract smoothly, eventually leading to a tonic contraction at approximately 35 to 50 pps.

Mode: This switch allows the user to select the type of waveform used in the treatment.

On-off rate: This feature allows the user to set the duty cycle for the treatment. Neuromuscular stimulation units have separate dials to independently adjust the number of seconds that the current is flowing and the number of seconds it is not. Other units have preset duty cycles that the user cannot alter. A CONSTANT mode (100% duty cycle) may be provided. This is useful for adjusting the other treatment parameters (intensity, pulse duration, etc.) without waiting for the duty cycle to switch to its ON mode.

External trigger: A hand-held device that allows the user to manually control the ON-OFF time of the stimulation. When the trigger is depressed, current is allowed to flow to the tissues.

Reciprocal rate: When two channels are being used, this feature selects the duration of time that the current is flowing to each channel.

Ramp: The RAMP parameter allows the user to determine the amplitude rise time until the peak current is obtained. Often the RAMP represents the percentage of the ON duty cycle time required to reach the maximum intensity. For example, a 20 percent RAMP with an ON duty cycle time of 5 seconds would require 1 second to reach the maximum intensity.

Interrupt switch: This device is held by the patient and is used to terminate the treatment if the intensity becomes too great or too painful.

Setup and Application

Initiation of the Treatment

1. *Prepare the generator:* Reduce the output intensity to zero and turn the unit on. If applicable, press the RESET button.
2. *Prepare electrodes:* Connect the leads to the unit and to the electrodes and secure the electrodes to the patient.
3. *Make interrupt switch available:* Give the patient the INTERRUPT SWITCH and provide instruction on its purpose and use.
4. *Set pulse variables:* Set the phase duration (WIDTH) and pulse frequency (RATE) to the midrange of the parameters to be used.
5. *Set current variables:* If the RAMP and ON-OFF parameters are manually adjustable on the unit, increase the RAMP to a rapid rise and adjust the ON-OFF controls to a 100 percent duty cycle. This configuration allows the INTENSITY to be increased without waiting for the generator to run through its duty cycle. If these parameters cannot be changed during the course of the treatment, adjust them to the desired settings now. (Certain generators may be designed to allow the intensity to be increased without adjusting these parameters.)
6. *Adjust frequency:* Adjust the output FREQUENCY to the appropriate level for this treatment (see step 11 below).
7. *Set treatment duration:* Set the TIMER for this session.
8. *Initiate treatment:* Press the START button to activate the unit.
9. *Increase intensity:* Begin the treatment by slowly increasing the INTENSITY until the desired tension is developed in the muscle.
10. *Adjust ramp for treatment goals:* If applicable, reset the RAMP time to match the treatment goals and patient needs.
11. *Adjust the DUTY CYCLE to match the treatment goals:* The following protocol may be used as an example:[111]
    - *Muscle strengthening:* ON = 10 seconds, OFF = 50 seconds.
    - *Muscle endurance:* ON and OFF have approximately equal durations (4 to 15 seconds). FREQUENCY equals 50 to 200 Hz.

Duration and Frequency of Treatment

Treatments used for muscular reeducation may be given daily, but as with any muscle-building program, the patient should be monitored for undue pain. Treatments for the delay of atrophy are given throughout the day with the use of a portable stimulator.

Precautions

- Improper use may result in electrode burns or skin irritation.
- Intense or prolonged stimulation may result in muscle spasm and/or muscle soreness.
- An electrically induced contraction can generate too much tension within the muscle (the function of the Golgi tendon organs is overridden).

Indications

- Maintaining range of motion
- Muscle reeducation
- Prevention of joint contractures
- Prevention of disuse atrophy
- Increasing local blood flow
- Decreasing muscle spasm

Contraindications

In addition to the contraindications presented in Table 5–1, contraindications to the use of NMES include:

- Musculotendinous lesions, in which the tension produced by the contraction will further damage the muscle or tendon fibers
- Cases in which there is not a secure bony attachment of the muscle

Microcurrent Electrical Stimulation

Although there is no universally accepted definition of microcurrent electrical therapy (MET or MENS), some common threads may be found. This form of electrical stimulation tends to be applied at the subsensory or very low sensory level with a current operating at less than 1000 μA. These devices deliver an electrical current to the body that has approximately 1/1000 the amperage of TENS but a pulse duration that may be up to 2500 times longer. Unlike the other electrical modalities described in this chapter, the distinguishing feature of microcurrent is that it does not attempt to excite peripheral nerves.[112] Microcurrent stimulators may deliver direct, alternating, or pulsed currents (in a wide range of waveforms), with each possessing a broad band of pulse durations, frequencies, and treatment durations. This range of currents makes it difficult to analyze the theoretical and clinical effects of MET.

The efficacy of this form of electrical stimulation has yet to be substantiated in professional literature, yet its accolades continue to be pronounced in lay journals and through anecdotal reports. Some referred articles report decreased pain, increased range of motion, and improved wound healing, but more often than not, these effects were greater in experimental subjects than those seen in a control group, but less than other modalities, or were conducted in an uncontrolled manner.[42,113,114] Likewise, notable research exists that does not support microcurrent's efficacy as a therapeutic modality.[67,115–119]

The following sections describe the theoretical effects of MET and its effect on traumatized tissues and discuss the potential limitations on this device's effectiveness.

Biophysical Effects

The theory supporting microcurrent's biophysical effects on the injury response process is based on the effect that a low amperage current has on adenosine triphosphate (ATP) levels. Currents below 500 μA increase the level of ATP, whereas higher amperages decrease the ATP level. Passing a low-amperage electrical current through mitochondria creates an imbalance in the number of proteins on either side of its cell membrane. As the protons move from the anode to the cathode, they cross the mitochondrial membrane, causing adenosine triphosphastase to produce ATP. The increased ATP production encourages amino acid transport and increased protein synthesis.[120]

Tissue trauma affects the electrical potential of the involved cells, the previously described **injury potential** or **current of injury**.[51] Resistance to electrical current flow increases after trauma, so the body's intrinsic bioelectrical currents take the path of least resistance around, rather than through, the involved tissues. As a result of the diminished bioelectrical activity within the traumatized area, cellular capacitance is decreased, and the cell's homeostasis is further disrupted.[121–123] Theoretically, re-establishing the body's natural electrical balance allows the cell's ATP supply to be replenished, thus providing the metabolic energy for healing to occur.

Although it seems that a DC would best produce the effects described in this section, many MET protocols use an alternating or pulsed current.[123,124] It is unlikely that a DC is sufficient to overcome the skin's capacitive resistance because of the low amperage at which MET is applied to the body. As you will recall, capacitive skin resistance decreases as the pulse frequency increases. Therefore, applying MET with an alternating or pulsed current lowers the current threshold required to overcome the skin's resistance. The distances used between the electrodes during treatment also serve to increase the amount of energy needed to complete the circuit.

Research has validated the effects of subthreshold electrical stimulation on cell membrane properties, neurological responses, and ionic responses.[112,125,126] These experimental designs most commonly use electrodes that are implanted within the tissues themselves. Other derivations have arisen from the benefits of sensory-level DC application. Unlike MET, the currents used in these studies did not have to overcome the resistance produced by the skin or have the electrical power needed to overcome the resistance posed by the tissues. Any interpolation between these effects and microcurrent may be considered to be inappropriate.

Electrode Placement

The electrodes should be placed so that a line drawn through them transects the target tissues. This, in concept, is similar to the contiguous electrode placement technique described earlier in this chapter. However, proponents of MET view electrode placement in a three-dimensional rather than the traditional two-dimensional manner. This view holds that electrodes should also be placed on opposite sides of the torso or extremity and the current will flow through them. Perhaps if electricity flowed in a perfectly straight line between opposing electrodes, this would be true. However, remember that electricity follows the path of least resistance, which would most likely course the current around the body's circumference rather than straight through the core. Also remember that the greater the distance between the electrodes, the greater the resistance and the more current required to overcome this resistance.

One technique for treating back pain places an electrode near the spinal cord at the same level as the painful tissues. The opposite electrode is then positioned on the contralateral side of the spinal cord on the anterior side of the body. When the axial skeleton is being treated, MET protocol suggests that treatment occur bilaterally.

The use of MET probes is described in the Setup and Application section of this unit.

Instrumentation

Power: When this switch is in its ON position, the current is allowed to flow to the internal components of the generator. Some units have a speaker that emits an audible sound when a certain electrical threshold is met. In this type of generator, the power switch often serves as a VOLUME control as well.

Timer: This control sets the duration of the treatment and subsequently displays the remaining time. On some units, the TIMER serves as the master power switch.

Start-stop: When this button is depressed to start the treatment, the circuit is closed, allowing the current to flow to the patient's tissues. When it is depressed again, the circuit is opened, interrupting the current flow. The START-STOP button may also set the treatment mode on some generators.

Amplitude: This control adjusts the current amperage from zero (OFF) to the maximal value of the unit. The output for each channel has its own AMPLITUDE control. The applied output is displayed on the OUTPUT meter.

Frequency (hertz): When a pulsed current is being applied, the FREQUENCY sets the number of pulses per second; when an AC is being administered, it sets the number of cycles per second. Each channel has its own output control.

Multiplier: A three-position switch that multiplies the output FREQUENCY by the value indicated. The output for each channel has its own multiplier control.

Polarity: This switch selects the output polarity in monophasic mode, or the rate at which the output polarity is alternated in biphasic mode.

Ramp: The ramp selects the rise time of the modulated output in biphasic mode.

Threshold: This button adjusts the level on the power meter at which audible output occurs.

Meter select: This control adjusts which channel is displayed on the power output meter.

Ohm meter: This device is used as a method of identifying stimulation points. When the probe is passed over an area of decreased electrical resistance (e.g., stimulation points, traumatized tissues), a tone, light, or numerical readout identifies the point on the skin at which stimulation should occur.

Setup and Application

Initiation of the Treatment

1. *Position the electrodes:* Most MET stimulators require the use of silver electrodes. Unapproved carbon-rubber electrodes may present too much resistance to current flow and render the treatment ineffective.

2. *Wet the electrodes:* If felt-tipped electrodes or probes are being used, wet them with saline solution. Tap water should not be used because of its potentially high mineral content. Note that medicinal saline solution requires a physician's prescription. If this type of saline solution is not readily available, a saline-based contact lens cleaner may be used to wet the electrodes.

3. *Select the output frequency:* Most MET treatment protocols employ a 0.5-Hz frequency. If this frequency proves to be ineffective, a 1.5-Hz output may be attempted. Other protocols suggest using a frequency between 80 to 100 Hz for inflammatory conditions.

4. *Increase the output intensity:* Increase the intensity to the highest comfortable level, keeping in mind that most treatment applications occur at the subsensory level. Some protocols suggest a series of 5- to 10-minute treatments using a range of output intensities and varying pulse frequencies.

5. *Reposition electrodes:* Each treatment bout with the electrode technique lasts from 5 to 10 minutes. At the end of each bout the electrodes are removed, rewetted, and repositioned around the painful area.

6. *Treat the contralateral side:* Many MET protocols suggest that the same treatment that was delivered to the injured extremity or injured side of the body be repeated on the noninjured side.

Probe Technique

1. *Set the timer:* If the MET generator has a PROBE setting, select this. Otherwise, each treatment bout should last approximately 10 seconds.

2. *Select output channel:* Only one channel is used during the probe technique.

3. *Identify target treatment area:* Localize the center of pain as accurately as possible. A grease pencil or dry-erase marker may be used to mark the area on the skin.

4. *Position probe:* The area surrounding the target tissues is treated in an "X" manner. For example, the first treatment bout may have one probe positioned in the upper left-hand quadrant and the opposite probe in the lower right-hand quadrant, relative to the mark identified in step 2. The next treatment bout would have the probes positioned in the upper right-hand and lower left-hand quadrant. The treatment progresses in this manner, with the probes being rotated around the target tissues in varying directions and distances, including anterior-posterior and medial-lateral placements.

5. *Determine number of bout sessions:* Each bout in a single session persists for 10 seconds, and each session lasts approximately 2 minutes. Up to four sessions may be used during a single treatment.

6. *Re-evaluate the patient:* The patient should be re-evaluated after each bout session, and treatment parameters adjusted accordingly.

Duration of Treatment

Most MET treatments range from 30 minutes to 2 hours and may be repeated up to four times per day.

Precautions

- The use of MET on dehydrated patients may result in nausea, dizziness, and/or headaches.
- Electrical "shocks" may be reported by the patient when MET is applied to scar tissue. This represents the amount of current required to overcome the scar's electrical resistance.

Indications

- Acute and chronic pain
- Acute and chronic inflammation
- Reduction of edema
- Sprains
- Strains
- Contusions
- Temporomandibular joint dysfunction
- Carpal tunnel syndrome
- Superficial wound healing
- Scar tissue
- Neuropathies

Contraindications

In addition to the contraindications presented in Table 5–1, the use of microcurrent electrical stimulation should not be used in:

- Pain or other symptoms of unknown origin
- *Osteomyelitis*

Iontophoresis

Iontophoresis is the introduction of medication ions into the human skin using a low-voltage DC. By adapting to fluctuations in tissue resistance, iontophoresis generators (iontophoresors) produce a constant voltage output by adjusting the amperage. The medication types most commonly used for iontophoresis include anesthetics, analgesics, and anti-inflammatory agents (Table 5–24). Experimental work has begun that explores the use of iontophoresis as a substitute for certain types of *dialysis* and repeated injections, such as insulin.

Based on the ionic reaction between the positive and negative poles of the generator, ionized medication molecules travel along the lines of force created by the current. At the positive electrode, positive ions are driven through the skin; negative ions are introduced through the skin at the negative pole. This technique has been shown to deliver the medication to depths of 6 to 20 mm below the skin.[127,128]

The transdermal introduction of medication has advantages over oral ingestion or injection of medication. An advantage over oral medication includes bypassing the liver, thus reducing the metabolic breakdown of the medication. The medication can also be concentrated in a localized area rather than be absorbed in the gastrointestinal tract, providing local rather than systemic delivery of the drug.[129] Most of these advantages also hold true with injected medication, but iontophoresis is less traumatic and less painful than injected medication. In addition,

---

Osteomyelitis: Inflammation of the bone marrow and adjacent bone.
Dialysis: An external device that is used to assist or replace the kidney's function of filtering blood.

TABLE 5–24 **Sample Medications, Their Indications, and Treatment Dosages Used during Iontophoresis*†**

Medication(s)	Pathology	Concentration	Dosage	Delivery Polarity
Acetic acid	Myositis ossificans	2% Mixed with distilled water	80 mA/min	Positive
Dexamethasone and lidocaine	Inflammation	4 mg Decadron (1 cm² suspension)	41 mA/min	Negative
	Pain control	4% Xylocaine (2 cm² suspension)	40 mA/min	Positive
Lidocaine and epinephrine	Pain control	4% Lidocaine 0.01 mL 1:50,000 epinephrine	30 mA/min	Positive Positive
Lidocaine and epinephrine	Pain control	4% Lidocaine and 0.25 cc of 1:1000 epinephrine	20 mA/min	Positive
Dexamethasone	Inflammation	2 cc 4 mg/mL dexamethasone	41 mA/min	Negative

*Refer to the physician's prescription for exact treatment parameters.
†Each size electrode has a maximum amperage that should not be exceeded. Consult the packaging information included with the electrodes.

the injection of medication can result in a high concentration of medication in a localized area, resulting in tissue damage.[127]

Iontophoresis also has its disadvantages. Unreliable results are obtained with certain medications, and there may be doubt to as how much medication is actually introduced into the tissues.[15] In children, the anxiety caused by iontophoresis was not significantly less than that of an injection, whereas injections appear to be more tolerable over time. Also, cutaneous anesthesia derived from an injection is more tolerable than that obtained through iontophoresis.[130]

Many of the medications used during iontophoresis are controlled substances requiring a physician's prescription. The use of the iontophoresor may also be regulated by state practice acts.

Iontophoresis Mechanisms

Traditional iontophoresors deliver a low-voltage, high-amperage DC to the body. The generator's output ranges from 0 to 5 mA at skin impedances ranging from 500 ohms to 100 kilohms.

As we will also see in the Phonophoresis section of the next chapter, the stratum corneum is the primary barrier to the transfer of substances across the skin into the subcutaneous tissues. The electrical charge of the medication helps complete the circuit by carrying the current between the two electrode poles. During iontophoresis, the primary path for current flow, and hence medication transfer, occurs through portals formed by hair follicles and skin pores.[131]

For iontophoresis to occur, the applied current must be sufficient to overcome the skin/electrode resistance and still have enough energy to drive the medication through the skin's portals.[131,132] As the treatment progresses, the portals' resistance to electrical current flow and medication entry into the body decreases.[133] Once they are within the tissues, the medication is spread locally through passive diffusion and is no longer affected by the current source. The rate of this diffusion is such that the medication tends to remain more highly concentrated within those tissues directly subcutaneous to the introduction site and progressively less concentrated in the deeper tissues and in tissues peripheral to the treatment site.[134]

Iontophoresis uses a monopolar electrode arrangement in which the electrode containing the medication serves as the active electrode. The increased current density under the delivery electrode also decreases the resistance to the iontophoretic current; the higher the current density, the less resistance to electrical flow.[135] Although this trait seems to contradict Ohm's law, the decreased resistance is an artifact of an increase in the size of the skin pores or the creation of new ones.[136,137]

Local blood flow is increased for 1 hour after the treatment, and the stratum corneum is hydrated for 30 minutes after treatment. Although this assists in the subcutaneous diffusion of the medication, it may result in a wider-than-normal diffusion, spreading the medication systemically and lowering its concentration in the intended treatment area. The increased blood flow may also explain the hyperemia after the treatment.[138]

Burns or severe skin irritation are problems inherent to the application of a DC on the human body. Either of these negative reactions is related to the hydrogen and hydroxide ions generated by the current. Experimental work using a low-frequency AC or a combination of alternating and direct currents has shown to be effective in delivering certain forms of medication to the body without the associated skin irritation.[139,140]

Medication Dosage

The medication dose delivered during the treatment is measured in terms of milliamperes per minute (mA/min) and is based on the relationship between the amperage of the current and the treatment duration:

Current amperage (milliamperes) × Treatment duration = mA/min

Most iontophoresors use a **dose-oriented** treatment protocol in which the user indicates the desired treatment dose and the generator calculates the duration and intensity of the treatment. A subsequent change in the output alters the treatment duration; increasing the amperage decreases duration and vice versa. If the treatment duration were shortened, the output intensity would be increased.

For example, if a medication were being used that called for a dose of 50 mA/min, the generator may default to an output of 5 mA and a treatment duration of 10 minutes (5 mA × 10 minutes = 50 mA/min). If this is the patient's first exposure to iontophoresis or if the patient has a history of sensitivity to this treatment, the operator would choose to decrease the intensity of the treatment. For this example, let's suppose the intensity was decreased to 3 mA. The generator would then recalculate the treatment duration to approximately 16 minutes and 40 seconds (3 mA × 16.67 minutes = 50 mA/min). The amperage should be immediately reduced when the patient reports any sensation other than tingling (e.g., reports of burning).

Medications

The type of medication used during iontophoresis depends on the type of pathology and the desired treatment outcome. Table 5–24 presents some common medications used during this treatment, indications for use, and typical treatment dosages. This information should not be viewed as recommended treatment protocols. For this information, refer to the physician's or pharmacist's recommended concentrations and treatment doses.

For the application of iontophoresis, water-soluble medications are dissolved in a carrier. The amount and rate of medication delivery are based on the total voltage applied, the duration of the treatment, the local pH, and the concentration of the medication in the delivery electrode. As the magnitude of each of these factors increases, the total dosage of the treatment increases.

Certain reactions occur that complicate the delivery of medication into the tissues. The medication competes with other ions having the same polarity as the delivery electrodes. There is an equal chance that the medication ions will be driven into the tissues as other ions having the same molecular weight and size. Medications of larger ionic weight and mass require an increased output intensity to drive them through the tissues. Because of the amount of work (energy) required, smaller ions tend to be preferentially moved relative to larger ones.

Passive iontophoresis also alters the amount, rate, and quality of the phoresis. Recall that ions that have unlike charges attract each other. As a charged *ion* enters the tissues, it tends to "pull" ions having the opposite charge. Consider a negatively charged ion being pushed into the skin by the negative charge of the electrode. A nearby positively charged ion may be within the negative ion's field of attraction. The positively charged ion is pulled behind the negative ion as it enters the tissue.

Different types of medications may be mixed together so long as their ionic charges do not change or significantly weaken. To achieve equal doses of one medication of a relatively large molecular size and weight and another one of smaller mass, the concentration of the larger, less mobile medication must be increased.[134]

Biophysical Effects

The exact biophysical effects obtained from the treatment depend on the type of medication(s) being used. Medications introduced into the body via iontophoresis can penetrate 6 to 20 mm below the skin and in most instances can reach the depth of tendinous structures and underlying cartilage. However, the exact dose of the medication reaching this depth is undetermined.[15,127,128]

When an anti-inflammatory or anesthetic mixture is used (e.g., dexamethasone [Decadron] and lidocaine [Xylocaine]), the onset of relief may take 24 to 48 hours, although immediate relief is sometimes reported. The latent effects may be attributed to a cumulative effect of the treatments.[15] Lidocaine, in concentrations of up to 50 percent, requires a minimum 10 minutes of electrical current before the skin is anesthetized.[141]

Electrode Placement

The delivery of iontophoresis involves the use of a **delivery electrode** ("drug electrode") that serves as the **active electrode** and a return electrode that serves as the

---

Ion: An atom, or group of atoms, that has a net charge other than zero.

dispersive electrode (Fig. 5–35). Many application procedures use only one delivery electrode, but most units allow two to be used. The delivery electrode is placed over the target tissues, whereas the return electrode is placed 4 to 6 inches way. When placing each electrode on the body, care should be taken to consider the underlying tissues. For example, if iontophoresis is being used to treat plantar fasciitis, the delivery electrode should be placed on the medial aspect of the arch, where the skin is relatively thin, rather than over the thick padding provided under the heel.

Instrumentation

Power: The POWER switch activates or deactivates the generator.

Reset: The RESET switch serves as an "emergency shutoff" in case of patient discomfort or a malfunction within the generator. At the conclusion of the treatment, pressing the RESET button decreases the dosage, output, and duration values to zero.

Dosage: This parameter sets the medication dosage, in milliamperes per minute, for this treatment. Some units allow for the dosage to be keyed in directly (e.g., if a keypad is used, the numerical value is typed in) or set using INCREASE and DECREASE buttons.

Intensity (amperage): By setting the DOSAGE, the amperage increases to a preset level. Increasing the INTENSITY decreases the treatment DURATION; decreasing this value increases the DURATION while keeping the dosage at the level indicated.

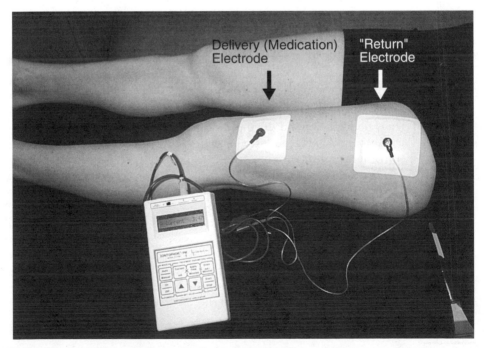

FIGURE 5–35 **Electrode Setup for Iontophoresis.** The appropriate medication is introduced into the delivery electrode and the return electrode is saturated with an electrically neutral buffering solution. The polarity of the delivery electrode must correspond with the medication being introduced to the body.

Treatment duration: Decreasing the DURATION increases the treatment INTENSITY and vice versa.

Polarity: The polarity of the delivery electrode must be the same as that of the medication currently being applied (i.e., if a medication has a negative polarity, the delivery electrode must have a negative polarity). Units having a POLARITY switch change the polarity of the delivery electrode to either positive or negative. Other units require that the electrode leads be physically plugged into the positive and negative jacks.

Start-Stop: Pressing this button the first time begins the current flow to the patient's body. For patient comfort, most generators are programmed so that the current is gradually ramped up from zero to the actual treatment duration. Pressing this button again either creates a pause in the treatment or terminates it, depending on the unit's design.

Setup and Application

Initiation of the Treatment

1. *Clean the treatment site:* Using alcohol, cleanse the area where the active and return electrodes are to be affixed to the body. The areas where the electrodes are to be placed should be free of cuts, abrasions, and other open wounds and of excess body hair. Shaving of the treatment area may be required.

2. *Prepare electrodes:* Fill the delivery electrode with the appropriate medication(s) in the manner applicable to the type of electrode being used. Wet the return electrode with an appropriate buffering solution.

3. *Position electrodes:* Place the DELIVERY electrode over the treatment site and the RETURN electrode 4 to 6 inches away.

4. *Set electrode polarity:* Depending on the type of generator being used, either attach the electrode leads to the generator so that the polarity of the DELIVERY electrode matches the medication's charge or attach the electrode leads as indicated and adjust the POLARITY selector as needed.

5. *Provide patient instructions:* Inform the patient that tingling and itching may be experienced during the treatment, but the treatment should not be uncomfortable. Advise the patient to inform you of any pain, burning, or other unpleasant sensations.

6. *Set treatment dose:* Indicate the treatment dose recommended by the physician and pharmacist. Do not exceed the recommended dose or intensity for the electrode being used.

7. *Adjust output parameters:* Normally the INTENSITY parameter is adjusted to suit the patient's comfort. If this is the patient's first treatment or if the patient has a history of sensitivity to this treatment or electrical stimulation in general, the output intensity should be decreased. The treatment intensity can be increased if indicated. Remember that decreasing the intensity increases the treatment duration and vice versa.

Myositis ossificans: Ossification or deposition of bone in muscle fascia, resulting in pain and swelling.

8. *Supplemental treatment:* Administer any appropriate follow-up treatments. Pulsed ultrasound (see Chap. 6) may be used after acetic acid iontophoresis for the reduction in the mass of traumatic *myositis ossificans.*[142]
9. *Repeat treatment with the opposite polarity:* If medications of different polarities are being used, repeat this procedure with the other medication using the appropriate polarity.
10. *Apply a soothing ointment:* A mild massage cream, aloe lotion, or skin-soothing ointment may be applied to the electrode sites to aid in reducing the amount of residual skin irritation associated with the treatment.
11. *Discard electrodes:* Iontophoresis electrodes may be used only for a single treatment.

Duration of Treatment

The duration of an individual treatment is based on the intensity of the treatment and the desired treatment dose (see Medication Dosage). Treatments are usually given every other day for up to 3 weeks. Consult the athlete's prescription for the exact treatment regimen.

Precautions

- Most medications require a physician's prescription. Pay close attention to any notes or instructions provided by the pharmacist.
- The exact dosage of the medication delivered to the body is unknown.
- Erythema under the electrodes is common after the treatment.
- A treatment dose that is too intense (in amperage or duration) can result in burns beneath the delivery and/or return electrode.
- Do not reuse an electrode because medications remain in it, contaminating it for future use.

Indications

- Acute inflammation
- Chronic inflammation
- Arthritis
- Myositis ossificans
- Myofascial pain syndromes
- As a vehicle for delivering local anesthetics before injection or other minor invasive procedures[130]
- Hyperhidrosis

Contraindications

In addition to the contraindications presented in Table 5–1, iontophoresis should not be used when:

- The patient has a history of adverse reactions or hypersensitivity to electrical stimulation
- The patient has contraindications to the medication(s) being administered
- Pain or other symptoms of unknown origin are present

Chapter Quiz

1. Electrons travel from the ———————————————, which has a ———————————
   of electrons, to the ———————————————, which has a ——————————— of
   electrons.
   A. Anode • high concentration • cathode • low concentration
   B. Anode • low concentration • cathode • high concentration
   C. Cathode • high concentration • anode • low concentration
   D. Cathode • low concentration • anode • high concentration

2. The ability of a material to store energy by means of an electrostatic field is called:
   A. Capacitance
   B. Inductance
   C. Impedance
   D. Work

3. What is the current flow in a 40-V circuit possessing 10 ohms of resistance?
   A. 0.25 A
   B. 50 A
   C. 4 A
   D. 30 A

4. What is the resistance found in a 40-V circuit possessing a current flow of 10 A?
   A. 4 ohms
   B. 400 ohms
   C. 0.25 ohms
   D. 30 ohms

5. What is the voltage of a circuit providing 4 ohms of resistance when 10 A are flow-
   ing?
   A. 0.4 V
   B. 2.5 V
   C. 6 V
   D. 40 V

6. What is the amount of power used by a device drawing 2 A from a 120-V source?
   A. 0.02 W
   B. 60 W
   C. 240 W
   D. Unable to calculate because the resistance is not provided

7. What is the total amount of resistance to current flow in a series circuit possessing
   two resistors, one of 10 ohms and another of 30 ohms?
   A. 4 ohms
   B. 7.5 ohms
   C. 20 ohms
   D. 40 ohms

8. What is the total amount of resistance to current flow in a parallel circuit possessing two resistors, one of 10 ohms and another of 30 ohms?
   A. 4 ohms
   B. 7.5 ohms
   C. 20 ohms
   D. 40 ohms

9. Monopolar stimulation involves the use of active and dispersive electrodes. The parameter that determines which pad(s) will be active is:
   A. The POLARITY adjustment
   B. The average current
   C. The pulse duration
   D. The current density

10. What is the percent duty cycle for an electrical current that flows for 30 seconds and has no flow for 10 seconds?
    A. 300 percent
    B. 25 percent
    C. 75 percent
    D. 3:1

11. All of the following are excitable tissues **except:**
    A. Muscle fiber
    B. Meniscal cartilage
    C. Sensory nerves
    D. Secretory cells

12. Which of the following would be the modality of choice to cause physiochemical changes within the tissues?
    A. High-voltage pulsed stimulation
    B. Interferential stimulation
    C. Low-voltage alternating current
    D. Low-voltage direct current

13. Under normal circumstances, which of the following nerves would be the **first** to be stimulated by an electrical current?
    A. A superficial large-diameter nerve
    B. A deep large-diameter nerve
    C. A superficial small-diameter nerve
    D. A deep small-diameter nerve

14. Most tissues provide capacitive resistance to electrical current flow. Which of the following currents would meet the **least** amount of capacitive resistance?
    A. 1 Hz
    B. 10 Hz
    C. 50 Hz
    D. 100 Hz

15. High-frequency stimulation possessing pulses of a short duration and applied at the sensory level is thought to activate which pain control mechanism?
    A. Gate mechanism
    B. Endogenous opiate
    C. Central biasing
    D. Specificity

16. The electrodes from lead (A) have an area of 10 square inches and 5 square inches, whereas the electrodes originating from lead (B) have an area of 7.5 square inches and 7.5 square inches. This type of stimulation would be classified as:
    A. Monopolar
    B. Bipolar
    C. Quadripolar
    D. Polypolar

17. Which of the following types of nerve fibers is most difficult to stimulate using most electrical modalities?
    A. A-beta
    B. A-delta
    C. A-gamma
    D. C fibers

CASE STUDY CONTINUATION

The following discussion relates to Case Study 3, found on pages 104 through 109 of Chapter 3.

Based on this patient's condition, the availability of other modalities, and the lack of contraindications to the use of therapeutic modalities and therapeutic exercise, the most probable acute use of electrical stimulation would be that of pain control and trigger point therapy. However, the lack of access to electrotherapeutic modalities probably would not hinder this patient's progress. Other types of modalities could adequately address and resolve the patient's problems.

Pain Control

The problem of acute pain control has been addressed by the use of thermal agents, and the patient has received a prescription for muscle relaxants. If these approaches fail to adequately reduce pain, electrical stimulation could be incorporated into the program.

The acute nature of this injury, the lack of radicular symptoms, and the fact that the patient is taking medication for the pain would make sensory-level pain control an appropriate choice, especially if the patient's symptoms are alleviated during the application of heat and cold. In this case, the use of a portable TENS unit should be considered and used as a part of the patient's home treatment program.

The electrodes would be positioned so that the current intersects over the primary area of pain. A short pulse duration, a high number of pulses per second, and a sensory-level intensity would be used. Because this unit would be used for long periods, its output must be modulated to help prevent accommodation. The patient would be instructed about how to connect and disconnect the unit, how to adjust the intensity, and if indicated, how to modify the pulse characteristics.

Trigger Point Therapy

If the patient's trigger points do not subside after the other treatment approaches, electrical stimulation could be used to target them. High-voltage pulsed stimulation, delivered with a probe, a Neuroprobe, brief-intense TENS, or noxious-level stimulation can be used to attempt to break down the trigger point. Interrupting the local pain-spasm-pain cycle, decreasing the pain response, and/or causing the trigger point's fibers to fatigue can bring about long-term relief. The electrodes could safely be worn under the patient's cervical collar.

REFERENCES

1. Kloth, LC and Cummings, JP: Electrotherapeutic Terminology in Physical Therapy. Section on Clinical Electrophysiology and the American Physical Therapy Association, Alexandria, VA, 1990.
2. Lake, DA: Neuromuscular electrical stimulation: An overview and its application in the treatment of sports injuries. Sports Med 13:320, 1992.
3. Robinson, AJ: Basic concepts and terminology in electricity. In Snyder-Mackler, L and Robinson, AJ (eds): Clinical Electrophysiology: Electrotherapy and Electrophysiologic Testing. Williams & Wilkins, Baltimore, 1989, pp 1–19.
4. Alon, G: Principles of electrical stimulation. In Nelson, RM and Currier, DP (eds): Clinical Electrotherapy. Appleton & Lange, Norwalk, CT, 1987, pp 29–80.
5. Kantor, G, Alon, G, and Ho, HS: The effects of selected stimulus waveforms on pulse and phase characteristics at sensory and motor thresholds. Phys Ther 74:951, 1994.
6. Cook, TM: Instrumentation. In Nelson, RM and Currier, DP (eds): Clinical Electrotherapy. Appleton & Lange, Norwalk, CT, 1987, pp 11–28.
7. Baker, LL: Neuromuscular electrical stimulation in the restoration of purposeful limb movements. In Wolf, SL (ed): Electrotherapy. Churchill Livingstone, New York, 1981, pp 25–48.
8. Urbschait, NL: Review of physiology. In Nelson, RM and Currier, DP (eds): Clinical Electrotherapy. Appleton & Lange, Norwalk, CT, 1987, pp 1–9.
9. Binder, SA: Application of low- and high-voltage electrotherapeutic currents. In Wolf, SL (ed): Electrotherapy. Churchill Livingstone, New York, 1981, pp 1–24.
10. DeVahl, J: Neuromuscular electrical stimulation (NMES) in rehabilitation. In Gersh, MR (ed): Electrotherapy in Rehabilitation. FA Davis, Philadelphia, 1992, pp 218–268.
11. Nolan, MF: Conductive differences in electrodes used with transcutaneous electrical nerve stimulation devices. Phys Ther 71:746, 1991.
12. Lieber, RL and Kelly, MJ: Factors influencing quadriceps femoris muscle torque using transcutaneous neuromuscular stimulation. Phys Ther 71:715, 1991.
13. Alon, G, Kantor, G, and Ho, HS: Effects of electrode size on basic excitatory responses on selected stimulus parameters. J Orthop Sports Phys Ther 20:29, 1994.
14. Gieck, JH and Saliba, EN: The athletic trainer and rehabilitation. In Kuland, DN: The Injured Athlete, ed 2. JB Lippincott, Philadelphia, 1988, pp 165–240.
15. Harris, PR: Iontophoresis: Clinical research in musculoskeletal inflammatory conditions. J Orthop Sports Phys Ther 4:109, 1982.
16. De Domenico, G: Interferential Stimulation (monograph). Chattanooga Group, Chattanooga, TN, 1988.
17. Baker, LL, Bowman, BR, and McNeal, DR: Effects of wave form on comfort during neuromuscular electrical stimulation. Clin Orthop 223:75, 1988.
18. Killian, CB: Electrical Stimulation Overview: Introduction to High Frequency Stimulation. Presented to the Physical Therapy Combined Section Meeting, Orlando, FL, 1985.

19. Lieber, RL, Silva, PD, and Daniel, DM: Equal effectiveness of electrical and volitional strength training for quadriceps femoris muscles after anterior cruciate ligament surgery. J Orthop Res 14:131, 1996.

20. Ferguson, JP, et al: Effects of varying electrode site placements on the torque output of an electrically stimulated involuntary quadriceps femoris muscle contraction. J Orthop Sports Phys Ther 11:24, 1989.

21. Delitto, A and Rose, SJ: Comparative comfort of three wave forms used in electrically eliciting quadriceps femoris muscle contractions. Phys Ther 66:1704, 1986.

22. Miller, CR and Webers, RL: The effects of ice massage on an individual's pain tolerance level to electrical stimulation. J Orthop Sports Phys Ther 12:105, 1990.

23. Durst, JW, et al: Effects of ice and recovery time on maximal involuntary isometric torque production using electrical stimulation. J Orthop Sports Phys Ther 13:240, 1991.

24. Belanger, AY, Allen, ME, and Chapman, AE: Cutaneous versus muscular perception of electrically evoked tetanic pain. J Orthop Sports Phys Ther 16:162, 1992.

25. Singer, K, et al: Electrical modalities. In Drez, D (ed): Therapeutic Modalities for Sports Injuries. Year Book Medical Publishers, Chicago, 1989, p 42.

26. Parker, MG, et al: Fatigue response in human quadriceps femoris muscle during high frequency electrical stimulation. J Orthop Sports Phys Ther 7:145, 1986.

27. Bowman, BR and Baker, LL: Effects of wave form parameters on comfort during transcutaneous neuromuscular electrical stimulation. Ann Biomed Eng 13:59, 1985.

28. Delitto, A and Snyder-Mackler, L: Two theories of muscle strength augmentation using percutaneous electrical stimulation. Phys Ther 70:158, 1990.

29. Miller, C and Thepaut-Mathieu, C: Strength training by electrostimulation conditions for efficacy. Int J Sports Med 14:20, 1993.

30. Trimble, MH and Enoka, RM: Mechanisms underlying the training effects associated with neuromuscular electrical stimulation. Phys Ther 71:273, 1991.

31. Sinacore, DR, et al: Type II fiber activation with electrical stimulation: A preliminary report. Phys Ther 70:416, 1990.

32. Draper, U and Ballard, L: Electrical stimulation versus electromyographic biofeedback in the recovery of quadriceps femoris muscle function following anterior cruciate ligament surgery. Phys Ther 71:455, 1991.

33. Currier, DP and Mann, R: Muscular strength development by electrical stimulation in healthy individuals. Phys Ther 63:915, 1983.

34. Garrison, DW and Foreman, RD: Decreased activity of spontaneous and noxiously evoked dorsal horn cells during transcutaneous electrical nerve stimulation (TENS). Pain 58:309, 1994.

35. Cox, PD, Kramer, JF, and Hartsell, H: Effect of different TENS stimulus parameters on ulnar motor nerve conduction velocity. Am J Phys Med Rehabil 72:294, 1993.

36. Taylor, K, et al: Effects of interferential current stimulation for treatment of subjects with recurrent jaw pain. Phys Ther 67:346, 1987.

37. Longobardi, AG, et al: Effects of auricular transcutaneous electrical nerve stimulation on distal extremity pain. Phys Ther 69:10, 1989.

38. Jensen, JE, et al: The use of transcutaneous neural stimulation and isokinetic testing in arthroscopic knee surgery. Am J Sports Med 13:27, 1985.

39. Lewers, D, et al: Transcutaneous electrical nerve stimulation in the relief of primary dysmenorrhea. Phys Ther 69:3, 1989.

40. Gersh, MR: Transcutaneous electrical nerve stimulation (TENS) for management of pain and sensory pathology. In Gersh, MR (ed): Electrotherapy in Rehabilitation. FA Davis, Philadelphia, 1992, pp 149–196.

41. French, S: Pain: Some psychological and sociological aspects. Physiotherapy 75:255, 1989.

42. Carley, PJ and Wainapel, SF: Electrotherapy for acceleration of wound healing: Low intensity direct current. Arch Phys Med Rehabil 66:443, 1985.

43. Feedar, JA, Kloth, LC, and Gentzkow, GD: Chronic dermal ulcer healing enhanced with monophasic pulsed electrical stimulation. Phys Ther 71:639, 1991.

44. Kloth, LC: Physical modalities in wound management: UVC, therapeutic heating and electrical stimulation. Ostomy Wound Management 41:18, 1995.

45. Falanga, V, et al: Electrical stimulation increases the expression of fibroblast receptors for transforming growth factor-beta (abstract). J Invest Dermatol 88:488, 1987.

46. Gentzkow, GD: Electrical stimulation to heal dermal wounds. Journal of Dermatology, Surgery, and Oncology 19:753, 1993.

47. Reich, JD, et al: The effect of electrical stimulation on the number of mast cells in healing wounds. J Am Acad Dermatol 25:40, 1991.
48. Snyder-Mackler, L: Electrical stimulation for tissue repair. In: Snyder-Mackler, L and Robinson, AJ (eds): Clinical Electrophysiology: Electrotherapy and Electrophysiologic Testing. Williams & Wilkins, Baltimore, 1989, pp 229–244.
49. Kloth, LC and Feedar, JA: Electrical stimulation in tissue repair. In Kloth, LC, McCulloch, JM, and Feedar, JA (eds): Wound Healing: Alternatives in Management. FA Davis, Philadelphia, 1990, pp 221–258.
50. Newton, R: High-voltage pulsed galvanic stimulation: Theoretical bases and clinical application. In Nelson, RM and Currier, DP (eds): Clinical Electrotherapy. Appleton & Lange, Norwalk, CT, 1987, pp 165–182.
51. Hart, FX: Changes in the electric field at an injury site during healing under electrical stimulation. Journal of Bioelectricity 10:33, 1991.
52. Litke, DS and Dahners, LE: Effects of different levels of direct current on early ligament healing in a rat model. J Orthop Res 12:683, 1994.
53. Fujita, M, Hukuda, S, and Doida, Y: The effect of constant direct electrical current on intrinsic healing in the flexor tendon in vitro: An ultrastructural study of differing attitudes in epitendon cells and tenocytes. J Hand Surg [Br] 17:94, 1992.
54. Bettany, JA, Fish, DR, and Mendel, FC: Influence of high voltage pulsed direct current on edema formation following impact injury. Phys Ther 70:219, 1990.
55. Mendel, FC and Fish, DR: New perspectives in edema control via electrical stimulation. Journal of Athletic Training 28:1, 1993.
56. Lilly-Masuda, D and Towne, S: Bioelectricity and bone healing. J Orthop Sports Phys Ther 7:54, 1985.
57. McLeod, KJ and Rubin, CT: The effect of low-frequency electrical fields on osteogenesis. J Bone Joint Surg [Am] 74:920, 1992.
58. Nash, HL and Rogers, CC: Does electricity speed the healing of non-union fractures. Physician and Sportsmedicine 16:156, 1988.
59. Stanish, WD, et al: The use of electricity in ligament and tendon repair. Physician and Sportsmedicine 13:110, 1985.
60. Pepper, JR, et al: Effect of capacitive coupled electrical stimulation on regenerate bone. J Orthop Res 14:296, 1996.
61. Chakkalaka, DA, et al: Electrophysiology of direct current stimulation of fracture healing in canine radius. IEEE Trans Biomed Eng 37:1048, 1990.
62. Newton, RA and Karselis, TC: Skin pH following high voltage pulsed galvanic stimulation. Phys Ther 63:1593, 1983.
63. Mohr, T, et al: The effect of high volt galvanic stimulation on quadriceps femoris muscle torque. J Orthop Sports Phys Ther 7:314, 1986.
64. Balogun, JA, et al: High voltage electrical stimulation in the augmentation of muscle strength: Effects of pulse frequency. Arch Phys Med Rehabil 74:910, 1993.
65. Mohr, T, et al: Comparison of isometric exercise and high volt galvanic stimulation on quadriceps femoris muscle strength. J Orthop Sports Phys Ther 65:606, 1985.
66. Ralston, DJ: High voltage galvanic stimulation: Can there be a "state of the art"? Athletic Training 20:291, 1985.
67. Wolcot, C, et al: A comparison of the effects of high volt and microcurrent stimulation on delayed onset muscle soreness. Phys Ther 71:S117, 1991.
68. Butterfield, DL, et al: The effects of high-volt pulsed current electrical stimulation on delayed-onset muscle soreness. Journal of Athletic Training 32:15, 1997.
69. Reed, BV: Effect of high voltage pulsed electrical stimulation on microvascular permeability to plasma proteins: A possible mechanism in minimizing edema. Phys Ther 68:481, 1988.
70. Taylor, K, et al: Effect of electrically induced muscle contractions on post traumatic edema formation in frog hind limbs. Phys Ther 72:127, 1992.
71. Michlovitz, S, Smith, W, and Watkins, M: Ice and high voltage pulsed stimulation in treatment of lateral ankle sprains. J Orthop Sports Phys Ther 9:301, 1988.
72. Griffin, JW, et al: Reduction of chronic posttraumatic hand edema: A comparison of high voltage pulsed current, intermittent pneumatic compression, and placebo treatments. Phys Ther 70:279, 1990.
73. Mohr, TM, Akers, TK, and Landry, RG: Effect of high voltage stimulation on edema reduction in the rat hind limb. Phys Ther 67:1703, 1987.

74. Taylor, K, et al: Effect of a single 30-minute treatment of high voltage pulsed current on edema formation in frog hind limbs. Phys Ther 72:63, 1992.

75. Fish, DR, et al: Effect of anodal high voltage pulsed current on edema formation in frog hind limbs. Phys Ther 71:724, 1991.

76. Walker, DC, Currier, DP, and Threlkeld, AJ: Effects of high voltage pulsed electrical stimulation on blood flow. Phys Ther 68:481, 1988.

77. Heath, ME and Gibbs, SB: High-voltage pulsed stimulation: Effects of frequency of current on blood flow in the human calf. Clin Sci (Colch) 82:607, 1992.

78. Tracy, JE, Currier, DP, and Threlkeld, AJ: Comparison of selected pulse frequencies from different electrical stimulators on blood flow in healthy subjects. Phys Ther 68:1526, 1988.

79. Agren, MS, Engle, MA, and Mertz, PM: Collagenase during burn wound healing: Influence of a hydrogel dressing and pulsed electrical stimulation. Plast Reconstr Surg 94:518, 1994.

80. Kincaid, CB and Lavoie, KH: Inhibition of bacterial growth in vitro following stimulation with high voltage, monophasic, pulsed current. Phys Ther 69:651, 1989.

81. Fitzgerald, GK and Newsome, D: Treatment of a large infected thoracic spine wound using high voltage pulsed monophasic current. Phys Ther 73:355, 1993.

82. Roeser, WM, et al: The use of transcutaneous nerve stimulation for pain control in athletic medicine. A preliminary report. Am J Sports Med 4:210, 1976.

83. Jette, DU: Effect of different forms of transcutaneous electrical nerve stimulation on experimental pain. Phys Ther 66:187, 1986.

84. Walsh, DM, et al: Transcutaneous electrical nerve stimulation: Relevance of stimulation parameters to neurophysiological and hypoalgesic effects. Am J Phys Med Rehabil 74:199, 1995.

85. Indergand, HJ and Morgan, BJ: Effects of high-frequency transcutaneous electrical nerve stimulation on limb blood flow in healthy humans. Phys Ther 74:361, 1994.

86. Walsh, DM, et al: A double-blind investigation of the hypoalgesic effects of transcutaneous electrical nerve stimulation upon experimentally induced ischaemic pain. Pain 61:39, 1995.

87. Widerström, EG, et al: Relations between experimentally induced tooth pain threshold changes, psychometrics and clinical pain relief following TENS. A retrospective study in patients with long-lasting pain. Pain 51:281, 1992.

88. Marchand, S, Li, J, and Charest J: Letter to the Editor: Effects of caffeine on analgesia from transcutaneous electrical nerve stimulation. N Engl J Med 333:325, 1995.

89. Levin, MF and Hui-Chan, CWY: Conventional and acupuncture-like transcutaneous electrical nerve stimulation excite similar afferent nerves. Arch Phys Med Rehabil 74:54, 1993.

90. Buxton, BP, et al: Self selection of transcutaneous electrical nerve stimulation (TENS) parameters for pain relief in injured athletes (Abstract). Journal of Athletic Training 29:178, 1994.

91. Tulgar, M, et al: Comparative effectiveness of different stimulation modes in relieving pain. I. A pilot study. Pain 47:151, 1991.

92. Tulgar, M, et al: Comparative effectiveness of different stimulation modes in relieving pain. II. A double-blind controlled long-term study. Pain 47:157, 1991.

93. Reib, L and Pomeranz, B: Alterations in electrical pain thresholds by use of acupuncture-like transcutaneous electrical nerve stimulation in pain-free subjects. Phys Ther 72:658, 1992.

94. Bechtel, TB and Fan, PT: When is TENS effective and practical for pain relief? Journal of Musculoskeletal Medicine 2:37, 1985.

95. Ottoson, D and Lundeberg, T: Pain Treatment by Transcutaneous Electrical Nerve Stimulation: A Practical Manual. Springer-Verlag, New York, 1988.

96. Denegar, CR and Huff, CB: High and low frequency TENS in the treatment of induced musculoskeletal pain: A comparison study. Athletic Training 23:235, 1988.

97. Gersh, MR and Wolf, SL: Applications of transcutaneous electrical nerve stimulation in the management of patients with pain. Phys Ther 65:314, 1985.

98. Denegar, CR, et al: Influence of transcutaneous electrical nerve stimulation on pain, range of motion, and serum cortisol concentration in females experiencing delayed onset muscle soreness. J Orthop Sports Phys Ther 11:100, 1989.

99. Paris, DL, Baynes, F, and Gucker, B: Effects of the neuroprobe in the treatment of second-degree ankle sprains. Phys Ther 63:35, 1983.

100. Snyder-Mackler, L: Electrical stimulation for pain modulation. In Snyder-Mackler, L and Robinson, AJ (eds): Clinical Electrophysiology: Electrotherapy and Electrophysiologic Testing. Williams & Wilkins, Baltimore, 1994, pp 205–227.

101. Kloth, LC: Electrotherapeutic alternatives for the treatment of pain. In Gersh, MR (ed): Electrotherapy in Rehabilitation. FA Davis, Philadelphia, 1992, pp 197–217.

102. Chen, XH, Geller, EB, and Adler, MW: Electrical stimulation at traditional acupuncture sites in periphery produces brain opioid-receptor-mediated antinociception in rats. J Pharmacol Exp Ther 227:654, 1996.

103. Nussbaum, E, Rush, P, and Disenhaus, L: The effects of interferential therapy on peripheral blood flow. Physiotherapy 76:803, 1990.

104. Kramer, JF: Effect of electrical stimulation frequencies on isometric knee extension torque. Phys Ther 67:31, 1987.

105. Hobler, CK: Case study: Reduction of chronic posttraumatic knee edema using interferential stimulation. Athletic Training 26:364, 1991.

106. Selkowitz, DM: Improvement in isometric strength of the quadriceps femoris muscle after training with electrical stimulation. Phys Ther 65:186, 1988.

107. Laughman, RK, et al: Strength changes in the normal quadriceps femoris muscle group as a result of electrical stimulation. Phys Ther 63:494, 1983.

108. Snyder-Mackler, L, et al: Strength of the quadriceps femoris muscle and functional recovery after reconstruction of the anterior cruciate ligament: A prospective, randomized clinical trial of electrical stimulation. J Bone Joint Surg Am 77:1166, 1995.

109. Currier, DP, Petrilli, CR, and Threlkeld, JA: Effect of graded electrical stimulation on blood flow to healthy muscle. Phys Ther 66:937, 1986.

110. Liu, H, Currier, DP, and Threlkeld, AJ: Circulatory response of digital arteries associated with electrical stimulation of calf muscle in healthy subjects. Phys Ther 67:340, 1987.

111. Selkowitz, DM: High frequency electrical stimulation in muscle strengthening: A review and discussion. Am J Sports Med 17:103, 1989.

112. Alon, G: "Microcurrent": Subliminal electric stimulation. Does the research support its clinical use? Sports Medicine Update 9:8, 1993.

113. Bertolucci, LE and Grey, T: Clinical comparative study of microcurrent electrical stimulation to mid-laser and placebo treatment in degenerative joint disease of the tempomandibular joint. Craniology 13:116, 1995.

114. Lerner, FN and Kirsch, DL: A double-blind comparative study of microstimulation and placebo effect in short-term treatment of chronic back patients. Journal of the American Chiropractic Association 15:S101, 1981.

115. Byl, NN, et al: Pulsed microamperage stimulation: A controlled study of healing of surgically induced wounds in Yucatan pigs. Phys Ther 74:201, 1994.

116. Leffmann, DL, et al: The effect of subliminal transcutaneous electrical nerve stimulation of the rate of wound healing in rats. Phys Ther 74:195, 1994.

117. Sinnreich, MJ, et al: Microcurrent electrical nerve stimulation (MENS) and coracoacromial arch pain: The effects after one treatment. Phys Ther 72:S68, 1992.

118. Ray, R, et al: Microcurrent therapy versus a placebo for the control of symptoms in mild and moderate acute ankle sprains. Unpublished manuscript, 1996.

119. Weber, MD, Servedio, FJ, and Woodall, WR: The effects of three modalities on delayed onset muscle soreness. J Orthop Sports Phys Ther 20:236, 1994.

120. Cheng, N, et al: The effects of electric currents on ATP generation, protein synthesis, and membrane transport in rat skin. Clin Orthop 171:264, 1982.

121. Becker, RO: The Body Electric. William Morrow, New York, 1985.

122. Becker, RO: Electrical control systems and regenerative growth. Journal of Bioelectricity 1:239, 1982.

123. Windsor, RE, Lester, JP, and Herring, SA: Electrical stimulation in clinical practice. Physician and Sportsmedicine 21:85, 1993.

124. Stromberg, BV: Effects of electrical currents on wound contraction. Ann Plast Surg 21:121, 1988.

125. Swadlow, HA: Monitoring the excitability of neocortical efferent neurons to direct activation by extracellular current pulses. J Neurophysiol 68:605, 1992.

126. Pubols, LM: Characteristics of dorsal horn neurons expressing subliminal responses to sural nerve stimulation. Somatosens Mot Res 7:137, 1990.

127. Hasson, SH, et al: Exercise training and dexamethesone iontophoresis in rheumatoid arthritis: A case study. Physiotherapy Canada 43:11, 1991.

128. Glass, JM, Stephen, RL, and Jacobson, SC: The quantity and distribution of radiolabeled dexamethasone delivered to tissue by iontophoresis. Int J Dermatol 19:519, 1980.

129. Henley, EJ: Transcutaneous drug delivery: Iontophoresis, phonophoresis. Physical and Rehabilitation Medicine 2:139, 1991.

130. Zeltzer, L, et al: Iontophoresis versus subcutaneous injection: A comparison of two methods of local anesthesia delivery in children. Pain 44:73, 1991.

131. Nimmo, WS: Novel delivery systems: Electrotransport. J Pain Symptom Manage 8:160, 1992.
132. Bertolucci, LE: Introduction of antiinflammatory drugs by iontophoresis: A double blind study. J Orthop Sport Phys Ther 4:103, 1982.
133. Scott, ER, et al: Transport of ionic species in skin: Contribution of pores to the overall skin conductance. Pharmacol Res 10:1699, 1993.
134. Bogner, RB and Ajay, KM: Iontophoresis and phonophoresis. US Pharmacist, August, 1994, p H-10.
135. Kalia, YN and Guy, RH: The electrical characteristics of human skin in vivo. Pharmacol Res 12:1605, 1995.
136. Pikal, MJ and Shah, S: Transport mechanisms in iontophoresis. II. Electroosmotic flow and the transference number measurements for hairless mouse skin. Pharmacol Res 7:213, 1990.
137. Inada, H, Ghanem, AH, and Higuchi, WI: Studies on the effects of applied voltage and duration on the human epidural membrane alteration/recovery and the resultant effects upon iontophoresis. Pharmacol Res 11:687, 1994.
138. Grossmann, M, et al: The effect of iontophoresis on the cutaneous vasculature: Evidence for current-induced hyperemia. Microvasc Res 50:444, 1995.
139. Howard, JP, Drake, TR, and Kellogg, DL: Effects of alternating current iontophoresis on drug delivery. Arch Phys Med Rehabil 76:463, 1995.
140. Reinauer, S, et al: Iontophoresis with alternating current and direct current offset (AC/DC iontophoresis): A new approach for the treatment of hyperhydrosis. Br J Dermatol 129:166, 1993.
141. Oshima, T, et al: Cutaneous iontophoresis application of condensed lidocaine. Can J Anaesth 41:667, 1994.
142. Wieder, DL: Treatment of traumatic myositis ossificans with acetic acid iontophoresis. Phys Ther 72:133, 1992.
143. Berlant, SR: Method of determining optimal stimulation sites for transcutaneous electrical nerve stimulation. Phys Ther 64:924, 1984.
144. Davson, H: A Textbook of General Physiology, vol 2, ed 4. Williams & Wilkins, Baltimore, 1970.
145. Griffin, JE and Karselis, TC: Physical Agents for Physical Therapists, ed 2. Charles C Thomas, Springfield, IL, 1988.

CHAPTER 6

Ultrasound

Ultrasound is presented in this chapter rather than in the thermal agents chapter because of its presence on the acoustical spectrum rather than on the electromagnetic spectrum. In addition, ultrasound is capable of producing mechanical, nonthermal effects in addition to its thermal properties.

Ultrasound is a deep penetrating modality capable of producing changes in tissue through both thermal and nonthermal (mechanical) mechanisms (Fig. 6–1). Unlike most other electrically driven modalities, ultrasonic energy is not a part of the electromagnetic spectrum but is located on the acoustical spectrum (Box 6–1). Depending on the frequency of the waves, ultrasound is used for diagnostic imaging, therapeutic tissue healing, or tissue destruction. This chapter focuses on its therapeutic effects. Many textbooks place the discussion of ultrasound in the section on thermal agents, but it is addressed separately in this text to reinforce the fact that its application results in both thermal and nonthermal effects. Although ultrasound can increase subcutaneous tissue temperature, it is not necessarily interchangeable with other forms of thermotherapy.

Traditionally, therapeutic ultrasound has been used in sports medicine primarily for its deep-heating effects, but the actual range of biophysiological effects is the property that makes ultrasound such a potentially useful modality. Depending on the output parameters, effects of ultrasound application can include increased rate of tissue repair and wound healing, increased blood flow, increased tissue extensibility, breakdown of calcium deposits, reduction of pain and muscle spasm through alteration of nerve conduction velocities, and changes in cell membrane permeability (Table 6–1). Ultrasonic energy is also used to deliver medications to the subcutaneous tissues and to assist in fracture healing.

The human ear is capable of hearing sound waves ranging from 16 to 20,000 Hz. Any sound wave above this range is considered ultrasound (Box 6–2). Therapeutic ultrasound ranges from 750,000 to 3,000,000 Hz (0.75 to 3 MHz). In the United States, the most frequently used ultrasound frequencies are 1 and 3 MHz.

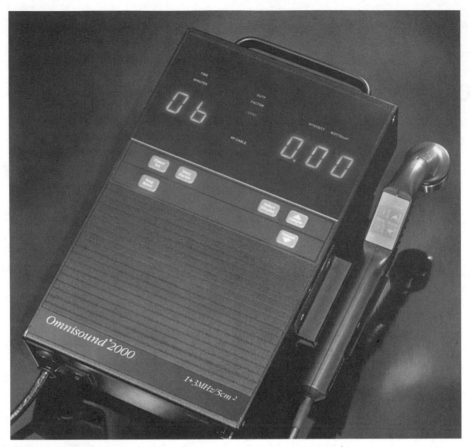

FIGURE 6–1 **An Ultrasound Unit Having a Sound Head Capable of Delivering Output at 1 MHz or 3 MHz.** (The Ominisound 2000, courtesy of PTI, Topeka, KS.)

PRODUCTION OF ULTRASOUND

Ultrasound is produced by an alternating current flowing through a piezoelectric crystal, such as quartz, barium titanate, lead zirconate, or titanate, housed in a *transducer*. Synthetic crystals have replaced natural ones, yielding a better, more consistent field of energy. Experimental work has begun on the development of a laser-driven ultrasound generator, potentially providing a more precise and more flexible ultrasonic output.[1]

Piezoelectric crystals produce positive and negative electrical charges when they contract or expand (Fig. 6–2). A reverse (indirect) piezoelectric effect occurs when an alternating current is passed through a piezoelectric crystal, resulting in contraction and expansion of the crystals. Ultrasound is produced through the reverse piezoelectric effect. The vibration of the crystals results in the mechanical production of high-frequency sound waves.

Transducer: A device that converts one form of energy to another.

BOX 6–1 **The Acoustical Spectrum**

The transmission of acoustical energy varies greatly from the transmission of electromagnetic energy. Although electromagnetic energy is capable of being transmitted through a complete vacuum, transmission of acoustical energy requires a medium and the denser the medium the better. Electromagnetic radiation involves the transmission of individual particles that prefer not to be hindered by a medium. The sun emits a particle of light that travels unhindered through the vast void of space. This particle stays in motion until it strikes a differing density, such as the earth or the earth's atmosphere.

In a uniform environment, sound travels at a constant speed, at which the velocity is calculated as: Velocity = Frequency × Wavelength. For sounds of different frequencies to travel at the same speed, their wavelengths must be different. Shorter wavelengths must have a higher frequency to match the velocity of longer wavelengths. This concept may be visualized by picturing two people walking side by side. One of these people is 7 feet tall and has a stride length of 3 feet. The other is 5 feet tall and has a stride length of 1.5 feet. After traveling 90 feet, the taller person has taken 30 steps; the shorter has taken 60 steps. In contrast to the emission of individual particles, acoustical energy is transmitted by mechanical waves (vibration) that deform the medium. Therefore, the transmission of acoustical energy is impossible in the vacuum of space. If you yell at a person across the street, your voice causes a deformation in the air. This wave travels through the air and is received by the other person's ear. The acoustical and electromagnetic spectra do share common features. Like electromagnetic energy, acoustical energy is capable of being reflected, refracted, and absorbed.

TABLE 6–1 **Ultrasound Output Parameters and Measures**

Parameter	Description
Beam nonuniformity ratio (BNR)	The BNR describes the consistency (uniformity) of the ultrasound output as a ratio. The lower the ratio, the more uniform the beam. A BNR greater than 8:1 is considered unsafe.
Duty cycle	A 100% duty cycle indicates a constant ultrasound output and results in primarily thermal effects within the body. A low duty cycle produces nonthermal effects.
Effective radiating area (ERA)	The area of the sound head that produces ultrasonic waves. Measured in square centimeters.
Frequency	The frequency determines the effective depth of penetration. A 1-MHz output targets tissues up to 5 cm deep; 3 MHz has a penetrating depth of 2 cm.
Intensity	The intensity describes the amount of power generated by unit.
Spatial average intensity (SAI)	Measured in watts per square centimeter, the SAI describes the amount of power per unit area of the sound head's ERA.
Time average intensity (TAI)	Only meaningful when delivering pulsed ultrasound, the TAI describes the average amount of energy delivered per second.
Treatment duration	The treatment duration is determined by the output intensity and the specific goals of the treatment.

BOX 6–2 **Contrast and Comparison of Ultrasound and Audible Sound**

The way in which piezoelectric crystals produce ultrasound bears some striking similarities to the way in which a stereo produces audible sound. When a stereo plays music, it detects the patterns of recorded sound impulses. These patterns are converted to electrical energy that is transferred to a speaker. Once the energy reaches the speaker, it activates a magnet, causing a cone to expand and contract. The vibration of the cone produces mechanical waves that are transmitted through the air and subsequently strike our eardrums.

Ultrasound generators operate on basically the same principle. An alternating current is passed through a crystal, causing it to expand and contract. The vibration of this crystal produces mechanical waves that are passed along to the body.

The difference between the production of these two sound waves lies in the frequency at which the "speaker" vibrates. Stereos use a much lower frequency than ultrasound, so the waves can be transmitted through air and detected by the human ear. Ultrasound units use such a high frequency so that the waves cannot be transmitted without the use of a dense medium and cannot be detected by the human ear.

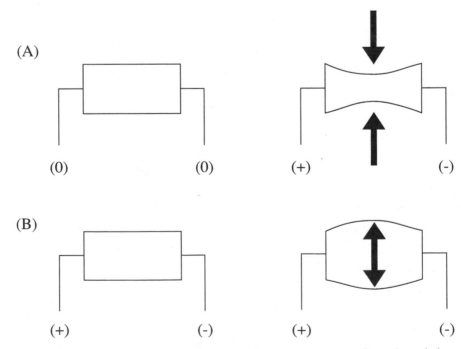

FIGURE 6–2 Piezoelectric Crystals. (*A*) The direct piezoelectric effect. Crystals possessing piezoelectric properties produce positive and negative electrical charges when they are compressed or expanded. (*B*) The reverse (indirect) piezoelectric effect. These same crystals expand and contract when an electrical current is passed through them.

TRANSMISSION OF ULTRASOUND WAVES

Because of the high frequencies involved, ultrasound requires a dense medium through which to travel and therefore is unable to pass through the air. Ultrasound has a sinusoidal waveform and displays the properties of wavelength, frequency, amplitude, and velocity (see Box 6–1).

Wave energy is transferred by one molecule jostling against its neighbor and exchanging kinetic energy without the actual displacement of molecules. Consider a leaf floating in a pond. If a pebble is dropped near it, the leaf bobs up and down as the ripples pass beneath it but does not change its position.

Longitudinal Waves

Particle displacement in longitudinal waves takes place parallel to the direction of the sound. A person dangling from the end of a bungee cord is an example of longitudinal waves. Longitudinal waves result in the elongation and contraction of the cord, causing the jumper to bob up and down. In this case the energy, as represented by the jumper, is transmitted parallel to the direction of the wave.

The alternation of high and low pressure exerted by the ultrasound beam results in regions of high particle density (compression) and low particle density (rarefaction) along the path of the wave (Fig. 6–3). These pressure fluctuations transmit the energy within the tissues and, as discussed in subsequent sections, produce physiological effects. Longitudinal waves are capable of traveling through both solid and liquid media, and ultrasound passes through soft tissue in this form.

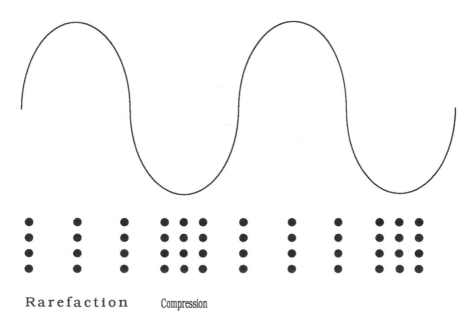

Rarefaction   Compression

FIGURE 6–3 **Rarefaction and Compression of Molecules.** An ultrasound wave passing through the tissues creates alternating periods of low and high pressure. Molecules in the low-pressure areas expand (rarefaction) and molecules in the high pressure area compress.

Transverse (Shear) Waves

Particles in transverse waves are displaced perpendicular to the direction of the sound wave. A vibrating guitar string is an example of this type of wave. Plucking a guitar string causes it to vibrate parallel to its length. Transverse waves cannot pass through fluids and are found in the body only when ultrasound strikes bone.

THE ULTRASOUND WAVE

Low-frequency sound waves, such as those produced by human speech, diverge in all directions, making it possible to hear the voice of a person behind you. The more the frequency of the sound wave increases, the less the sound beam diverges.[2] The frequencies used in therapeutic ultrasound produce cylindrical beams that have a width somewhat smaller than the diameter of the sound head. Like all sound waves, ultrasound waves are capable of reflection, refraction, penetration, and absorption (Box 6–3).

As ultrasound waves travel through a medium, there is some degree of divergence, but it is not as pronounced as sound waves within the range of human hearing. Consider the difference between a beam of light produced by a spotlight and the light produced by an ordinary light bulb. If the spotlight and lamp were held 1 foot from a wall, the spotlight would concentrate the light within an area approximately the same diameter as the lens. The light produced from the bare bulb would illuminate an area significantly larger than the bulb itself. As the distance between each source of light and the wall is increased, the diameter of each beam would increase, but much more so with the bare bulb than with the spotlight. Likewise, the treatment area effectively exposed to the ultrasonic energy is limited to the diameter of the sound head.

Close to the transducer head, the pressure of the sound field is nonuniform, forming peaks of high intensity and valleys of low intensity (Fig. 6–4). This area, the **near field,** is the portion of the ultrasound beam used for therapeutic purposes. The pressure variations occur because the transducer head acts as if it were made up of many smaller heads, each producing its own sound wave. Close to the transducer, these areas are individually distinguishable. As the distance from the head is increased, the waves begin to interact to produce a more unified beam. An example of this can be found in a television set. If you look very closely at the screen, individual colored elements are seen. As the distance between your eye and the screen is increased, the dots lose their individuality and a complete picture is formed.

Ultrasound heads are available in different sizes and with different crystal *resonating* frequencies (Fig. 6–5). Each transducer head must be labeled with its frequency, effective radiating area, and the beam nonuniformity ratio (covered later). Large-diameter heads produce a beam that is more *collimated,* whereas smaller ultrasound heads yield a more divergent beam. Low-frequency (1 MHz) ultrasound has a beam that diverges more than high-frequency (3 MHz) ultrasound.

Resonating: Vibrating.
Collimated: Possessing a beam of parallel rays or waves that form a column of energy.

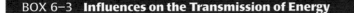

BOX 6–3 **Influences on the Transmission of Energy**

Reflection	Refraction	Absorption

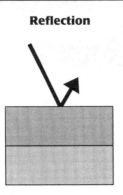 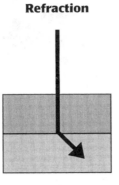 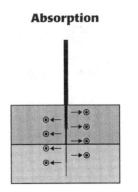

Reflection occurs when the wave cannot pass through the next density. The wave strikes the object and reverses its direction away from the material. Reflection may be complete, as when all energy is precluded from entering the next density layer, or it may be partial. An echo is an example of reflection that involves acoustical energy.

Refraction is the bending of waves as a result of a change in the speed of a wave as it enters a medium of different density. When the energy leaves a dense layer and enters a less dense layer, its speed increases. When moving from a low-density to a high-density layer, the energy decreases. A prism refracts light rays. As the light is bent within the prism, the velocity of the light slows to the point at which each of the seven color bands becomes visible.

Absorption occurs through the medium collecting the wave and changing it into kinetic energy. The tissues may absorb part or all of the energy being delivered to the tissue. Any energy not reflected or absorbed by one tissue layer continues to pass through the tissue until it strikes another density layer. At this point, it may again be reflected, refracted, absorbed, or passed on to the next tissue layer. Each time the wave is partially reflected, refracted, or absorbed, the remaining energy available to deeper tissue is reduced.

Most energy prefers to travel in a straight line. However, when traveling through a medium, its course is influenced by changes in density. Energy striking the interface between two different densities may be reflected, refracted, or absorbed by the material, or continue through the material unaffected by the change.

The effective radiating area (ERA) of the ultrasound head represents the portion of the transducer's surface area that actually produces ultrasound waves. Measured 5 mm from the face of the sound head, the ERA represents all areas producing more than 5 percent of the maximum power output of the transducer. Based on this calculation, the ERA is always of lesser area than the actual size of the sound head.[3]

Frequency

The output frequency of an ultrasound generator is measured in megahertz (MHz) and describes the number of waves occurring in 1 second. Often, chang-

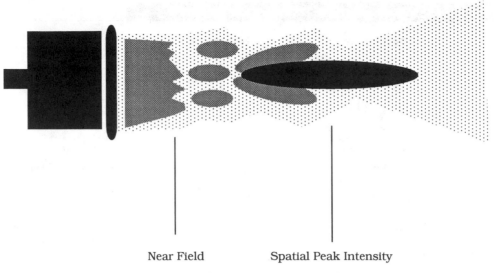

Near Field   Spatial Peak Intensity

FIGURE 6–4   **A Schematic Representation of an Ultrasound Beam.** Note the irregular intensity of the near field and the spatial peak intensity.

ing the output frequency requires changing the sound head (see Fig. 6–5). Some units have transducers that are capable of delivering output of varying frequencies through the same crystal (see Fig. 6–1). Each crystal is calibrated to its generator, so do not attempt to replace the sound head on units that are not specifically designed to do so.

The output frequency of the ultrasound determines the energy's depth of penetration, with a linear correlation between the frequency of the ultrasound and the

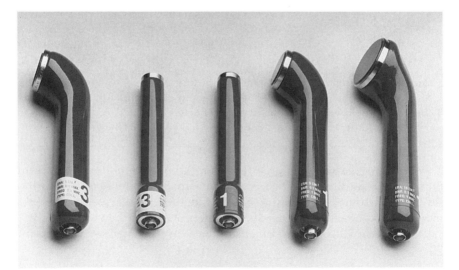

FIGURE 6–5   **Variety of Ultrasound Heads.** Ultrasonic transducers are available in a range of sizes and frequencies. Note the labels indicating the effective radiating area (ERA), beam nonuniformity ratio (BNR), and frequency (1 or 3 MHz). (Courtesy of Mettler Electronics Corporation, Inc., Anaheim, CA.)

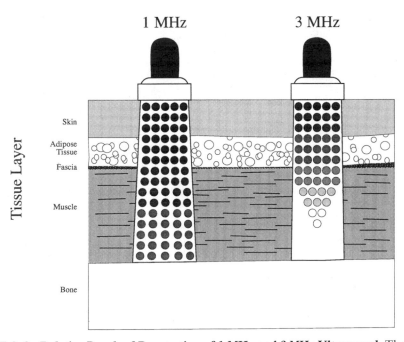

FIGURE 6–6 **Relative Depth of Penetration of 1-MHz and 3-MHz Ultrasound.** The effects of 1-MHz ultrasound occur more deeply within the tissues than 3-MHz ultrasound, which attenuates in the superficial tissues. Note that the 1-MHz beam has a greater degree of divergence than the 3-MHz beam. The actual depth of penetration is based on the half-layer value of the ultrasonic energy.

tissue depth at which energy is absorbed.[4] The rate of absorption, and therefore attenuation, increases as the frequency of the ultrasound is increased because of the molecular friction that the sound waves must overcome in order to pass through the tissues.[5] Because of this, less energy is available to pass deeper into the tissues.[2]

High-frequency (3 MHz) ultrasound generators provide treatment to superficial tissues because the energy is rapidly absorbed (Fig. 6–6). The commonly used 1-MHz generator offers a compromise between deep penetration and adequate heating because of the relatively low frequency used.[2]

Power and Intensity

The power produced by an ultrasound generator is measured in watts (W) and represents the amount of energy being produced by the transducer. Intensity describes the strength of the sound waves at a given location within the tissues being treated. There are two primary measures of intensity: the spatial average intensity and the temporal (time) average intensity.

Another important measure of the amount of ultrasonic energy produced by the generator is the **half-layer value.** This describes the depth at which 50 percent of the ultrasonic energy has been absorbed by the tissues. If ultrasound is applied at 1 W/cm² and loses 50 percent of its energy at a depth of 2.3 cm, the beam intensity is now 0.5 W/cm². At twice this depth (4.6 cm), the ultrasound intensity is reduced to 0.25 W/cm².[6] The effect of the half-layer value, coupled with the penetrating effects of 1- and 3-MHz output frequencies, should be kept in mind when attempting to target deep tissues (e.g., use 1-MHz ultrasound for deep structures).

Spatial Average Intensity

Spatial average intensity (SAI) describes the amount of energy passing through a specified area, in this case, the area of the sound head (the ERA). Expressed in watts per square centimeter (W/cm²), the SAI provides a measure of the power per unit area of the sound head. This value is calculated by dividing the power of the output (watts) by the ERA of the transducer head (square centimeters). For example, if 10 W were being delivered through a transducer head with an ERA of 5 cm², the spatial average intensity would be 2 W per square centimeter.

Ultrasonic generators can express their output as either total watts or watts per square centimeter. Standard treatment doses range from 0.5 to 5 watts per square centimeter. If the radiating area of the sound head is smaller than specified, or if a portion of the sound head is obstructed from transmitting sound, a higher spatial average intensity is produced than that indicated on the meter.

As seen with electrical current density, altering the size of the sound head affects the power density. Passing 10 W of energy through a transducer of 10 cm² results in a lower density than if a head of 5 cm² is used (Table 6–2).

Temporal Average Intensity

Temporal average intensity measures the power of ultrasonic energy delivered to the tissues over a given period and is meaningful only for the application of pulsed ultrasound. The energy delivered to the tissues per unit time with ultrasound operating at a 50 percent duty cycle is half of that delivered in a continuous mode. If we take a spatial average intensity of 2 W per square centimeter and pulse it with a 50 percent duty cycle, the temporal average density of the treatment would be 1 W per square centimeter (2 W/cm² × 0.5 = 1 W/cm²). It is important to distinguish between the temporal average intensity, the average amount of power delivered during a single cycle, and the temporal peak intensity, the maximum amount of energy delivered by a single pulse (Fig. 6–7).

Ultrasound Beam Nonuniformity

The degree to which the intensity within the ultrasound beam varies is measured by the beam nonuniformity ratio (BNR). This is the ratio of the highest intensity

TABLE 6–2   **Effect of Ultrasound Radiating Area on the Total Amount of Energy Produced**

Intensity (W/cm²)	Effective Radiating Area (ERA) of the Sound Head (cm²)	Total Power Produced (W)
1.5	5	7.5
1.5	6	9.0
1.5	10	15.0

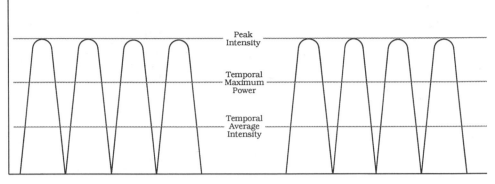

FIGURE 6–7 **Peak Intensity, Temporal Maximum Power, and Temporal Average Intensity of a Pulsed Ultrasound Beam.** The peak intensity represents the amplitude of a single wave. The temporal maximum power is the average amount of energy delivered by a single pulse. The temporal average intensity is the average amount of energy delivered to the tissues during the application of pulsed ultrasound.

within the beam, the spatial peak intensity (Fig. 6–8), to the average intensity reported on the output meter. The optimal, though clinically unobtainable, BNR is 1:1, a BNR greater than 8:1 may be considered unacceptable. The Food and Drug Administration (FDA) requires that the BNR must be indicated on the ultrasound unit.[7]

If the BNR is indicated as 3:1 and the meter displays an output of 2 W per square centimeter, then at some point in the beam the actual intensity is 6 W per centimeter squared (3 × 2 W = 6 W). The existence of high-intensity areas in the beam, "hot spots," is the primary reason for keeping the sound head moving during the treatment.

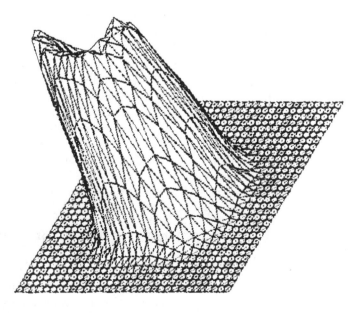

FIGURE 6–8 **Ultrasound Beam Profile.** This topographical map of an ultrasound beam was plotted from the intensities produced from various points on the transducer. The peak on the left side represents the beam's peak intensity. (Courtesy of IAPT. Used with permission.)

TABLE 6–3 **Rate of Ultrasound Heating per Minute Based on a Treatment Area Two to Three Times the Effective Radiating Area**

Intensity (W/cm²) Tissue Depth	1 MHz 5 cm	3 MHz 1.2 cm
0.5	0.04°C	0.3°C
1.0	0.2°C	0.6°C
1.5	0.3°C	0.9°C
2.0	0.4°C	1.4°C

Source: Adapted from Draper and Ricard.[19]

Treatment Duration

The length of the treatment depends on the size of the area being treated, the output intensity, and the therapeutic goals of the treatment. In all circumstances, the area for any particular treatment should be no larger than two to three times the surface area of the sound head's ERA.[3] Rather than attempting to treat a large area during a single ultrasound administration, the area can be divided into smaller treatment zones.

When vigorous heating effects are desired, the treatment duration should be in the range of 10 to 12 minutes for 1-MHz output and 3 to 4 minutes for 3-MHz ultrasound.[3] Table 6–3 should be used as a guide for determining the actual treatment duration based on the frequency of the ultrasound being applied and the goals of the treatment. Ultrasound treatments are generally delivered for a 10- to 14-day period, at which time the efficacy of the treatment approach is re-evaluated.

Dose-Oriented Treatments

As previously discussed, the amount of temperature increase is based on the output intensity and the treatment duration (see Table 6–3). Although this method of determining treatment dosage has traditionally been used with ultrasound, it is at best an inexact technique. The body area being treated and the depth of the target tissue, the ultrasound unit's BNR, the duty cycle, and even the coupling medium used influence the rate and degree of temperature increase.

Improvements in the quality of ultrasound generators, microprocessors, and research regarding the heating effects of ultrasound have led to the development of dose-oriented treatment parameters. Here the clinician indicates the desired amount of temperature increase and the characteristics of the target tissues. The ultrasound unit then calculates the best parameters for the treatment. The clinician may still adjust the treatment intensity, but the treatment duration would change inversely. Decreasing the intensity would increase the duration and vice versa.

TRANSFER OF ULTRASOUND THROUGH THE TISSUES

Ultrasound passes through soft tissue in the form of longitudinal waves until it strikes bone, when some of the energy is reflected and the rest is converted into transverse waves. The propagation of ultrasonic energy depends on the frequency

TABLE 6–4 **Percent Reflection of Ultrasonic Energy at Various Interfaces**

Interface	Energy Reflected (%)
Water–Soft tissue	0.2
Soft tissue–Fat	1
Soft tissue–Bone	15–40
Soft tissue–Air	99.9

Source: Adapted from Williams,[10] p 113.

of the sound waves and the density of the tissues. Passage of ultrasound through the body causes the tissues to acquire kinetic energy, resulting in cellular vibration.

When the ultrasound beam strikes an *acoustical interface* (such as different tissue layers), some of the energy is reflected or refracted. The amount of reflection depends on the degree of change in density at the junction between the two tissues (Table 6–4). Ultrasound meeting with air produces almost total reflection of the energy. The interface between soft tissue and bone is also highly reflective. Other highly reflective interfaces include the musculotendinous junction and intermuscular interfaces. Unlike infrared energy, ultrasound is not greatly affected by adipose tissue and easily passes through it.[8]

If a reflected wave meets the incoming incident wave, a *standing wave* is created, increasing the intensity of the energy by creating areas of high and low pressure. Free-floating gas bubbles move toward the low-pressure areas, whereas freely moving cells collect at the high-pressure centers.[9] Because of this, a high level of energy is formed in a limited amount of space, increasing the risk of tissue damage. Standing waves can be avoided by keeping the sound head moving.

Reflecting intense ultrasonic energy off bone can produce periosteal pain (a deep-seated burning or aching), an unwanted effect. Caution must be used when applying ultrasound to areas having bony protuberances, such as the elbow's olecranon process. The intensity used to treat the muscle or tendon can produce periosteal pain if applied over these protuberances.

Any energy not reflected or absorbed is passed on to the underlying tissues (see Law of Grotthus-Draper, Appendix B). The intensity of ultrasonic energy decreases as the distance it travels through the tissues increases. This process, attenuation, occurs through the scattering and absorption of the waves within the tissues. Absorption of the sound waves transfers energy from the beam into the surrounding tissues through conversion of mechanical energy into thermal energy. The amount of absorption that occurs depends on the protein content of the tissues (especially collagen). Tissues such as bone, cartilage, and tendon absorb much more ultrasonic energy than muscle, fat, or blood.[2] Ultrasound tends to reflect as it strikes bone and refract as it passes through joint spaces.[8]

Acoustical interface: A surface where two materials of different densities meet.

Standing wave: A single-frequency wave formed by the collision of two waves of equal frequency and speed traveling in opposite directions. The energy with a standing wave cannot be transmitted from one area to another and is focused in a confined area.

MODES OF ULTRASOUND APPLICATION

As we learned in the first few paragraphs of this chapter, depending on the type of output therapeutic ultrasound is capable of producing thermal or nonthermal physiological changes within the body's tissues. Continuous (100 percent) output causes primarily thermal effects, whereas the application of low pulses (e.g., 20 percent) primarily produces nonthermal effects. Based on this range of effects, the injury being treated should be thoroughly evaluated to determine the stage of healing, inflamma-

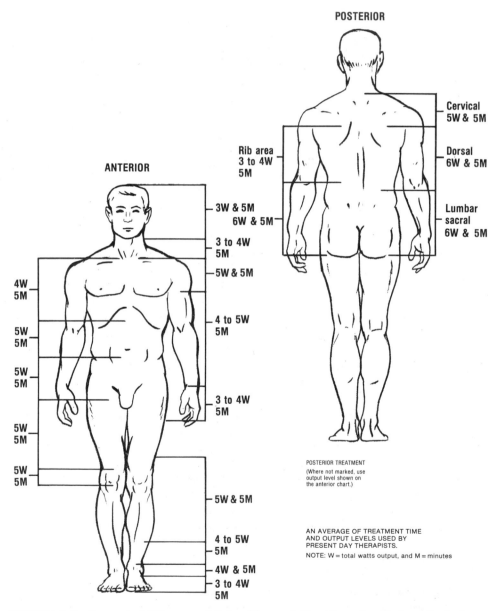

FIGURE 6–9 **Suggested Ultrasound Intensities and Durations for Various Body Areas.** The duration of the treatment depends on the desired physiological outcomes and the intensities used during the treatment.

tory state, and therapeutic goals of the treatment. With this information, the proper duty cycle, duration, and intensity for the treatment can be established.

Continuous Output

Continuous ultrasound application can effectively heat tissues located 5 (or more) cm deep, depending on the frequency used. Because the output is being delivered 100 percent of the time, the ultrasonic energy is measured in terms of the spatial average intensity (watts per square centimeter). The spatial peak intensity, as determined by the BNR, should not be allowed to exceed 8 W per square centimeter (metered output × BNR).

Pulsed Output

Pulsing the ultrasound beam decreases the temporal average intensity of the output, reducing the thermal effects while still allowing for the nonthermal effects of ultrasound. The ratio between the pulse length and the pulse interval is expressed as a percentage duty cycle:

$$\text{Duty cycle} = \frac{\text{Pulse length}}{(\text{Pulse length} + \text{Pulse interval})} \times 100$$

The closer the duty cycle is to 100 percent, the greater the net thermal effects of the treatment; lower duty cycles produce greater proportions of nonthermal effects, although a proportion of thermal and nonthermal effects occur at all duty cycles. The output of pulsed ultrasound is measured by the temporal maximal intensity, but the actual amount of energy delivered to the tissue is dependent on the duty cycle. The average treatment doses are presented in Figure 6–9. Note that this chart indicates the output in terms of total watts.

COUPLING AGENTS AND METHODS

Ultrasonic waves cannot pass through the air; a coupling agent must be used to allow the waves to pass out of the transducer into the tissues. A good medium is characterized by the ability to transmit a significant percentage of the ultrasound; therefore, it should be nonreflective. The optimal medium for transmission is distilled water, which reflects only 0.2 percent of the energy.[10]

Attempting to pass ultrasound through a nonconductive medium can damage the crystal. For this reason, only approved conducting agents should be used, and the intensity of the unit should not be increased without the sound head in proper contact with the body. When large, regularly shaped body areas (such as the quadriceps group) are being treated, proper coupling is relatively easy. However, irregularly shaped areas decrease the contact area between the transducer and the skin, causing uneven amounts of energy to be delivered to the tissues, and therefore require modified coupling methods.

Most modern ultrasound generators automatically shut down if application is attempted without a medium, if an unacceptable medium is used, or if sufficient contact is not made with the skin. Operating an improperly coupled ultrasound head causes its temperature to increase. Many generators have a built-in thermostat that shuts down the unit if a predetermined temperature is exceeded.

Direct Coupling

In this method of ultrasound application, the transducer is applied directly to the skin, with a gel serving to exclude air between the skin and the sound head. Coupling gels consist of distilled water and an inert, nonreflective material that increases the viscosity of the mixture. This gel should be applied liberally to the area to ensure that a consistent coat with no large air bubbles is available throughout the treatment. Not all substances efficiently transfer the ultrasonic energy from the transducer to the tissues, and many block the energy all together. For this reason, only approved transmission media should be used (Table 6–5).

The effectiveness of gels is decreased if the body part is hairy or irregularly shaped. Each of these conditions can increase the spatial average intensity by decreasing the contact area between the transducer and the tissues. The application of gels causes air bubbles to cling to hair. The greater amount of hair on the body part, the greater the reduction of ultrasound delivered to the tissues. Consideration should be given to shaving the treatment area if body hair is excessive. Every effort should be made to eliminate these bubbles while spreading on the coupling agent.

Firm, constant pressure should be used to hold the sound head in contact with the skin.[11] Too little pressure creates an insufficient couple, whereas too much pressure decreases the amount of energy transferred to the tissues, and the pressure may cause the patient discomfort. The use of 0.44 to 1.32 pounds of pressure has been recommended.[11]

Water Immersion

When treating irregularly shaped areas such as the distal extremities, a more uniform dose of ultrasound can be given using water as the transmission medium.

TABLE 6–5   **Coupling Ability of Potential Ultrasound Media**

Substance	Transmission Relative to Water (%)
Saran Wrap	98
Lidex gel, fluocinonide 0.05%	97
Thera-gesic cream, methyl salicylate	97
Mineral oil	97
Ultrasound transmission gel	96
Ultrasound transmission lotion	90
Chempad-L	68
Hydrocortisone powder (1%) in US gel	29
Hydrocortisone powder (10%) in US gel	7
Eucerine cream	0
Myoflex cream, trolamine salicylate 10%	0
White petrolatum gel	0

Source: Adapted from Cameron and Monroe,[42] with permission
US = ultrasound.

The body part is immersed in a tub of water (*degassed water* is the ideal medium but is seldom used). The transducer is then placed in the water with the sound head facing the body part approximately 1 inch away (Fig. 6–10). The operator's hand should not be immersed in the water. Although this is not necessarily dangerous in a single treatment, immersion could unnecessarily expose the hand to ultrasonic energy over repeated exposures.

The use of a ceramic tub for underwater ultrasound application has been recommended.[10] The ceramic sides make an excellent reflective surface, creating an "echo chamber" that allows the sound waves to strike the body part from all angles. If nondistilled water is being used, the intensity of the ultrasound can be increased by approximately 0.5 W per square centimeter to account for attenuation caused by air and minerals in the water. Tap water immersion, using ultrasound delivered at 3 MHz, is less effective in increasing subcutaneous tissue temperatures than the direct coupling method.[12]

Bladder Method

This technique typically uses a water-filled balloon or plastic bag (bladder) coated with a coupling gel. The bladder can conform to irregularly shaped areas such as

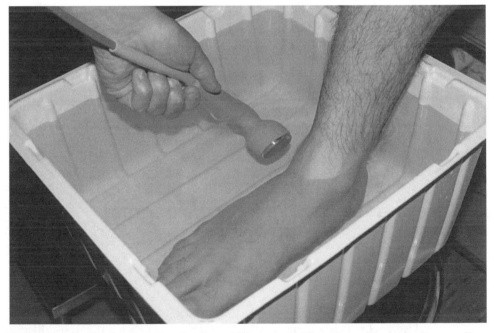

FIGURE 6–10   **Underwater Application of Ultrasound.** Water is used as a coupling medium to evenly distribute the energy over irregularly shaped areas. The sound head does not come into contact with the body part.

Degassed water: Water that has been allowed to sit undisturbed for 4 to 24 hours, allowing the gaseous bubbles to escape.

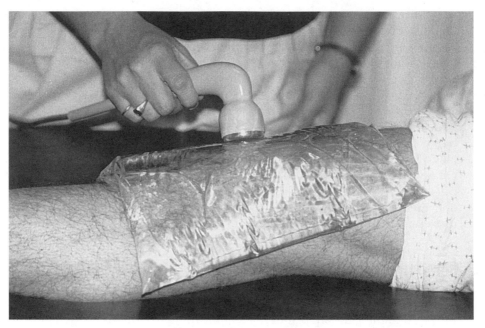

FIGURE 6–11 **Ultrasound Application Using the Bladder Coupling Method.** This method is used to deliver ultrasound to irregularly shaped areas when the underwater area is not practical.

the acromioclavicular or talocrural joints (Fig. 6–11). After a transmission medium has been applied to the skin, the bladder is held against the body part and the sound applicator is moved over the gel-coated bladder. Because balloons are relatively fragile, condoms may be used.

Regardless of the type of bladder used, all air pockets must be removed before sealing. If the ultrasound wave comes into contact with a large air pocket, the energy will not be transmitted.

BIOPHYSICAL EFFECTS OF ULTRASOUND APPLICATION

The physiological changes within the tissues associated with ultrasound application can be grouped into two classifications, and some overlap exists between the two (Table 6–6):

- Nonthermal effects: changes within the tissues resulting from the mechanical effect of ultrasonic energy
- Thermal effects: changes within the tissues as a direct result of ultrasound's elevation of the tissue temperature

Thermal and nonthermal effects are not exclusive of each other. Both effects occur within the body, but the proportion and magnitude of each are based on the duty cycle and the output intensity. The higher the duty cycle, the greater are the thermal effects; the higher the output intensity, the greater is the magnitude of the effects.

TABLE 6–6 **Physiological Effects of Ultrasound Application**

Nonthermal Effects	Thermal Effects
Increased cell membrane permeability	Increased sensory nerve conduction velocity
Altered rates of diffusion across the cell membrane	Increased motor nerve conduction velocity
Increased vascular permeability	Increased extensibility of collagen-rich structures
Secretion of chemotactics	Increased collagen deposition
Increased blood flow	Increased blood flow
Increased fibroblastic activity	Reduction of muscle spasm
Stimulation of phagocytosis	Increased macrophage activity
Production of healthy granulation tissue	Enhanced adhesion of leukocytes to damaged endothelial cells
Synthesis of protein	
Reduction of edema	
Synthesis of collagen	
Diffusion of ions	
Tissue regeneration	
Formation of stronger, more deformable connective tissue	

Nonthermal Effects

Pulsing ultrasonic energy leads to two related events—**cavitation** and **acoustical streaming,** which give rise to ultrasound's nonthermal ("mechanical") effects. The individual pulses delivered by the ultrasound generator cause cells and molecules in the beam's path to oscillate in a cyclical manner and in direct proportion to the unit's output intensity. These oscillations encourage the formation of gas-filled bubbles. **Stable cavitation** occurs when the bubbles compress during the high-pressure peaks as ultrasonic energy followed by expansion of the bubbles during the low-pressure troughs. **Transient cavitation** (unstable cavitation) involves the compression of the bubbles during the high-pressure peak, but is followed by a total collapse during the trough. Transient cavitation is an unwanted, deleterious effect of ultrasound being applied at too great of an intensity and can damage immobile tissue, free-floating blood cells, or other biological structures in the area.[4]

Stable cavitation leads to acoustical streaming (microstreaming), the one-directional flow of tissue fluids, and is most marked around the cell membranes and its *organelles*. The flow of bubbles in the acoustical streams causes changes in cell membrane permeability and diffusion rates across the cell membrane. This effect facilitates the passage of calcium, potassium, and other ions and metabolites into and out of the cell. So long as the cell membrane is not damaged by this process, the response to cavitation and acoustical streaming can be synthesis of collagen,

---

Organelle: A specialized portion of a cell that performs a specific function, such as the mitochondria and the Golgi apparatus.

secretion of chemotactics, increased uptake of calcium in fibroblasts, and increased fibroblastic activity (essential for the production of functional, healthy granulation tissue and scar tissue), all of which assist the healing process (see Table 6–6).[9]

Pulsed ultrasound, often delivered at a relatively high intensity and for a very brief duration, may trigger a series of physiological events that stimulate the healing process. Application in this mode stimulates phagocytosis (assisting in the reduction of chronic inflammation),[13] increases the number of *free radicals* in the area (increasing ionic conductance and acting on the cell membrane),[14] and accelerates *fibrinolysis*.[15,16]

Cycloaminoglycan, the primary component needed for the proper remodeling of collagen, and hydroxyproline, one of the essential amino acids of collagen, are increased following low-dose pulsed ultrasound.[17] These events lead to the healing connective tissue being stronger and more deformable, and thus able to withstand greater loads.

Thermal Effects

The amount of temperature increase during an ultrasound treatment depends on the mode of application (continuous or pulsed), the intensity and frequency of the output, the vascularity and type of tissues, and the speed with which the sound head is moved over the tissues. The physiological changes within the tissues are based on the amount of temperature increase and are the greatest when ultrasound is applied in the continuous mode (Table 6–7). Ultrasound applied with a 1-MHz output frequency can affect tissues located up to 5 cm deep; 3-MHz ultrasound is effective on tissues located up to 2 cm deep.

To achieve a therapeutic effect through ultrasound heating, the tissue temperatures must be elevated for a minimum of 3 to 5 minutes.[9,18] As shown in Table 6–3, 3-MHz ultrasound heats three to four times faster than 1-MHz ultrasound, although the thermal effects of low-frequency ultrasound may last longer.[6,19] The relationship between the output intensity and treatment duration cannot be understated. Lower treatment output intensities require a longer duration to elevate the tissue temperature to the desired level.

Heat production is related to the amount of attenuation of the sound waves in the tissues.[20] The process involved in attenuation, absorption, and scattering creates friction between the molecules and results in a temperature increase. Collagen-rich tissues, such as tendon, joint menisci, superficial bone, large nerve roots, intermuscular fascia, and scar tissue, are preferentially heated.[9] Tissues that are largely fluid-filled, such as the fat layer, are relatively transparent to ultrasonic energy.[8]

Temperatures in poorly vascularized tissues increase by 0.8°C per minute during the application of continuous ultrasound with a frequency of 1 MHz.[4] In highly vascularized areas like muscle, the temperature rise is not as great because incoming, cooler blood continually washes out the local warmer blood. Tempera-

---

Free radical: A highly reactive molecule having an odd number of electrodes. Free radical production plays an important role in the progression of an ischemic injury.

Fibrinolysis: Pathological breaking up of fibrin.

TABLE 6–7 **Temperature Increases Required to Achieve Specific Therapeutic Effects during Ultrasound Application**

Classification of Ultrasound Thermal Effects	Temperature Increase	Used for
Mild	1°C	Mild inflammation Accelerating metabolic rate
Moderate	2°–3°C	Decreasing muscle spasm Decreasing pain Increasing blood flow Reducing chronic inflammation
Vigorous	3°–5°C	Tissue elongation, scar tissue reduction Inhibition of sympathetic activity

Source: Adapted from Draper et al.[6]

ture increases of up to 4.9°C have been documented 2.5 cm deep within the muscle after the application of ultrasound at 1.5 w/cm² for 10 minutes.[8]

Reflected waves also increase the amount of heating. When ultrasound waves are reflected, the energy passes through the tissues more than once, increasing the thermal effects. Standing waves greatly exaggerate the rise in temperature.

EFFECTS ON THE INJURY RESPONSE CYCLE

The effects of ultrasound application are dependent on the mode of application (continuous or pulsed), the frequency of the sound, the size of the area treated, and the tissues being treated (vascularity and density). The deep thermal effects are similar to those described in the thermotherapy section. Mechanical changes resulting from the nonthermal effects are discussed, where relevant, in each of the following sections.

Because of similarities in the biophysical effects, the use of laser energy has been suggested as an alternative to ultrasound. Currently, laser energy is available only for experimental use as a therapeutic modality in the United States, although more powerful surgical lasers are commonplace (Box 6–4).

Blood Flow

Continuous ultrasound can increase local blood flow for up to 45 minutes after treatment,[21] although these findings are not universally accepted.[22] It is reasonable to expect increased blood flow during and after the application of continuous ultrasound simply because of its thermal effects. Other physiological factors may promote increased blood flow as well.[23] Alteration of cell membrane permeability (a result of acoustical streaming) could result in decreased vascular tone, thus leading to a dilation of the vessels, and histamine released in the treated area could also produce a vasodilation, further increasing blood flow.

BOX 6–4 **Laser Therapy**

Laser, an acronym for **l**ight **a**mplification by **s**timulated **e**mission of **r**adiation, uses highly organized light to elicit physiological changes in the tissues. Therapeutic "cold" lasers, which do not normally result in tissue destruction, have been introduced in European countries as an alternative to ultrasound.[53] Material such as helium-neon (HeNe) gas is electrically energized to produce an output of photon radiation to stimulate areas such as acupuncture and trigger points and to assist in superficial wound healing.

The energy produced by therapeutic lasers has a wavelength ranging from 1 *nanometer* (nm) to 1 millimeter (mm). This range includes ultraviolet, visible, and infrared light, and lasers are considered an electromagnetic modality. Lasers in the ultraviolet range produce photochemical effects within the tissues, whereas lasers in the infrared range produce deeper thermal effects. Visible lasers, like the HeNe laser, produce wavelengths that fall between ultraviolet and infrared lasers and possess characteristics of both.[54]

The effects of laser energy in the tissues are similar to the effects of ultrasound. Laser energy can effectively stimulate tissues at depths up to 15 mm below the surface of the skin.[55,56] When the energy is absorbed by the tissues, it is converted into thermal vibration or may produce a photobiological effect similar to the way in which plants use light.

Application of laser energy is thought to activate many events at the molecular level, including short-term stimulation of the electron transport chain, increased synthesis of adenosine triphosphate (ATP), and a reduction in *intracellular* pH. These actions are theorized to affect pain-producing tissue, such as areas of muscle spasm, by restoring the normal properties of muscle tissue via the increased formation of ATP and increased enzyme activity.[56] Extreme exposure to cold lasers can result in tissue destruction through *thermolysis*.

Pain reduction is thought to occur as a result of decreasing muscle spasm or altering nerve conduction velocity, whereas tissue healing is believed to occur through increased collagen production. Recent studies investigating the effect of low-level laser therapy on musculoskeletal pain and skin disorders strongly suggest that low-level laser energy is not an effective modality in the treatment of these conditions.[57–59]

Laser therapy is tightly controlled in the United States. An investigational device exemption from the Food and Drug Administration is required for its use. For this reason, therapeutic laser devices are not available for general use. The use of high-powered destructive surgical lasers is becoming commonplace.

Clinicians have long attempted to alter blood flow by applying moist heat, ice massage,[21] and ice packs[18] before the administration of ultrasound. In one study, the application of moist heat before ultrasound greatly diminished the increase in blood flow in the treatment area. In one study, the application of ice massage before ultrasound maintained the increased blood flow at the level found with ultrasound application alone. Cold pack application, long thought to increase the thermal effects of ultrasound, greatly decreased intramuscular temperature increase at a depth of 5 cm below the skin after ultrasound, 1.8°C compared with the 4°C rise in tissues that were not cooled before treatment.[18]

Nanometer: One-billionth (10^{-9}) of a meter.
Intracellular: Within the membrane of a cell.
Thermolysis: Chemical decomposition caused by heating.

Tissue Healing

Ultrasound application accelerates the inflammatory phase of tissue healing.[24] The application of continuous ultrasound has been shown to positively influence macrophage activity[25] and to increase the adhesion of leukocytes to the damaged endothelial cells.[26] When applied during the proliferation phase, ultrasound stimulates cell division.[27]

Low-frequency (0.75 MHz) continuous ultrasound enhances the release of preformed fibroblasts, whereas high-frequency (3 MHz) ultrasound increases the cell's ability to synthesize and secrete the building blocks of fibroblasts.[24,25,27]

This response appears to be localized to areas with a high collagen content, especially tendons. Studies on animals have shown that the application of continuous ultrasound increased the rate of collagen synthesis in tendon fibroblasts[27] and tendon healing[28] and increased the tensile strength of tendons.[29]

Superficial wounds also respond favorably to ultrasound application. The use of continuous ultrasound delivered at 1.5 W/cm² for a 5-minute treatment over a 1-week period has been demonstrated to increase the breaking strength of incisional wounds. The same protocol, except applied at 0.5 W/cm² for a 2-week duration, produced the same results of increased breaking strength after 1 week, and facilitation of collagen deposition was demonstrated during the second week.[30] (*Note:* The preceding studies were performed with a 1-MHz output frequency; the results of the same protocol using a 3-MHz output are unknown.)

In the acute stage of injury, the use of continuous ultrasound output is contraindicated because of the increased tissue temperature and the associated increased need for oxygen. For this reason, ultrasound application during the acute and subacute inflammatory stages should be delivered with a low duty cycle and at a low intensity.

Tissue Stretching

The thermal effect of increased extensibility in collagen-rich tissues may be used advantageously by incorporating range-of-motion exercises after the application of continuous ultrasound. Gentle passive or active stretching is needed to elongate these tissues. As scar tissue possesses a high concentration of collagen, these areas are preferentially heated with ultrasound.

To promote the elongation, the temperature of the target tissues must be elevated 5°C. After ultrasound application, this opportunity, Draper's "stretching window," is short-lived.[19] The thermal effects associated with vigorous heating (see Table 6–7), when applied at 3 MHz, have an effective stretching time of just over 3 minutes after the termination of the treatment, although the window may be slightly longer when 1-MHz ultrasound is used.[19] When the goal of the ultrasound treatment is to promote tissue elongation, place the tissues on stretch during the treatment. Any subsequent stretching should be performed immediately after the treatment ends.

Pain Control

Ultrasound may control pain through the direct effect that the energy has on the peripheral nervous system, or pain control may be the result of the other tissue changes with ultrasound application. Ultrasound directly influences the transmission of painful impulses by eliciting changes within the nerve fibers themselves. Cell membrane permeability to sodium ions is changed, altering the electrical activity of the nerve fiber[9] and elevating the pain threshold.[31] Nerve conduction velocity is increased as a result of the thermal effects of ultrasound application and may produce a counterirritant effect as well.[2]

Indirect pain reduction results from the other effects of ultrasound application. Increased blood flow and increased capillary permeability augment the delivery of oxygen to hypoxic areas, reducing the activity of chemosensitive pain receptors. Input from mechanical pain receptors is reduced because of a reduction in the amount of muscle spasm and increased muscular relaxation.[31]

PHONOPHORESIS

Ultrasonic energy can be used to deliver medication into tissues through the process of phonophoresis. The philosophy behind phonophoresis is similar to that of iontophoresis (see Chap. 4), but this technique does not require that the medication be electrically charged.[32] Although it is easiest to visualize phonophoresis as the process of the ultrasound waves physically driving the medication through the skin, this does not occur. The effects of the ultrasonic energy open pathways that allow the medication to diffuse through the skin and pass deeper into the tissues.

The advantage of introducing these medications into the body through phonophoresis rather than by injection is that the medication is spread over a larger area, and this technique is noninvasive.[33] Medication that has entered the tissues through this manner bypasses the liver, thus lessening the metabolic elimination of the substances.

For transdermally introduced medications to be absorbed by the viable subcutaneous tissues, they must first pass through the enzymatic barrier of the epidermis and the stratum corneum, the rate-limiting barrier to diffusion.[34] This layer of skin determines the rate and amount of medication that is transmitted to the deeper tissues. With this in mind, the type and consistency of the skin overlying the treatment area are perhaps the most important elements in determining the success of the treatment. Factors such as skin composition, hydration, vascularity, and thickness combine to encourage or prohibit medication diffusion through the skin and, therefore, into the deeper tissues (Table 6–8).

Some substances can be moved past the skin's barriers simply by massaging them into the skin (e.g., medicated lotions). However, some medications have been shown to be delivered to depths of 6 cm into the tissues with the assistance of ultrasound.[35,36] The thermal and nonthermal effects associated with standard ultrasound application may increase the rate and amount of medication absorbed. The thermal effects of ultrasound increase the kinetic energy of both the local cells and the medication, dilating the points of entry (hair follicles, sweat glands, etc.), increasing circulation, increasing capillary permeability, and disordering the structured lipids in the stratum corneum.[37,38] Nonthermal effects enhancing diffusion across the membranes include altering the cell's resting potential, affecting the permeability of ionized and un-ionized molecules, and increasing cell membrane permeability.[37,39,40]

Preheating the treatment area with a moist hot pack to increase local blood flow and kinetic energy can further enhance delivery of the medication into the tissues. After the treatment, leave the remaining mixture on the skin and cover the area with an occlusive dressing to further encourage diffusion of the remaining medication. Systemic effects may be promoted by again heating the area after treatment to encourage vascular absorption and distribution of the medication.[37]

TABLE 6–8 Skin Factors Determining the Rate of Medication Diffusion during Transdermal Application

Factor	Effect
Hydration	The higher the water content, the more permeable the skin to the passage of medications.
Age	Dehydration occurs as skin ages; circulation and lipid content are also decreased.
Composition	The easiest passage of medication through the skin is near hair follicles, sebaceous glands, and sweat ducts.
	Although hair follicles encourage the passage of medication through the skin, excessive hair should be shaved off the area being treated.
Vascularity	Highly vascular areas are more apt to allow for the transfer of the medication into the deep tissues. Constricted vessels localize the effects, whereas dilated vessels enhance the systemic delivery of the medication.
Thickness	Thick skin presents a much more cumbersome barrier to medication than does thinner skin. When applying phonophoresis to an area, attempt to administer it over areas of low skin density (e.g., when treating an individual suffering from plantar fasciitis, apply the medication to the medioinferior aspect of the calcaneus rather than on its plantar surface).

Adapted from Byl.[37]

In the application of phonophoresis, a gel or cream containing medication, which is quite varied and may require a physician's prescription, replaces the standard coupling gel. Traditional phonophoresis techniques allow only molecules of relatively small size and of low molecular weight to be introduced into the tissues.[41] A wide range of substances is commonly used during phonophoresis, with perhaps the most common being *hydrocortisone* (Table 6–9).

The use of medication mixtures not specifically designed for phonophoresis should be avoided. Research has shown that the majority of commonly used phonophoresis coupling agents reflect most of the ultrasonic energy; some of the most popular bases that have been used for years result in 100 percent reflection.[32,40] The majority of thick, white, corticosteroid creams are poor conductors of ultrasound, whereas topical gel-mixed media, such as commercially available transmission gels, are good conductors.[42] Another approach to administration of phonophoresis is the **"invisible method,"** in which, rather than mixing the substance within another base, the medication is first directly massaged into the skin, followed by a traditional ultrasound application.

The efficacy of phonophoresis has not been fully substantiated, and confusion still exists.[33,36,40,43] Many of the contradictions in the results of these studies can be related to the type of coupling agent used and the concentration of the medication. For example, one study examined the subcutaneous absorption of a commercially available *salicylate,* Myoflex, and found no difference in the level of salicylates in the bloodstream with or without the use of ultrasound.[40] A later

Hydrocortisone: An anti-inflammatory drug that closely resembles cortisol.
Salicylates: A family of compounds that includes aspirin.

TABLE 6–9   **Substances Commonly Administered via Phonophoresis**

Classification	Indication	Target Tissues	Examples
Corticosteroids	Inflammatory conditions	Subcutaneous tissues Nerves Muscle	Hydrocortisone Dexamethasone
Salicylates	Inflammatory conditions Pain	Subdermal tissues	Myoflex*
Anesthetics	Pain Trigger points	Nerves Circulatory system	Lidocaine

*Does not transmit ultrasonic energy.

study revealed that Myoflex transmitted no ultrasonic energy compared to water (see Table 6–5).[42]

Still, the actual amount of medication that penetrates to the viable tissues and the effect that ultrasonic energy has on the absorption is unknown. Hydrocortisone is thought to be delivered into the subcutaneous tissues, where it slowly diffuses into the deeper tissues, but increased serum cortisol levels have not been substantiated after treatment.[44] Likewise, dexamethasone has not been proved to produce a measurable effect in the submuscular or subtendinous tissue[45] or in any amount sufficient to impair adrenal function.[46]

The following recommendations have been made to provide the most optimal phonophoresis application:[37]

- Use only approved ultrasound transmission media.
- Ensure that the skin is well moistened; areas of dry skin should be avoided.
- Apply ultrasound or moist heat or shave the area before treatment to improve the medication's ability to diffuse through the skin and into the tissues.
- Position the extremity to encourage circulation.
- Use a continuous output to maximize the effect of phonophoresis (unless the thermal effects of ultrasound are contraindicated).
- After treatment, cover the remaining medication with an occlusive dressing.

Many of the limitations found in traditional phonophoresis techniques may be circumvented through the use of new, low-frequency sound generators. These devices, still in their experimental stage, use a 20-kHz frequency (at the upper range of human hearing), 125 mW/cm², pulsed output to enhance the introduction of medication into the deep tissues. The lower frequency allows medications of a larger molecular size and weight, including insulin and *interferon gamma*, to penetrate deeper into the tissues. Initial reports on this technique indicate that low-frequency sonophoresis is capable of delivering a wide range of medications up to 1000 times more effectively than those produced with the traditional ultrasound method.[41,46,47]

Interferon gamma: A group of proteins released by white blood cells and fibroblasts when devouring the unwanted tissues. The gamma classification is also referred to as "angry macrophages" because of their heightened phagocytic activity.

FRACTURE HEALING

Although active fracture sites are a contraindication to ultrasound use, a technique using a 1.5-MHz output, low-intensity (30 mW per square centimeter), pulsed beam applied in one 20-minute session per day has shown great promise in accelerating acute fracture healing. These output parameters are *not* available on standard therapeutic ultrasound units.

Many of the accolades that this technique has received are anecdotal and found primarily on the sports pages. However, a controlled study of low-dose ultrasonically assisted fracture healing has helped to substantiate the claims of success. This study examined two groups of patients, each suffering from acute tibial fractures. The group receiving ultrasound treatments required less clinical healing time (86 days compared to 144 days for the control group) and radiographic healing time (96 days; control group equals 154 days), an outcome which was found to be both statistically significant and, perhaps most important, clinically significant.[48,49]

Ultrasound and Electrical Stimulation

Ultrasound and electrical stimulation have long been applied concurrently for treatment of trigger points and other superficial painful areas, although research supporting the benefits of this combined treatment approach is lacking. In this technique, the ultrasound head serves as an electrode for an electrical stimulating current (Fig. 6–12). Theoretically, this application method would provide the same benefits as ultrasound (thermal and mechanical) and electrical stimulation if they were applied separately, namely, improved circulation, reduction of muscle spasm, and decreased adhesion of scar tissue.

Recall that trigger and other stimulation points display a decreased resistance to electrical current flow (see Chap. 5). When a moderate pulse duration and moderate pulse frequency are applied at an intensity sufficient to produce a strong muscle contraction, the muscle fibers within the trigger point may fatigue

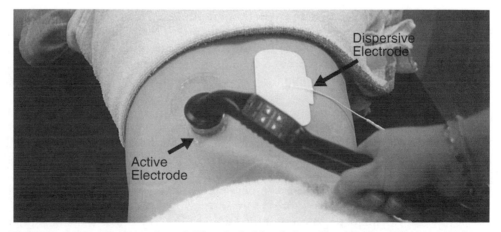

FIGURE 6–12 **Ultrasound and Electrical Stimulation Combination Therapy.** Using a sound/stimulation combination unit, one electrode is attached to the patient's body while the ultrasound head serves as the active electrode.

to the point where they no longer have the biochemical ability to spasm. Low-amperage electrical stimulation is capable of increasing adenosine triphosphate activity within the cells, in turn increasing their ability to repair themselves. Increased phagocytosis and increased circulation would assist in the collection and removal of cellular wastes from the treatment area.[50]

Wide ranges of combined ultrasound and electrical stimulation units are being marketed. The electrical stimulation part of these units delivers a monophasic, biphasic, or alternating current. Each of these parameters would affect the target tissues differently. Likewise, many ultrasound generators in this configuration, especially older ones, deliver only a 1-MHz output. In most instances, a 3-MHz output would be needed to target the stimulation points.

A slowly moving sound head is needed to produce the required amount of subcutaneous tissue temperature increase, approximately 4° to 5°C. Placing the target tissues on stretch during treatment could assist the reduction of trigger points and muscle spasm.

CLINICAL APPLICATION OF ULTRASOUND

Ultrasound application has evolved from what was once a rote, "cookbook" approach to a clinical science. Determining the proper output parameters (indeed, determining if ultrasound is even the proper modality) requires knowledge of the type of tissues involved, the depth of the trauma, the nature and inflammatory state of the injury, and consideration of the skin and tissues overlying the treatment area.

To ensure safe application of this modality, ultrasound units should be calibrated at least once a year (many manufacturers recommend that this be done twice a year). The FDA requires that the output frequency, BNR, ERA, and date of last calibration be indicated on the generator or the transducer if the unit has interchangeable sound heads.

Instrumentation

Power: Allows the source current to flow into the internal components of the generator. On many units, a POWER light goes on, or the WATT METER illuminates.

Timer: Sets the duration of the treatment. The time remaining is displayed on the console, or the timer rotates to display the time remaining.

Start-Stop: Initiates or terminates the production of ultrasound from the transducer.

Pause: Interrupts the treatment but retains the remaining amount of treatment time when the treatment is reinstated.

Intensity: Adjusts the intensity of the ultrasound beam. The WATT METER displays the output in either total watts or watts per square centimeter.

Duty cycle: Adjusts between continuous and pulsed ultrasound application. Most units display the duty cycle as a percentage, with 100 percent representing continuous ultrasound.

Watt meter: Displays the output of ultrasound in total watts or watts per square centimeter. Digital meters may require that the user manually switch between the two displays. Most analog meters display the total watts on an upper scale while simultaneously displaying output in watts per square centimeter on the lower scale. These typically have a sound head with a fixed ERA.

Maximum head temperature: Sets the maximum heat tolerance in the sound head in case the head is not properly coupled.

Setup and Application

Patient Preparation

1. Establish that no contraindications are present.
2. Determine the method and mode of ultrasound application to be used during this treatment.
3. Clean the area to be treated to remove any body oils, dirt, or grime.
4. Determine the type of coupling method to be used. The efficacy of phonophoresis for the bladder and immersion methods has not been established.
5. If the direct coupling method is used, spread the gel over the area to be treated. Use the sound head to evenly distribute the gel.
6. Explain the sensations to be expected during the treatment. During the application of continuous ultrasound, a sensation of mild to moderate warmth (but not pain or burning) should be expected.[3] No subcutaneous sensations should be felt during the application of pulsed ultrasound. Advise the patient to inform you of any unexpected sensations.
7. For phonophoresis, preheating of the area to be treated is recommended to decrease skin resistance and increase the absorption of the medication.[35]

Initiation of the Treatment

1. Reduce the INTENSITY to zero before turning on the POWER.
2. Select the appropriate mode for the output. Use CONTINUOUS to increase the thermal effects of ultrasound application or PULSED output for nonthermal effects. The more acute the injury or the more active the inflammation process, the lower the duty cycle that is used.
3. Ensure that the WATT METER displays the appropriate output for the type of treatment.
4. Set the TIMER to the appropriate treatment length, but treat an area no larger than two to three times the size of the unit's ERA. The actual duration of the treatment depends on the desired effects of the treatment, the output intensity, and the body area being treated. Nonthermal effects require a shorter treatment duration than thermal effects. Refer to Tables 6–3 and 6–6 for the approximate times required to reach various therapeutic heating levels.
5. Begin slowly moving the sound head over the medium and depress the START button to begin the treatment session. Units having low BNR may be moved at a slower rate than those with a higher BNR.
6. Slowly increase the INTENSITY to the appropriate level while keeping the sound head moving (see step 4).
7. The sound head is moved at a moderate pace with overlapping strokes. Firm, yet not strong, pressure should be applied to the sound head.[11]

8. If periosteal pain is experienced, move the sound head at a faster rate, use a reduced duty cycle, and/or lower the intensity. If the pain continues, discontinue the treatment.
9. If the gel begins to wear away or if the sound head begins sticking on the skin, depress the PAUSE button and apply more gel.

Termination of the Treatment

1. Most units automatically terminate the production of ultrasound when the time expires. If this is not the case, or if the treatment is being terminated prematurely, the intensity must be reduced before removing the transducer from the medium.
2. Remove the remaining gel or water from the patient's skin.
3. To ensure continuity of treatment sessions, record the parameters used for this treatment in the individual's file; specifically, record the output frequency, intensity, duration, and duty cycle. A running count of ultrasound treatments given for this condition should also be made.
4. Immediately initiate any post-treatment stretching.

Duration and Frequency of Treatment

The treatment time is from 3 to 12 minutes, depending on the size of the area being treated, the intensity of the treatment, and the goal of the treatment. Ultrasound is normally given once a day for 10 to 14 days, at which time the efficacy of the treatment protocol should be evaluated.

Precautions

- Symptoms may increase after the first two treatments because of an increase in inflammation in the area. If the symptoms do not improve after the third or fourth treatment, the use of the modality should be discontinued.[51]
- Caution should be used when applying ultrasound around the spinal cord, especially after *laminectomy*. Many manufacturers list this as a contraindication to ultrasound application. The various densities provided by the spinal cord and its covering may result in a rapid temperature rise, causing trauma to the spinal cord.
- The use of ultrasound over metal implants is not contraindicated as long as the sound head is kept moving and the treatment area has normal sensory function.
- The use of ultrasound over the epiphyseal plates of growing bone should be performed with caution. Many authors cite this as a contraindication to ultrasound use.

Laminectomy: Surgical removal of the lamina from a vertebra.

Indications

- Joint contractures
- Muscle spasm
- Neuroma
- Scar tissue
- Sympathetic nervous system disorders
- Trigger areas
- Warts
- Spasticity
- Postacute reduction of myositis ossificans
- Acute inflammatory conditions (pulsed output)
- Chronic inflammatory conditions (pulsed or continuous output)

Contraindications

- Acute conditions (continuous output)
- Ischemic areas
- Tendency to hemorrhage
- Areas around the eyes, heart, skull, or genitals
- Pregnancy when used over the pelvic or lumbar areas
- Over cancerous tumors (Therapeutic doses applied over tumors have been shown to increase mass and weight of the tumor.[52])
- Over the spinal cord or large nerve plexus in high doses
- Anesthetic areas
- Over a fracture site before healing is complete
- Stress fracture sites
- Over sites of active infection
- Over the pelvic or lumbar area in menstruating female patients
- Areas of impaired circulation

SUMMARY

Ultrasound can produce both thermal and nonthermal changes within the tissues. Because of this, pulsed ultrasound—producing nonthermal effects—can be used for acute conditions, whereas continuous ultrasound is reserved for chronic conditions. The depth of effective penetration of the ultrasonic energy is based on the output frequency, with 1 MHz penetrating approximately 5 cm into the tissues and 3 MHz penetrating less than 2 cm. The relationship between the treatment intensity and treatment duration depends on the amount of heating required and the inflammatory stage of the injury being treated. Ultrasound is also used to assist in delivering medications into the subcutaneous tissues (phonophoresis), and recently a specific form of ultrasound has shown promise in speeding the rate of acute fracture healing.

Chapter Quiz

1. When applying ultrasound with a metered output of 4 W and an indicated beam nonuniformity ratio (BNR) of 4, the highest intensity in the beam is:
   A. 4 W
   B. 8 W
   C. 16 W
   D. 32 W

2. Which of the following is **not** an indication for the use of ultrasound?
   A. Scar tissue
   B. Infection
   C. Warts
   D. Trigger points

3. The spreading of an ultrasound beam is a result of:
   A. Attenuation
   B. Collimation
   C. Thermal synthesis
   D. Divergence

4. A metered reading of 2 W per square centimeter passing through a sound head having an effective radiating area of 10 cm² produces an output of _____ total watts.
   A. 5 W
   B. 10 W
   C. 15 W
   D. 20 W

5. Reflection of ultrasonic energy occurs **least** between:
   A. Water and soft tissue
   B. Soft tissue and fat
   C. Soft tissue and bone
   D. Soft tissue and air

6. All of the following are nonthermal (mechanical) effects of ultrasound **except:**
   A. Increased extensibility of collagen-rich structures
   B. Increased blood flow
   C. Synthesis of protein
   D. Increased cell membrane permeability

7. When treating the patellar tendon with ultrasound, what output frequency should be used?
   A. 1 MHz.
   B. 2 MHz.
   C. 3 MHz.
   D. It does not matter.

8. When cells are exposed to high-pressure ridges, their size
   A. Increases
   B. Decreases

9. Ultrasound that is pulsed so that it flows for 0.5 seconds and does not flow for 1 second is operating at a ———— percent duty cycle.
   A. 33
   B. 50
   C. 66
   D. 133

10. Determining the treatment duration is most closely dependent on what other output characteristic?
    A. Duty cycle
    B. Frequency
    C. Coupling method
    D. Intensity

11. To promote extensibility the tissues must be stretched within ———— minute(s) after the conclusion of the treatment.
    A. 1
    B. 3
    C. 10
    D. 30

12. What four factors determine a medication's ability to diffuse through the tissues?
    A.
    B.
    C.
    D.

13. Standard therapeutic ultrasound generators can be employed to assist in the healing of fractures.
    A. True
    B. False

14. Which of the following substances transmits the highest percentage of ultrasonic energy relative to water?
    A. Saran Wrap
    B. Eucerine Cream
    C. Ultrasound transmission gel
    D. Hydrocortisone powder (1%) in US gel

CASE STUDY CONTINUATION

The following discussion relates to Case Study 3, found on pages 104 through 109 of Chapter 3. Pulsed ultrasound (20 percent duty cycle) could be incorporated into our patient's program to reduce pain and promote tissue extensibility. Alterations in the cell membrane permeability bring about changes in the nerves' electrical activity, reportedly increasing the pain threshold, and assist in the healing process.

When applied with a continuous output (100 percent duty cycle), ultrasound preferentially heats collagen-rich tissues and assists in reducing muscle spasm. When vigorously heated (3° to 5°C increase), tissue extensibility can be increased. To obtain the maximal benefits of tissue elongation, the trapezius must be placed on stretch during the treatment and any flexibility exercises must be performed within 3 minutes after the conclusion of the treatment.

The treatment area would be limited to an area two to three times the size of the sound head; the output frequency would depend on the depth of our patient's trauma. The intensity and duration of the treatment would be sufficient to produce a vigorous heating effect. Recall that use of ultrasound is a precaution to ultrasound application, so extra care must be taken when applying these treatments.

REFERENCES

1. Chen, QX: A new laser-ultrasound transducer for medical applications. Ultrasonics 32:309, 1994.
2. Ziskin, MC, McDiarmid, T, and Michlovitz, SL: Therapeutic ultrasound. In Michlovitz, S (ed): Thermal Agents in Rehabilitation, ed 2. FA Davis, Philadelphia, 1990, pp 134–169.
3. Draper, DO: Ten mistakes commonly made with ultrasound use: Current research sheds light on myths. Athletic Training: Sports Health Care Perspectives 2:95, 1996.
4. Ter Haar, G: Basic physics of therapeutic ultrasound. Physiotherapy 73:110, 1987.
5. Kitchen, SS and Partridge, CJ: A review of therapeutic ultrasound: I. Background, physiological effects and hazards. Physiotherapy 76:593, 1990.
6. Draper, DO, Castel, JC, and Castel, D: Rate of temperature increase in human muscle during 1 MHz and 3 MHz continuous ultrasound. J Orthop Sports Phys Ther 22:142, 1995.
7. Ferguson, BH: A Practitioner's Guide to the Ultrasonic Therapy Equipment Standard. U.S. Department of Health and Human Services, Public Health Service, Food and Drug Administration, Rockville, MD, 1985.
8. Draper, DO and Sunderland, S: Examination of the law of Grotthus-Draper: Does ultrasound penetrate subcutaneous fat in humans? Journal of Athletic Training 38:246, 1993.
9. Dyson, M: Mechanisms involved in therapeutic ultrasound. Physiotherapy 73:116, 1987.
10. Williams, R: Production and transmission of ultrasound. Physiotherapy 73:113, 1987.
11. Klucinec, B, Denegar, C, and Mahmood, R: The transducer pressure variable: Its influence on acoustic energy transmission. Journal of Sport Rehabilitation 6:47, 1997.
12. Draper, DO, et al: A comparison of temperature rise in human calf muscles following applications of underwater and topical gel ultrasound. J Orthop Sports Phys Ther 17:247, 1993.
13. De Deyne, P and Kirsch-Volders, M: In vitro effects of therapeutic ultrasound on the nucleus of human fibroblasts. Phys Ther 72:629, 1995.
14. Adinno, MA, et al: Effect of free radical scavengers on changes in ion conductance during exposure to therapeutic ultrasound. Membrane Biochemistry 10:237, 1993.
15. Blinc, A, et al: Characterization of ultrasound-potentated fibrinolysis in vitro. Blood 81:2636, 1993.
16. Francis, CW, et al: Enhancement of fibrinolysis in vitro by ultrasound. J Clin Invest 90:2063, 1992.
17. Byl, NN, et al: Low-dose ultrasound effects on wound healing: A controlled study with Yucatan pigs. Arch Phys Med Rehabil 73:656, 1992.

18. Draper, DO, et al: Temperature changes in deep muscle of humans during ice and ultrasound therapies: An *in vivo* study. J Orthop Sports Phys Ther 21:153, 1995.
19. Draper, DO and Ricard, MD: Rate of temperature decay in human muscle following 3 MHz ultrasound: The stretching window revealed. Journal of Athletic Training 30:304, 1995.
20. Weinberger, A and Lev, A: Temperature elevation of connective tissue by physical modalities. Critical Reviews in Physical and Rehabilitation Medicine 3:121, 1991.
21. Baker, RJ and Bell, GW: The effect of therapeutic modalities on blood flow in the human calf. J Orthop Sports Phys Ther 13:23, 1991.
22. Robinson, SE and Buono, MJ: Effect of continuous-wave ultrasound on blood flow in skeletal muscle. Phys Ther 75:147, 1993.
23. Fabrizio, PA, et al: Acute effects of therapeutic ultrasound delivered at varying parameters on the blood flow velocity in a muscular distribution artery. J Orthop Sports Phys Ther 24:294, 1996.
24. Kitchen, SS and Partridge, CJ: A review of therapeutic ultrasound: II. The efficacy of ultrasound. Physiotherapy 76:595, 1990.
25. Young, SR and Dyson, M: Macrophage responsiveness to therapeutic ultrasound. Ultrasound Med Biol 16:809, 1990.
26. Maxwell, L, et al: The augmentation of leukocyte adhesion to endothelium by therapeutic ultrasound. Ultrasound Med Biol 20:383, 1994.
27. Ramirez, A, et al: The effect of ultrasound on collagen synthesis and fibroblast proliferation in vitro. Med Sci Sports Exerc 29:326, 1997.
28. Jackson, BA, Schwane, JA, and Starcher, BC: Effect of ultrasound therapy on the repair of achilles tendon injuries in rats. Med Sci Sports Exerc 23:171, 1991.
29. Enwemeka, CS: The effect of therapeutic ultrasound on tendon healing: A biomechanical study Am J Phys Med Rehabil 68:283, 1989.
30. Byl, NN, et al: Incisional wound healing: A controlled study of low and high dose ultrasound. J Orthop Sports Phys Ther 18:619, 1993.
31. Downing, DS and Weinstein, A: Ultrasound therapy of subacromial bursitis. A double blind trial. Phys Ther 66:194, 1986.
32. Henley, EJ: Transcutaneous drug delivery: Iontophoresis, phonophoresis. Physical and Rehabilitation Medicine 2:139, 1991.
33. Davick, JP, Martin, RK, and Albright, JP: Distribution and deposition of tritiated cortisol using phonophoresis. Phys Ther 68:1672, 1988.
34. Steinstrasser, I and Merkle, HP: Dermal metabolism of topically applied drugs: Pathways and models reconsidered. Pharm Acta Helv 70:3, 1995.
35. Quillen, WS: Phonophoresis: A review of the literature and technique. Athletic Training 15:109, 1980.
36. Ciccone, CD, Leggin, BG, and Callamaro, JJ: Effects of ultrasound and trolamine salicylate phonophoresis on delayed-onset muscle soreness. Phys Ther 71:666, 1991.
37. Byl, NN: The use of ultrasound as an enhancer for transcutaneous drug delivery: Phonophoresis. Phys Ther 75:539, 1995.
38. McElnay, JC, et al: Phonophoresis of methyl nicotinate: A preliminary study to elucidate the mechanism of action. Pharm Res 10:1726, 1993.
39. Machluf, M and Kost, J: Ultrasonically enhanced transdermal drug delivery. Experimental approaches to elucidate the mechanism. J Biomater Sci Polym Ed 5:147, 1993.
40. Oziomek, RS, et al: Effect of phonophoresis on serum salicylate levels. Med Sci Sports Exerc 23:397, 1991.
41. Mitragotri, S, Blankschtein, D, and Langer, R: Transdermal drug delivery using low-frequency sonophoresis. Pharm Res 13:411, 1996.
42. Cameron, MH and Monroe, LG: Relative transmission of ultrasound by media customarily used for phonophoresis. Phys Ther 72:142, 1992.
43. Bensen, HAE, McElnay, JC, and Harland, R: Use of ultrasound to enhance percutaneous absorption of benzydamine. Phys Ther 69:113, 1989.
44. Bare, AC, McAnaw, MB, and Pritchard, AE: Phonophoretic delivery of 10% hydrocortisone through the epidermis of humans as determined by serum cortisol concentrations. Phys Ther 76:738, 1996.
45. Byl, NN, et al: The effects of phonophoresis with corticosteroids: A controlled pilot study. J Orthop Sports Phys Ther 18:590, 1993.
46. Franklin, ME, et al: Effect of phonophoresis with dexamethasone on adrenal function. J Orthop Sports Phys Ther 22:103, 1995.
47. Mitragotri, S, Blankschtein, D, and Langer, R: Ultrasound-mediated transdermal protein delivery. Science 269:850, 1995.

48. Heckman, JD, et al: Acceleration of tibial fracture-healing by non-invasive, low-intensity pulsed ultrasound. J Bone Joint Surg Am 76:26, 1994.

49. Cook, SD, et al: Acceleration of tibia and distal radius fracture healing in patients who smoke. Clinical Orthop 337:198, 1997.

50. Cheng, N, et al: The effects of electric currents on ATP generation, protein synthesis, and membrane transport in rat skin. Clin Orthop 171:264, 1982.

51. McDiarmind, T and Burns, PN: Clinical application of therapeutic ultrasound. Physiotherapy 73:155, 1987.

52. Sicard-Rosenbaum, L, et al: Effects of continuous therapeutic ultrasound on growth and metastasis of subcutaneous murine tumors. Phys Ther 75:3, 1995.

53. Bischko, JJ: Use of the laser beam in acupuncture. Acupunct Electrother Res 5:29, 1980.

54. Kitchen, SS and Partridge, CJ: A review of low level laser therapy: I. Background, physiological effects and hazards. Physiotherapy 77:161, 1991.

55. Greathouse, DG, Currier, DP, and Gilmore, RL: Effects of clinical infrared laser on superficial radial nerve conduction. Phys Ther 65:1184, 1985.

56. King, CE, et al: Effect of helium-neon laser auriculotherapy on experimental pain threshold. Phys Ther 70:24, 1990.

57. Mulcahy, D, et al: Low level laser therapy: a prospective double blind trial of its use in an orthopaedic population. Injury 26:315, 1995.

58. Gam, AN, Thorsen, H, and Lnnberg, F: The effect of low-level laser therapy on musculoskeletal pain: A meta-analysis. Pain 52:63, 1993.

59. Beckerman, H, et al: The efficacy of laser therapy for musculoskeletal and skin disorders: A criteria-based meta-analysis randomized clinical trials. Phys Ther 72:483, 1992.

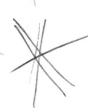

CHAPTER 7

Mechanical Modalities

This chapter presents therapeutic modalities that use mechanical energy to elicit involuntary responses within the human body.

INTERMITTENT COMPRESSION UNITS

These devices use mechanical pressure to encourage venous and lymphatic return from the extremities. Intermittent compression units consist of a nylon appliance designed to fit the body part (e.g., foot and/or ankle, half leg, full leg) that is connected to the unit through a series of hoses (Fig. 7–1). The compression is then formed by the flow of air or cold water into the appliance.

Intermittent cold compression units are ideal for the treatment of acute injuries because of their ease of use and their ability to provide cold and compression while the limb is elevated (ICE). However, this device should not be used until the possibility of a fracture or *compartment syndrome* has been ruled out by a physician. In subacute conditions, intermittent compression is used to reduce edema and decrease ecchymosis from the area.

Effect on the Injury Response Cycle

The movement of fluids out of the extremity is caused by the formation of a number of pressure gradients. When external compression is applied, the gradient between the tissue hydrostatic pressure and the capillary filtration pressure is re-

---

Compartment syndrome: A condition in which nerves, blood vessels, or tendons are constricted within a confined space (e.g., the anterior compartment of the lower leg).

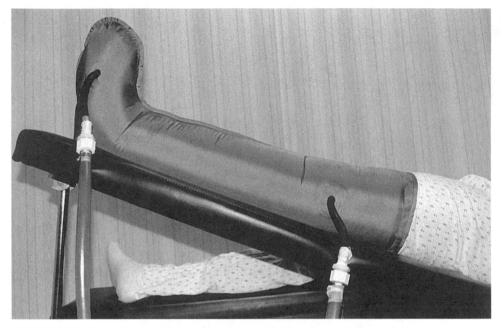

FIGURE 7–1 **Intermittent Compression Applied to the Lower Extremity.** Elevating the extremity assists in venous return. The amount of pressure applied to the extremity should not exceed the patient's diastolic blood pressure.

duced, thus encouraging the reabsorption of interstitial fluids. Because the tissues are being compressed, a second pressure gradient is formed between the distal portion of the extremity (high pressure) and the proximal portion (low pressure), forcing the fluids to move from the high-pressure area to a lower-pressure area. If the extremity is elevated during this treatment, both of these pressures are enhanced by gravity, speeding venous drainage. During the compression sequence, blood flow to the treated area is decreased because of the external pressure on the extremity.

The compression applied to the tissue is either circumferential or sequential. Circumferential compression simultaneously applies an equal amount of pressure to all parts of the extremity. This pressure is built up to a level determined by the operator and is held at this level for a preset time. The pressure then drops and the process repeats. Through this cycle, fluids are forced up the venous and lymphatic return systems. Sequential compression increases the distal-to-proximal gradient through the sequential filling of pressure chambers within the appliance. The most distal compartment inflates, followed by the next compartment, and so on, until pressure is applied to the length of the appliance (Fig. 7–2). This method massages the fluids through the venous and lymphatic systems.

Both circumferential and sequential compression units have been shown to significantly reduce the amount of edema in an injured body part. During the treatment of lower-leg edema, low pressure (35 to 55 mm Hg) increases the venous flow velocity 175 percent. When this pressure is increased to the range of 90 to 100 mm Hg, the venous flow accelerates to 336 percent of resting values.[1] Because extracellular debris is removed, the fresh blood flow to the area has been shown to significantly increase after the treatment.[2] Curiously, a study of post-

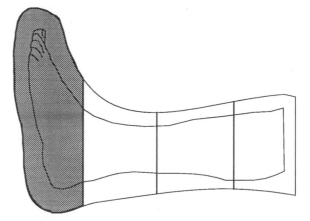

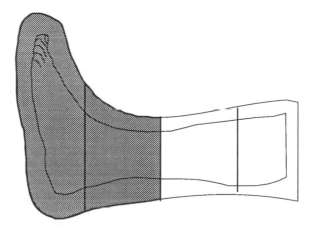

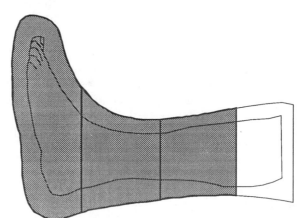

FIGURE 7–2 **Sequential Compression.**
Compartments within the appliance fill
distal to proximal, forcing the fluids toward the torso. Following the cycle, all
the compartments deflate and the process repeats.

acute ankle sprains that displayed *pitting edema* found not only that simple elevation was more effective in reducing edema than intermittent compression and
elastic wraps but also that the last two techniques actually increased the amount of
edema.[3]

Another form of compression therapy, controlled cold therapy units, is described in Chapter 4.

Clinical Application of Intermittent Compression

Instrumentation

Power: Turns the unit on or off.

Temperature: With cold compression units, regulates the temperature of the fluid
flowing through a refrigeration device to the appliance. Some portable cold
compression units use ice cubes for this purpose. The temperature of the fluid is
displayed in the TEMPERATURE GAUGE.

Pressure: Adjusts the amount of compression in millimeters of mercury (mm Hg)
applied to the extremity. This value must not exceed the patient's *diastolic blood
pressure.*

On-off time: Controls the proportion of the time that the compression is on and off.
This control may be a single switch with selectable duty cycles, or the ON and
OFF times may be adjusted individually.

Pump: Turns on the pressure to the appliance.

Drain: Removes the pressure and deflates the appliance.

Setup and Application

Preparation for the Treatment

1. Establish the absence of contraindications.
2. Determine the patient's diastolic blood pressure.
3. For sanitary purposes, cover the area to be treated with Stockinette or similar material. Care must be taken to ensure that this inner layer is free of
   wrinkles.
4. Select the appropriate size of appliance for the extremity being treated.
5. Insert the injured limb into the appliance.
6. For best results, elevate the limb. (On some fluid-filled units, it is easier to
   allow the appliance to initially fill and then to elevate the body part.)
7. Connect the appliance to the compression unit. Note that these units have
   an input and exhaust tubes. The hoses must be properly connected to the
   appliance and the unit.

Pitting edema: An exudate-rich form of edema that is characterized by being easily indented by pressure (hence, "pitting").

Diastolic blood pressure: The lowest level of pressure in the arteries. For example,
when a blood pressure reading is given as 120/80, 80 represents the diastolic
value.

Initiation of the Treatment

1. If the intermittent compression unit uses a cold fluid, select the TEMPER-ATURE to be used, generally between 50° and 55°F.
2. Select the maximal PRESSURE for the treatment. This pressure must not exceed the diastolic blood pressure. Normal pressure ranges are 40 to 60 mm Hg for the upper extremity and 60 to 100 mm Hg for the lower extremity.
3. Select the ON-OFF times. Normally a 3:1 duty cycle (e.g., 45 seconds ON, 15 seconds OFF) is used.
4. Select the appropriate TREATMENT TIME.
5. Inform the individual about the sensations to be expected during the treatment. Instruct the patient to contact you if any unusual sensations, such as pain or a "tingling" feeling, are experienced during the treatment.
6. Encourage the patient to perform gentle range-of-motion (ROM) exercises during the off cycle, if appropriate.

Termination of the Treatment

1. Reduce ON time or select the DRAIN mode to remove the air or fluid from the appliance.
2. Gently remove the body part from the appliance.
3. Apply a compression wrap and any appropriate supportive devices.

Duration and Frequency of Treatment

Intermittent compression can be applied once or twice a day for 20 minutes to several hours. If the unit uses cold fluid, increase the temperature as the treatment duration increases.

Precaution

- Care must be taken when treating the lower leg with any compression device. Even in the absence of a compartment syndrome, inflation devices can elevate intramuscular pressure to a level sufficient to cause ischemia.[4]
- Wrinkling of Stockinette may cause high-pressure areas and subsequent bruising as the pressure in the appliance increases.

Indications

- Post-traumatic edema
- Postsurgical edema
- Primary and secondary *lymphedema*
- *Venous stasis ulcers*

Lymphedema: Swelling of the lymph nodes caused by blockage of the vessels.
Venous stasis ulcer: Ischemic necrosis and ulceration of tissue, especially that overlying bony prominences caused by prolonged pressure. Also referred to as decubitus ulcers or "bedsores."

Contraindications

- Acute conditions in which the possibility of a fracture has not been eliminated
- Conditions in which the pressure would further damage the structures (e.g., compartment syndromes)
- Peripheral vascular disease
  - Arteriosclerosis
  - Edema secondary to congestive heart failure
  - Ischemic vascular disease
- Gangrene
- Dermatitis
- Deep vein thrombosis
- Thrombophlebitis

CONTINUOUS PASSIVE MOTION

The concept of applying continuous passive motion (CPM) to an injured or repaired joint is the antithesis of immobilization, a common postsurgical management technique. To thwart the deleterious effects of immobilization, CPM devices are used to deliver gentle stresses to the healing tissues. Still predominantly used for knee injuries (Fig. 7–3), CPM units have been designed for the hand, wrist, hip, shoulder, elbow, and ankle. Although passive motion can be applied through a dedicated CPM unit, it can be delivered manually by the clinician. Many isokinetic units incorporate "robotics" to deliver short-term passive motion treatments.

Robert Salter,[5] a Canadian physician, originally proposed the use of CPM to assist in the healing of synovial joints. On the basis of his clinical observations,

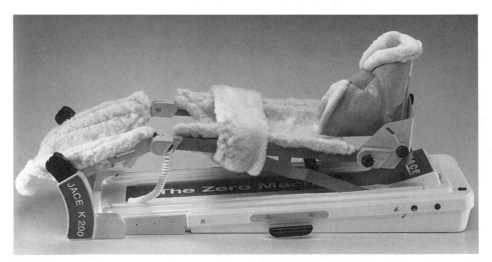

FIGURE 7–3 **A Continuous Passive-Motion Device for the Knee.** (The JACE K200 model manufactured by JACE Systems, Inc. Courtesy of Thera Kinetics, Inc., Mount Laurel, NJ.)

TABLE 7–1 **Characteristics of Different Classifications of Continuous Passive Motion Designs**

Parameter	Continuous Passive Motion Linkage Design		
	Free Linkage	**Anatomic Design**	**Nonanatomic Design**
Joint stability	Very poor	Good	Fair
Control of ROM	Very poor	Excellent	Fair
Total ROM	Poor	Excellent	Good
Multiaxis motion	Good	Poor	Fair
Adjustable to the patient	Excellent	Poor	Fair

Source: Adapted from Saringer.[7]

Salter hypothesized that the application of CPM would be beneficial for three reasons:

- Nutrition and metabolic activity of articular cartilage would be enhanced
- Articular cartilage regrowth would be achieved by stimulating tissue remodeling
- Healing of articular cartilage, tendons, and ligaments would be accelerated

The CPM devices are categorized into three types: free linkage, nonanatomic, and anatomic designs.[6,7] The free linkage design is similar to a clinician moving a limb by grabbing it proximal and distal to the joint. Because the joint itself is not supported, free linkage units are not suitable for unstable joints.[7] The CPM devices that incorporate an anatomic design attempt to mimic the natural movements of the involved joints, as well as the proximal joint, and are considered to be the most suitable for the knee. Nonanatomically designed CPM units make no attempt to replicate the natural joint motion, with compensatory movement occurring between the patient's extremity and the CPM's carriage. The difference between the ROM indicated on the CPM and the actual movement of the limb may be in excess of 20°.[7] Table 7–1 summarizes the advantages and disadvantages of each of these styles of CPM units. Regardless of the type of CPM unit being used, care must be taken to avoid placing unwanted stress on the joint's structures.

Incorporation of motion early into the patient's rehabilitation routine does not have to involve the use of CPM devices. Manual (passive) ROM progressing through active-assisted to fully active motion can decrease hospitalization time (thus decreasing hospital charges) and increase long-term range of motion 1 year after total knee *arthroplasty*.[8–10]

Effects on the Injury Response Cycle

The philosophy regarding the effects of CPM may be summarized as follows: "Motion that is never lost need never be regained. It is the regaining of movement

---

Arthroplasty: Surgical reconstruction or replacement of an articular joint.

that is painful."[11] Constant, gentle stresses applied to the injured structure encourage the remodeling of collagen along the lines of force and reduce the negative effects of joint immobilization.[12] When the injured joint is kept in motion, the unwanted effects of immobilization on muscle, tendons, ligaments, articular and hyaline cartilage, blood supply, and nerve supply are reduced.

Under the stress of motion, collagen that would normally be deposited in a random order aligns along the line of applied stress. This realignment reduces functional shortening and capsular adhesions, thus maintaining the range of motion,[6,8] enhancing the tensile strength of tendons and *allografts*,[5] and stimulating repair of articular cartilage.[13]

Range of Motion

In most cases, the benefits of CPM increasing the joint's ROM are seen early in the patient's rehabilitation program, with the differences relative to patients not receiving CPM equalizing over time (assuming that both groups receive proper therapy). When given free rein to control the ROM, patients, using comfort as their guide, increase their range of motion by 6° to 7° per day.[14] Introducing CPM early into the rehabilitation scheme allows active motion and strength training routines to be incorporated earlier in the patient's program, an important consideration when dealing with an athletic population.[15–17]

Joint Nutrition

Both meniscal and articular cartilage are relatively avascular and derive most of their nutrients from synovial fluid. Meniscal cartilage is like a sponge and is nourished by being expanded and compressed so that by the natural movement of the joint the synovial fluid is alternately absorbed by and squeezed out of the cartilage. During immobilization, synovial fluid is not distributed throughout the joint. The application of CPM stimulates the circulation of synovial fluids and causes the meniscal cartilage to increase its uptake of nutrients. The delivery and the subsequent absorption of nutrients assist both types of cartilage in the healing process.[18,19]

Edema Reduction

The effectiveness of CPM in the reduction of edema is not clearly understood and varies according to the body part and condition being treated.[20] The passive movements of the limb and the elevation of the body part should assist in venous and lymphatic return by milking the muscle (Table 7–2).[21] Significant edema reduction after arthroplasty of the knee and ankle,[17,22] after anterior cruciate ligament (ACL) surgery, for knee inflammatory conditions,[26] and hand edema[27,28] have been documented.

Allograft: A replacement or augmentation of a biological structure with a synthetic one.

TABLE 7–2 **Rate of Femoral Vein Flow Arising from the Application of Various Modalities**

Technique	Femoral Vein Blood Flow (mL/min)
Passive straight-leg raises	1524
Anatomic CPM	1199
Nonanatomic CPM	836
Active ankle dorsiflexion	640
Pneumatic sleeve	586
Manual calf compression	532
Passive dorsiflexion	385

Source: Adapted from von Schroeder et al.[21]

Pain Reduction

The movement of the joint activates afferent nerves located in the muscle, joint, and skin, and possibly provides pain control through the gate mechanism. Any associated reduction in edema or muscle spasm, as well as deterrence of functional shortening, aids in limiting pain. An undocumented benefit of the early application of CPM may be its assistance in helping the patient overcome the apprehension of moving the knee after surgery.

Post–Anterior Cruciate Ligament Surgery

The physiological benefits of CPM application post–ACL surgery are not as promising as its use with other conditions. The ACL does not receive the same nutritional benefits from CPM as meniscal or articular cartilage.[29] The ACL is surrounded by its own synovial lining, which shields the ligament from gaining nutrition from the joint's synovial fluid. Instead, the ligament must rely on its intrinsic blood vessels.

Although initial ROM immediately after surgery is increased in patients who receive CPM, as long as proper therapy is received, there is no long-term difference in the joint's ROM.[23,24,30]

Many knee CPM units having a proximal posterior tibial bar cause an excessive amount of *translation* of the tibia on the femur. In procedures such as ACL repair, this movement could produce stress sufficient to damage the healing tissue and graft.[31] After surgery, a properly fitted CPM can be used without increasing anterior ACL laxity.[9,32]

Clinical Application of Continuous Passive Motion

Instrumentation

Power: This switch activates the internal circuits of the CPM unit.
Reset: This button clears all previous settings from the CPM unit's memory.

Translation: Sliding or gliding of opposing articular surfaces.

Timer: This control sets the duration of the treatment. A CONTINUOUS setting is provided for long-term treatments

ROM: This control adjusts the ROM from slight hyperextension (approximately + 5°) to full flexion (approximately 130°). Some units have separate controls to adjust the amount of flexion and extension

Speed: This knob adjusts the rate of motion between 10° and 120° per second. Increased speed (cycles per second) has been theorized to produce better tensile properties of healing tendons than lower speeds.[33]

Pause: This button stops the motion at the extreme ROM (flexion and/or extension) to allow a passive stretching of the fibers to occur

Interrupt: This control allows the patient to discontinue the CPM.

Trigger jack: Some units allow synchronization of CPM and electrical stimulation. The TRIGGER JACK allows the neuromuscular electrical stimulation unit to be activated during the PAUSE function.

Setup and Application

Often the CPM unit is applied in the recovery room after surgery by a CPM technician. The following protocol is provided as an example for a post–ACL reconstructive surgery.

1. Most CPM devices can be adjusted to fit the involved extremity even when the patient is wearing a brace or surgical bandages.
2. Measure the length of the patient's thigh from the ischial tuberosity to the joint line of the knee. Adjust the proximal carriage so that the proximal end meets the bottom of the buttocks.
3. Determine the length of the lower leg by measuring from the joint line of the knee to approximately 1/4 inch beyond the heel. Adjust the distal portion of the carriage accordingly.
4. Place the lower extremity in the unit with the joint line of the knee aligning to the articular hinge of the CPM unit.
5. Adjust the foot in the footplate so that the tibia is placed in the neutral position. Internally or externally rotating the tibia can result in increased stress on the ACL.
6. Set the ROM as prescribed by the physician. Generally this protocol is started with a limited ROM (0° to 60°) and progresses to the full ROM as healing occurs.
7. Set the SPEED of the treatment (e.g., cycle time of 4 minutes; 15 cycles per hour).
8. Give the patient the hand-held control and provide instruction on how and when to use it, including increasing speed and ROM and terminating the treatment.
9. The patient may be instructed to increase the ROM at regular intervals as tolerated.

Termination of the Treatment

1. Clean the mechanical housings with soap. The use of a 10 percent solution of household bleach and water is required if the unit becomes soiled with blood, synovial fluid, and so on.
2. Dispose of the carriage cover or wash it according to the manufacturer's instructions.

Duration and Frequency of Treatment

Continuous passive motion may be applied in long-term bouts where the patient is continuously attached to the unit, or the device may be applied in 1-hour treatment bouts three times a day. After surgery, use is for 6 to 8 hours a day, although the duration preferred by patients is 4 to 8 hours.[14] Patients may also be instructed in the use of CPM for in-home treatments, or a home-care visit by a physical therapist or physical therapist assistant may be required.

Precautions

- The use of continuous passive motion in conjunction with anticoagulation therapy may produce an intracompartmental hematoma.[34]
- Skin irritation from the straps or carriage cover may develop.

Indications

- After surgical repair of stable intra-articular or extra-articular joint fractures
- After joint surgery, including surgery on the ACL[32]
- After knee arthroplasty
- After surgery or chronic pathology to the knee extensor mechanisms
- For joint contractures
- After menisectomy
- After knee manipulations
- After joint debridement
- For tendon lacerations
- After osteochondral repair
- For enhancing the reabsorption of a *hemarthrosis*
- For *thrombophlebitis*

Contraindication

Cases in which the device causes an unwanted translation of opposing bones, overstressing the healing tissues

BIOFEEDBACK

The process of biofeedback involves "tapping into" the body's physiological processes. The body's electrical activity is amplified by the biofeedback unit and converted into auditory and/or visual signals that the patient can then use to model further activity. It is important to note that biofeedback does not monitor the actual response, but rather the conditions associated with response. For instance, when biofeedback is used to monitor muscle contractions, it is the electrical activity associated with the contraction that is being measured, not the actual force of the contraction. With orthopedic patients, biofeedback is most often

---

Hemarthrosis: Blood in a joint.
Thrombophlebitis: Inflammation of the veins.

used as an adjunct to muscle reeducation and training or to encourage the relaxation of a muscle group.

Biofeedback units operate on one (or sometimes more) of four biophysical principles. Electromyographic (EMG) units measure the amount of electrical activity in skeletal muscle through the use of either implanted or surface-mounted electrodes. Peripheral temperature units measure changes in the temperature of the distal extremities, most commonly the fingers or toes. Increased temperature caused by increased blood flow indicates systemic relaxation, whereas decreased temperature denotes stress, fear, or anxiety. The relative size of blood vessels is also the basis for photoplethysmography, which measures the amount of light reflected by subcutaneous tissues. The body's production of sweat is used in galvanic skin response biofeedback. Microcurrents are applied to the body (generally the fingers and palm), and the amount of electrical resistance is monitored. Sweaty skin contains more salt and is therefore a better conductor than dry skin.

Singly or in combination, these responses can be used to assist in developing the strength of muscular contractions, facilitating muscular relaxation, controlling blood pressure and heart rate, and decreasing the physical manifestation of emotional stress. It also forms the basis of lie detection tests.

Because the EMG technique of biofeedback using superficial electrodes is most prevalent in sports medicine, it is the focus of this text (the reader should be mindful that biofeedback is also used in the athletic population to reduce anxiety and improve performance). Conceptually, the tasks of any biofeedback unit are as follows[35]:

- Monitoring the physiological process
- Objectively measuring the process
- Converting what is being monitored into feedback that optimizes the desired effects

The electronic and physiological mechanisms associated with biofeedback are covered in the next section. At this point a clarification must be made between "monitoring" and "measuring" the electrical activity. Monitoring involves determining whether neuromuscular activity is present and, if so, whether it is increasing or decreasing. Measuring the activity involves placing an objective scale on the monitored readout.

Consider the two analog meters depicted in Figure 7–4. The meter in Figure 7–4A shows that activity is taking place, and we can tell if it is increasing, decreasing, or holding steady by observing the relative position of the needle. When a scale is placed on the meter in Figure 7–4B, the degree of activity, and therefore the degree of change, can be objectively measured. The scale on a biofeedback unit may use the number of microvolts as the measure, or there can be a simple 0-to-10 scale. Because of the lack of a standard biofeedback scale, measures made on a unit of one brand cannot be compared to measurements on a unit of another brand.[35] Also, placement of skin electrodes from treatment to treatment affects the measurement's reliability.

The meter is only one form of meaningful information that biofeedback units can provide. Most units can convert the signals into sound waves, an advantage because they do not require that visual attention be focused on the unit. The pitch of the sound increases and decreases based on the amount of neuromuscular activity.

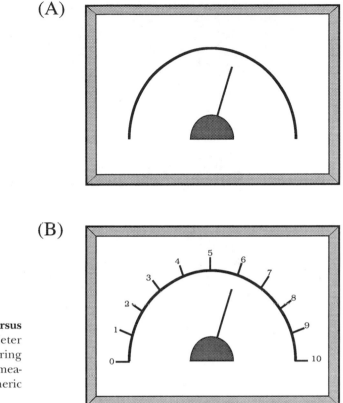

(A)

(B)

Biophysical Processes and Electrical Integration

Application of EMG biofeedback involves the use of three electrodes positioned over the muscle or muscle group that is the focus of the session (Fig. 7–5). As motor units are recruited into the contraction, the amount of electrical activity within the muscle increases. These signals are then picked up by the electrodes, amplified, and converted into visual and auditory signals.

Although this process seems rather simple, it is complicated by the presence of other electrical activity in our environment. We are always being bombarded by electromagnetic energy. A small portion of this energy is absorbed by the body and is consequently detected by the biofeedback unit. This unwanted energy, known as "noise," must be filtered out before the meaningful activity can be determined.

Referring to Figure 7–5, you will notice that the electrodes on each end are white and that the one in the middle is black. This black electrode serves as a point of reference for a very small current passed between the two white "active" electrodes. This results in two sources supplying input to a differential amplifier within the unit. Here, the meaningful information is separated from the useless noise. Because the extraneous noise is produced by electromagnetic sources, it occurs at a constant frequency and is detectable anywhere in the body. The differential amplifier compares the input from two sources and eliminates any activity that is common to both. In theory, the remaining activity represents neuromuscu-

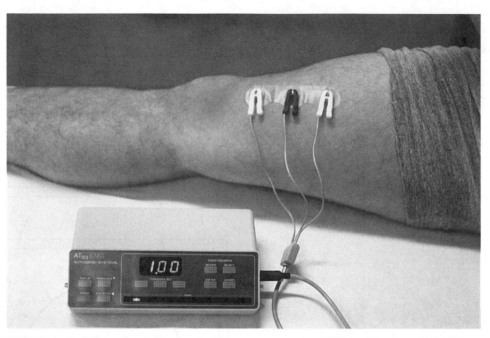

FIGURE 7–5 **Biofeedback Electrode Placement over the Oblique Portion of the Vastus Medialis.** Note the two white "active" electrodes and the black "reference" electrode. (The AT 33 Biofeedback Unit, courtesy of the Autogenic Corp.)

lar activity. However, the integrity of the final signal is dependent on the quality of the unit and the number of filters used.

Effects on the Injury Response Cycle

Electromyographic biofeedback itself does not affect the injury response process. Unlike other modalities presented in this text, this device assists voluntary functions to produce the desired results. Other types of biofeedback units monitor functions that are controlled by the autonomic nervous system. Because of this, the effectiveness of biofeedback is judged on a case-by-case basis. Clearly, however, proper use of this unit does facilitate muscle reeducation or promote relaxation and increase ROM. In turn, these effects can lead to a reduction in pain and/or an increase in function.

During neuromuscular rehabilitation, EMG is most effective when it is incorporated early in the patient's program, especially when active motions are involved.[36] The injured tissues must be able to withstand the tension and stresses associated with the motion, and there must be some level of nerve supply to the target muscle or muscle groups.

The benefits of biofeedback are enhanced by fully instructing the individual on the concept of biofeedback, incorporating learning strategies, and setting goals for the patient to achieve.[37,38] External, verbal feedback from the clinician can reinforce the neuromuscular learning as well as providing positive cognitive reinforcement to the patient. However, this type of feedback during the bout can distract the patient from the task at hand, so refrain from providing feedback until the exercise has been completed.[39]

Neuromuscular Effects

Biofeedback is most often incorporated into an orthopedic treatment and rehabilitation program after surgery or long-term immobilization. After surgical intervention, edema, pain, and decreased input from joint receptors make voluntary muscle contraction difficult, if not impossible. The use of biofeedback shapes the response that enables the central nervous system to re-establish sensory-motor loops "forgotten" by the patient.[40,41] On reaching the brain, afferent stimuli, in this case sound or visual cues, stimulate cerebral areas that normally receive proprioceptive information. These artificial signals, combined with the visual cue of actually watching the muscle contract, assist in reopening a neural loop that sends efferent signals to the appropriate muscle(s).

Biofeedback is used to augment the input lost from these receptors by providing other types of information. The normal proprioceptive, and perhaps kinesthetic, input is amplified through the use of sound, light, or meters. This concept applies not only to restoring the function of an injured body part but also to increasing the strength of healthy muscle.[42]

The cognitive process of neuromuscular relaxation is similar to that of evoking muscle contractions. However, rather than attempting to re-establish neural loops, these pathways are inhibited. The goal of relaxation therapy is to decrease the number of motor impulses being relayed to the spasming muscle. This technique is best used with cases of subconscious muscle guarding.

The use of relaxation biofeedback does not significantly increase flexibility in healthy individuals when compared with standard flexibility exercises. However, athletes combining flexibility with biofeedback displayed a greater retention of improvement than those training without the aid of biofeedback.[43]

It is best to try regaining deficits first through voluntary contractions. If this method is ineffective, biofeedback may then be introduced. Dramatic results can be seen after a single treatment bout.

Pain Reduction

The primary benefit of pain reduction stems from restoring normal function of the body part. Reeducating muscle removes the unwanted stress associated with abnormal biomechanics. Facilitating reduction of muscle spasm reduces the amount of mechanical pressure placed on nociceptors.

Although its mechanism is beyond the scope of this book, inhibitory biofeedback has also been successfully used in the reduction of myofascial pain, the pain associated with migraine and tension headaches, as well as in general stress reduction.[44] Most inhibitory pain-control approaches also involve cognitive and behavioral aspects that build on the biofeedback sessions.[45]

Clinical Application of Biofeedback

Instrumentation

Biofeedback units range from the very simple to the ultracomplex and may be in the form of clinical models or portable, "take-home" units. The following description is of the typical "midrange" unit. Consult the user's manual of your particular unit for a more detailed description of its operation.

Sensitivity range: This control provides coarse adjustments on the threshold necessary to acquire feedback.

Tuner: This knob allows fine adjustments on the threshold required to obtain feedback.

Output: This device determines the type of feedback available. Visual feedback appears by way of a meter or bar graph. The audio output is normally adjustable between various frequencies. Advanced units allow for a computer interface that stores results of the session.

Statistics: Some biofeedback units calculate statistics of the patient's muscular activity for assessment of the rehabilitation program. Measures such as the mean, maximum, and standard deviation provide quantitative information for evaluating the patient's progress.

Setup and Application

Patient Preparation

1. Have the patient shave the area if applicable.
2. Remove any dirt, oil, or makeup in the area where the electrodes are to be applied, by wiping the skin with alcohol. These substances impede the conduction of the bioelectric signals.
3. Very sensitive biofeedback units may require that the electrode site be mildly abraded with an emery cloth.
4. Apply a suitable conductive gel to the electrodes.
5. Secure the electrodes over the belly of the muscle targeted in this therapy. Note that the active electrodes must be applied over the target muscle. The reference electrode may be secured anywhere on the body, but by convention, it is normally placed between the two active electrodes (see Fig. 7–5).
6. Plug the common electrode lead(s) into the INPUT jack(s) on the unit.
7. Turn the unit ON.
8. Adjust the OUTPUT to the desired mode of feedback (visual, audio, or both).
9. Provide instructions to the individual regarding the proper use of biofeedback, including goal setting.
10. The patient should be free of visual and auditory distractions during the course of the session.

Facilitation of Isometric Muscle Contraction

1. Instruct the patient to relax the body part as much as possible.
2. Adjust the SENSITIVITY RANGE to the lowest value that does not provide feedback.
3. Place the body part in the desired position.
4. Instruct the patient to maximally contract the muscle and keep the meter (be it visual or audio) peaked.
5. Hold the isometric contraction for 6 seconds.
6. Complete relaxation should be obtained before the next contraction. Instruct the patient to completely relax the muscle so that the meter resets to the baseline.

7. Repeat the contractions as indicated. If the muscle group is severely atrophied, the number of contractions is normally limited to 10 to 15 contractions because of fatigue.
8. By decreasing the sensitivity, the patient will have to elicit a stronger contraction to receive feedback.
9. If the individual is unable to evoke a contraction, two strategies can be implemented:
    a. Have the patient contract the muscle on the opposite limb, then attempt to contract the involved muscle.
    b. Apply the biofeedback unit to the opposite limb so that the person will "learn" the biofeedback technique.

    Other strategies include having the person

    Watch and/or touch the contracting muscle

    Contract surrounding or opposing muscles

    Contract the proximal portion of the muscle to facilitate neuromuscular activity in the distal motor units

Termination of the Procedure

1. Remove the electrodes and wipe away any excess gel.
2. To avoid dependency on biofeedback, have the patient perform additional sets of contractions without the aid of the unit to "remember" how to perform the contractions.

Duration and Frequency of Treatment

Biofeedback can be performed daily as needed either in the clinical setting or at home. Be aware of any muscle soreness that may occur after exercise and adjust the treatment protocol accordingly.

Precautions

- Do not exceed the prescribed ROM.
- Avoid undue muscle tension that may affect grafts or other tissue restrictions.

Indications

- To facilitate muscular contractions
- To regain neuromuscular control
- To decrease muscle spasm
- To promote systemic relaxation

Contraindication

- Conditions in which muscular contractions would insult the tissues

CERVICAL TRACTION

Cervical traction is a technique that applies a longitudinal force to the cervical spine and associated structures. This force can be applied with continuous or intermittent tension. Continuous traction maintains the cervical region in an elongated position and is applied with a small force for an extended period. This method of application stimulates the supporting and stabilizing functions of the cervical structures and, by assisting in support of the head, allows the cervical musculature to "rest."

Intermittent cervical traction alternates periods of traction force with intervals of relaxation in the tension. During the traction, the cervical structures are elongated and the posterior articulating surfaces widen. The relaxation phase allows a decrease in the amount of cervical neuromuscular activity. Intermittent cervical traction is most commonly applied through the use of a motorized system (Fig. 7–6).

Continuous cervical traction may be applied through a weight-and-pulley system, pneumatic system, motorized device, or patient positioning. Another type of spinal traction, lumbar (or pelvic) traction, is used for the treatment of lumbar spine dysfunction (Box 7–1). Both lumbar and cervical traction may also be applied manually (Fig. 7–7).

The amount of tension applied to the body can be expressed in terms of pounds or as a percentage of the patient's body weight. Although the human head accounts for approximately 8.1 percent of the total body weight, a greater amount of force is needed to produce widening of the vertebral structures because of the cervical musculature and other soft tissues.[46] In most pathologies, when the patient is reclining, separation of the cervical spine begins to occur with an applied force equal to about 20 percent of the body weight. When the patient is placed in a seated position, a greater proportion of the total body weight is required before separation occurs. Specific styles of halters have been designed that allow for specificity of spinal separation. This specificity allows spinal separation to occur at a lower percentage of the body weight.[47]

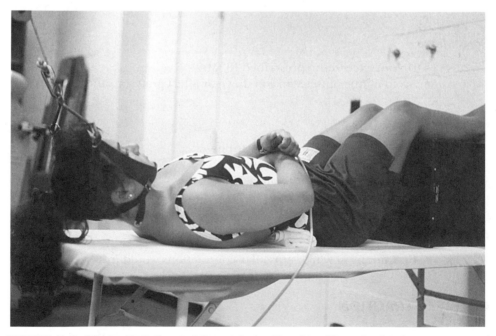

FIGURE 7–6 **Mechanical Cervical Intermittent Traction.** Note the lumbar support and flexion of the knees.

BOX 7–1 Lumbar Traction

Traction applied to the lumbar area is useful in treating many of the same conditions as cervical traction is used for, and is especially useful in the treatment of *spondylolisthesis*. Increasing the amount of separation between the vertebrae can reduce impingement of the lumbar nerve roots. Likewise, nerve entrapment as a result of a herniated disk is reduced by allowing the disk to return to its original shape, decompressing the nucleus pulposus to below –100 mm Hg.[83]

This method of traction can be applied manually or through the use of a pelvic halter and chest straps in a manner similar to cervical traction. An adjunct method of delivering lumbar traction uses a split table that reduces the amount of frictional force placed on the lumbar spine.

Biophysical Effects

The effectiveness of cervical traction has been linked to five mechanical factors[48]:

- The position of the neck
- The force of the applied traction
- The duration of the traction

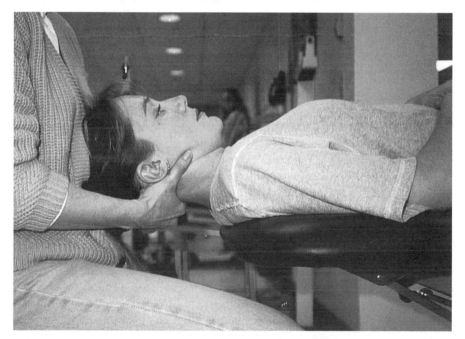

FIGURE 7–7 **Manual Cervical Traction.** The clinician cradles the patient's occiput to apply traction along the length of the entire cervical spine. Segmental traction (i.e., between C5 and C6) can be performed by grasping the transverse processes of the appropriate cervical vertebrae and applying traction while stabilizing the inferior vertebrae.

Spondylolisthesis: Forward slippage of the lower lumbar vertebrae on the vertebrae above.

BOX 7–2 **The Intervertebral Disk**

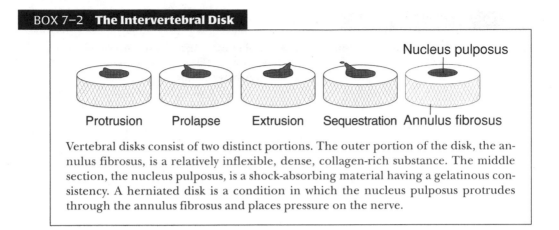

Protrusion   Prolapse   Extrusion   Sequestration   Annulus fibrosus

Nucleus pulposus

Vertebral disks consist of two distinct portions. The outer portion of the disk, the annulus fibrosus, is a relatively inflexible, dense, collagen-rich substance. The middle section, the nucleus pulposus, is a shock-absorbing material having a gelatinous consistency. A herniated disk is a condition in which the nucleus pulposus protrudes through the annulus fibrosus and places pressure on the nerve.

- The angle of pull
- The position of the patient

During the application of cervical traction, the neck is placed in approximately 25° to 30° of flexion. This position straightens the normal *lordosis* of the cervical spine and allows the posterior articulations to open, widening the intervertebral *foramen* and stretching the posterior soft tissue. The anterior portion of an intervertebral disk (Box 7–2) is compressed, and the posterior portion elongates when the neck is placed in flexion. When the cervical spine is placed in extension, the opposite effect occurs. To separate the facet joint surfaces, the traction must be administered in at least 15° of extension (Table 7–3).[49]

The force applied to the cervical spine during traction has been suspected of being transmitted to the lumbar area through the dural covering of the spinal cord. This can lead to residual lumbar nerve root impingement and subsequent pain, especially when the patient has a history of lumbar osteoarthritis or other lumbar degenerative changes.[48] Care must be taken to question the patient about sensations not only within the cervical area but also in the thoracic and lumbar regions and lower extremity.

Although treatment bouts with cervical traction can last for hours, the mechanical benefits appear to occur in the first few minutes of treatment.[50] Cervical traction may be applied with the patient in one of several positions, but the two most common are the seated and supine positions. When the patient is in a seated position, the traction must first overcome the force of gravity before therapeutic forces are placed on the cervical region. The supine position has several advantages. With the patient lying down, the cervical musculature is allowed to relax because it is not supporting the weight of the head. Therefore, a lower amount of tension is required to obtain therapeutic effects.

Lordosis: The forward curvature of the cervical and lumbar spine.
Foramen: An opening (e.g., in a bone) to allow the passage of blood vessels or nerves.

TABLE 7–3 **Amount of Cervical Intervertebral Separation Based on the Angle of Traction**

Structure	Spinal Segment	Traction Angle		
		Neutral	30° Flexion	15° Extension
Anterior intervertebral separation	C2-3	6%	21%	2%
	C3-4	8%	10%	–1%
	C4-5	12%	16%	–1%
	C5-6	5%	15%	–2%
	C6-7	0%	9%	–2%
Posterior intervertebral separation	C2-3	15%	5%	4%
	C3-4	22%	4%	–14%
	C4-5	19%	17%	–26%
	C5-6	19%	19%	–37%
	C6-7	37%	20%	–50%
Facet joint separation	C2-3	2%	–12%	7%
	C3-4	2%	–14%	3%
	C4-5	5%	–19%	15%
	C5-6	3%	–10%	17%
	C6-7	10%	–5%	6%

Source: Adapted from Wong et al.[49]
Negative percentages indicate a decrease in the intervertebral space.

Effects on the Injury Response Cycle

Intermittent cervical traction is incorporated into the treatment plan to reduce the pain and paresthesia associated with cervical nerve root impingement, muscle spasm, or articular dysfunction. This passive treatment can be combined with active exercise to enhance the benefits of the treatment.

Application of cervical traction reduces the amount of pressure on nerve roots as a result of mechanical pressure from bony protuberances or intervertebral disks. Elongating the cervical spine allows separation of the vertebrae and results in decompression of the disk.

Muscle Spasm

Traction is often applied in an effort to interrupt the pain-spasm-pain cycle through lengthening of the affected musculature. However, after treatment bouts of intermittent cervical traction, an analysis of *electromyograms* showed no decrease in the amount of spasm in the treated tissues when compared with pretreatment activity.[46,51,52]

Electromyogram: A recording of the electrical charges associated with the contraction of a muscle.

The reduction of cervical muscle spasm is contingent on finding the optimal amount of traction force. Too little force will not sufficiently elongate the musculature or open the intervertebral foramen, and little or no benefit will be gained. If too much force is applied, an unwanted muscle contraction will ensue as the body attempts to protect itself, resulting in the opposite effect of that desired.

Pain Reduction

In addition to breaking the pain-spasm-pain cycle, as described in the previous section, several other factors have been linked to the reduction of pain. Traction can reduce pain by decreasing the amount of mechanical pressure placed on the cervical nerve roots. The rhythmic pressure is thought to improve blood flow and to decrease myofascial adhesions. This same rhythm may also stimulate joint and muscular sensory nerves and inhibit the transmission of pain through the gate mechanism.[53]

If the pain results from a disk lesion, the bulging nucleus pulposus is encouraged to centralize or return to its normal position. Although a disk lesion is not normally responsive to intermittent traction, continuous traction can provide the time necessary for reabsorption of the nucleus pulposus.

Clinical Application of Cervical Traction

Instrumentation

Mode: This setting allows the traction to be applied intermittently or continuously.

Hold time: This control adjusts the duration of the traction phase (in seconds).

Rest time: This control adjusts the duration of the relaxation phase (in seconds). Applicable only to intermittent traction.

Tension: This knob controls the amount of tension, in pounds, applied to the halter.

Duration: This knob selects the total duration of the treatment.

Halter (harness): The "standard" halter applies force to the mandible and *occiput.* Modified halters have been designed that reduce the amount of force applied to the chin, allow specificity regarding the cervical level where the separation occurs, and decrease the forces placed on the temporomandibular joint (TMJ).

Spreader bar: This device connects the halter to the traction device through a pulley cable.

Safety switch: This switch allows the patient to interrupt the treatment and decrease tension.

Setup and Application

The following protocol describes the setup and application of motorized intermittent cervical traction with the patient in a reclined position.

Occiput: The posterior base of the skull.

Patient Preparation

1. Determine the presence of any contraindications.
2. Determine the patient's weight.
3. The cervical musculature may be pretreated with moist heat to decrease muscle spasm.
4. Instruct the patient to remove any earrings, glasses, or other clothing that may interfere with the placement of the halter.
5. Lay the patient on the treatment table in the supine position.
6. Place a pillow or two under the patient's knees.
7. Position the unit so that the line of pull is aligned with the midline of the body (i.e., so that the head is not laterally flexed).
8. Secure the halter to the cervical region according to the manufacturer's instructions. Normally the pressure points are the occipital processes and, to a lesser degree, the chin.
9. Connect the halter to the spreader bar.
10. Align the unit so that the angle of pull places the cervical spine in approximately 25° of flexion.

Initiation of the Treatment

1. Remove any slack in the pulley cable.
2. Reset all controls to zero and turn unit ON.
3. Adjust the RATIO to the appropriate on-off sequence, normally a 3:1 or 4:1 ratio.
4. Adjust the TENSION to approximately 10 percent of the person's body weight. If this is the patient's first exposure to intermittent cervical traction, or if the person is displaying apprehension about the treatment, the TENSION can be initiated at its lowest value.
5. Instruct the patient as to what to expect during the treatment and to inform you if any discomfort is experienced. Explain that the force of the pull is felt at the occiput and not at the chin.
6. Set the appropriate treatment DURATION, and initiate the treatment.
7. Allow the unit to cycle through its first tension cycle. The TENSION may be gradually increased during subsequent cycles. If pain is experienced at any time during the treatment, decrease the amount of force or discontinue the treatment.
8. Instruct the patient to remain relaxed during both the on and off cycles.
9. If the pressure placed on the mandible causes discomfort in the teeth or TMJ joint, gauze or a mouthpiece may be placed between the teeth to dissipate the force.

Termination of the Treatment

1. If the traction unit does not automatically do so, gradually reduce the TENSION over a period of three or four cycles.
2. Gain some slack in the cable and turn the unit off.
3. Remove the SPREADER BAR and HALTER.
4. Question the patient regarding any perceived benefit or complications derived from the treatment.

5. Have the patient remain sitting or lying supine for 5 minutes after the conclusion of the treatment.
6. Record the pertinent information (tension, duration, duty cycle) in the patient's medical file.

Duration and Frequency of Treatment

The duration of cervical traction can range from minutes to hours, but it is most commonly given for periods of 10 to 20 minutes. Cervical traction applied for a herniated disk has a duration of 5 to 10 minutes.

Precautions

- Cervical traction should never be attempted in conditions that have not been evaluated by a physician.
- The patient must be closely monitored throughout the treatment, and the treatment should be immediately discontinued if symptoms increase or if pain or paresthesia is experienced.
- Improper extension traction can result in a rupture of the cervical esophagus.[54]
- Excessive duration and/or traction weight can cause thrombosis of the internal jugular vein.[55]

Indications

- Cervical or lumbar muscle spasm
- Certain degenerative disk diseases
- Herniated or protruding intervertebral disk
- Nerve root compression
- Osteoarthritis
- Capsulitis of the vertebral joints
- Pathology of the anterior or posterior longitudinal ligaments

Contraindications

- Unstable spine
- Diseases affecting the vertebra or spinal cord, including cancer and *meningitis*
- Vertebral fractures
- Extruded disk fragmentation
- Spinal cord compression
- Conditions in which vertebral flexion and/or extension is contraindicated
- Conditions that worsen after traction treatments
- *Osteoporosis*

Meningitis: Inflammation of the membranes of the brain or spinal cord.
Osteoporosis: A porous condition resulting in softening of bone. Most commonly (but not exclusively) seen in postmenopausal women.

THERAPEUTIC MASSAGE

Massage, the systematic manipulation of the body's tissues, is one of the oldest healing techniques still used in modern medicine. Dating back at least to the ancient Olympics, massage has been present in most cultures. Regional variations have contributed to the different forms of massage used today, and it is this diverse background that leads to inconsistencies in application protocols.

Because it is a time-consuming task that requires the full attention of the clinician, the popularity of massage as a therapeutic technique has faded. Still, massage is a very effective treatment method for promoting local and systemic relaxation or invigoration, increasing local blood flow, breaking down adhesions, and encouraging venous return.

Because massage is a skill-based technique, and because the possibility of abuse is high, many states provide for licensure of massage therapists. Most other healing professions, including physical therapy and athletic training, incorporate massage techniques into their professional preparation.

Massage Strokes

There are several different types of massage strokes, and each may be varied by adding more or less pressure, using different parts of the hand, or changing the direction of the stroke. These elements may then be sequenced to produce different effects. The following sections describe the basic elements of each stroke and discuss how they can be varied (Table 7–4).

Effleurage

Effleurage, the stroking of the skin, is performed with the palm of the hand to stimulate deep tissues, or with the fingertips to stimulate sensory nerves (Fig. 7–8).

TABLE 7–4 Summary of Massage Strokes and Their Physiological Effect

Stroke	Technique	Effect
Effleurage	Stroking of the skin	Deep stroking: stimulates deep tissues, forces fluids in the direction of the stroke Superficial stroking: 　Slow strokes: promotes relaxation 　Fast strokes: stimulates tissues and encourages blood flow
Pétrissage	Lifting and kneading of the skin	Stretches and separates muscle fiber, fascia, and scar tissue
Friction	Deep pressure	Effects muscle mobilization, tissue separation, including the breakup of scar tissue
Tapotement	Tapping or pounding the skin	Promotes relaxation and the desensitization of nerve endings
Vibration	Rapid shaking of the tissues	Increases blood flow and provides systemic invigoration

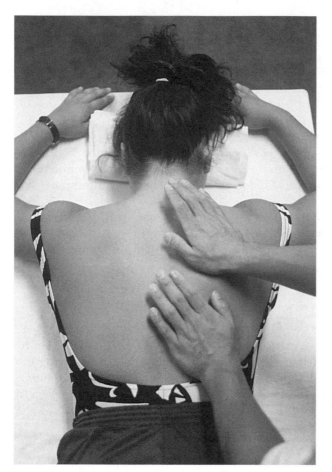

FIGURE 7–8 **Effleurage (Stroking) of the Spinal Erector Group.** The deep pressure is applied with the palm of the hands and runs the length of the muscle group.

This stroke is categorized as being either superficial or deep. Superficial stroking may either follow the contour of the body itself, or it may relate to the direction of the underlying muscles. Deep stroking should follow the course of veins and lymph vessels to force fluids in these vessels back toward the heart.

The strokes may be performed slowly to promote relaxation or rapidly to encourage blood flow and stimulate the tissues. In either case, the strokes are done in a rhythmic manner. Ideally, at least one hand should be in contact with the skin at any given point. This may be achieved by stroking the skin in one direction and lightly gliding the hands back to the starting point. Another method involves staggering the strokes. The stroke of one hand begins just before the other hand leaves the surface of the skin.

Light effleurage is generally done at both the beginning and end of the massage and may be used between pétrissage strokes. During the initial stages of the treatment, effleurage relaxes the patient and indicates the areas that will be massaged. At the conclusion of the treatment, this stroke "calms down" any nerves that may have become irritated during the massage.

Pétrissage

This method of massage involves the lifting and kneading of the skin, subcutaneous tissue, and muscle with the fingers or hand (Fig. 7–9). The skin is gently

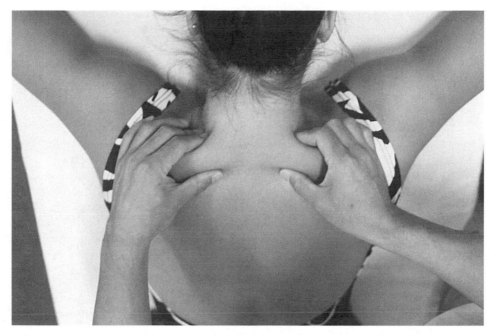

FIGURE 7–9 **Pétrissage (Kneading) of the Trapezius Muscle Groups.** The skin and underlying tissue is lifted and rolled in the hand.

lifted between the thumb and fingers or the fingers and palm and gently rolled and kneaded in the hand. For this reason, pétrissage is often performed without the use of a lubricant. This process frees adhesions by stretching and separating muscle fiber, fascia, and scar tissue while also assisting in venous return and milking the muscle of waste products.

Friction

The goal of friction massage is to mobilize muscle and separate adhesions in muscle, tendon fibers, or scar tissue that restrict movement and cause pain, and is used to facilitate local blood profusion.[56] There are two basic types of friction massage: circular and transverse. Circular friction massage is applied with the thumbs working in circular motion and is often effective in the treatment of muscle spasm and trigger points. In transverse friction massage, the thumbs or fingertips stroke the tissue from opposite directions, and it is particularly effective in the treatment of tendinitis or other forms of joint adhesions. When treating a large muscle mass, the elbow can be used in place of the thumb (Fig. 7–10). In each case, sufficient force is applied so that the pressure will reach deep into the tissues. Begin lightly and gradually progress to firmer, deeper strokes. To achieve the optimal effects of friction massage, the muscle should be placed in a relaxed position. The area may be preheated using a moist heat pack or ultrasound.

This method of massage is to be avoided in conditions in which the underlying tissues would be further injured by the pressure, such as acute injuries. Friction massage differs from the other massage strokes in that this is not necessarily pleasing to receive. Indeed, friction massage is often painful, especially when trigger points are the target of the treatment. Friction massage can be followed by a stretching routine to further facilitate the ROM.

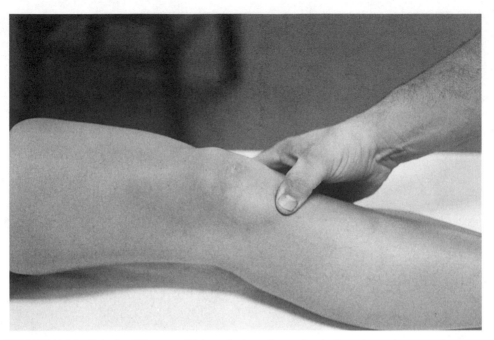

FIGURE 7–10   **Friction Massage.** This technique is used to isolate deep tissue, such as scar tissue.

Tapotement

Tapotement involves the gentle tapping or pounding of the skin. The most common form of tapotement uses the ulnar side of the wrist to contact the skin, in a manner similar to a "karate chop" (Fig. 7–11). This stroke is performed with the wrist and fingers limp so that the hand more or less "slaps" the skin. In an alternate form of tapotement, a cupped hand is used.

A tapotement variation that promotes relaxation and desensitization of irritated nerve endings is called "raindrops." The fingers lightly touch the skin in an alternating manner, as if you were typing on a keyboard.

Vibration

This method involves the rapid shaking of the tissue and serves to sooth peripheral nerves. Although a skilled masseur or masseuse is quite capable of achieving therapeutic effects manually, less skilled individuals often use a mechanical vibrator.

Myofascial Release

Myofascial release involves the traditional effleurage, pétrissage, and friction massage strokes with stretching of the muscles and fascia to obtain relaxation of tense and/or adhered tissues. Abnormalities of the myofascial system are thought to be linked to *fibromyalgia*, chronic fatigue syndrome, and myofascial pain syndrome.[57–59]

Fibromyalgia: Chronic inflammation of a muscle or connective tissue.

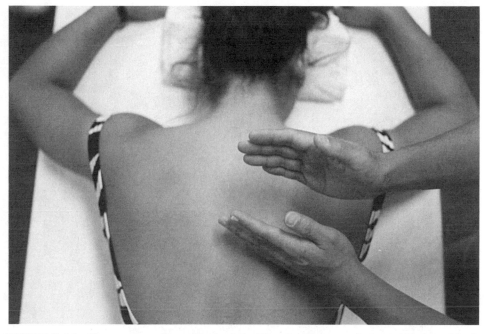

FIGURE 7–11 **Tapotement (Pounding) of the Muscle.** The muscle is rapidly hit with the ulnar side of the hand.

The true existence of myofascial pain syndrome and its related conditions have not been universally accepted.[60]

The actual delivery of myofascial release techniques tends not to follow a structured pattern. Rather, the clinician receives cues and feedback from the patient's tissues indicating what strokes and stretches are appropriate. The basic myofascial release techniques involve pulling the tissues in opposite directions, stabilizing the proximal or superior position with one hand while applying a stretch with the opposite hand, or using the patient's body weight to stabilize the extremity while a longitudinal stress is applied. Advanced techniques can involve more than one clinician applying opposing traction forces across the body (Fig. 7–12).

A discussion of the complex range of myofascial techniques and theories is beyond the scope of this text.

Massage Media

Most massages incorporate some type of medium to decrease the friction between the patient's skin and the hand; however, massage can be given without any medium being used. Lubricants, including massage lotion, peanut oil, powder, and even counterirritant, allow the hands to glide smoothly over the skin and focus the effects on the underlying muscle. If the massage is being given over hairy areas, lubricants are needed to keep from pulling body hair.

Various massage application techniques are enhanced when performed without the use of a lubricant. In strokes such as pétrissage, lubricants can interfere with the lifting and kneading of the skin. In addition, friction assists in mobilizing

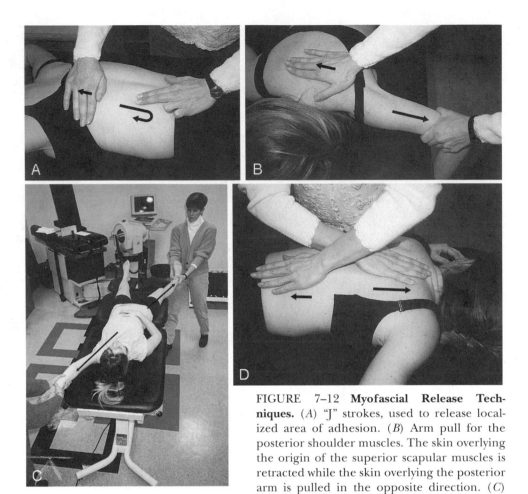

FIGURE 7–12 **Myofascial Release Techniques.** (*A*) "J" strokes, used to release localized area of adhesion. (*B*) Arm pull for the posterior shoulder muscles. The skin overlying the origin of the superior scapular muscles is retracted while the skin overlying the posterior arm is pulled in the opposite direction. (*C*) Two-person diagonal release. The opposite arm and leg are aligned and a traction force is placed on each extremity. (*D*) Focused stretching. The hands move the skin and fascia in opposite directions. In the case pictured, the force is parallel to the line of the muscles, but this technique can also be performed perpendicular to the muscle fibers.

the skin over the underlying tissues, making the use of lubricants contraindicated with this style of massage.

Frozen ice cups, described in Chapter 4, are also used during massage to produce numbness.

Effects on the Injury Response Cycle

Massage has been said to evoke a number of responses within the body. Many of these reputed effects, such as the mobilization of adipose tissue and increased muscle tone, have never been substantiated. This section attempts to separate fact from fiction.

In general, massage strokes can produce various responses, depending on the amount of pressure applied and the speed of the stroke. Light, slow stroking of the skin results in systemic relaxation. Fast, deep strokes cause an increase in blood flow to the area, invigorating the patient.

It is difficult to differentiate between the physiological and the psychological effects of massage. Athletes who believe that massage will improve their performance, or individuals who believe that massage will assist in the healing process, often will see improvement simply through the power of suggestion.

Cardiovascular Changes

Deep friction or vigorous massage is thought to produce vascular changes similar to those of inflammation, with the treated area being marked by increased blood flow, histamine release, and an increased temperature. Scientific studies have failed to support these theories. Massaging the forearm and quadriceps muscle groups with effleurage, pétrissage, and tapotement failed to increase the arterial blood flow supplying these groups.[61] Massage before submaximal treadmill testing revealed no significant differences in cardiac output, blood pressure, and lactic acid concentration in a treatment group compared with a group receiving no massage before testing.[62]

Massage applied for the purpose of inducing system relaxation does produce physiological changes in the cardiovascular system. Decreased heart rate, respiratory rate, and blood pressure have been observed in patients after 30 minutes of massage.[63]

Neuromuscular Changes

Pétrissage has been shown to decrease neuromuscular excitability, but only during the duration of the massage, and the effects are confined to the muscle(s) being massaged.[64–66] A study examining the effects of massage before competition concluded that this technique does not significantly increase the stride frequency of sprinters.[67]

A massage routine, consisting of deep effleurage, circular friction, and transverse friction applied to the hamstrings, has been shown to increase hamstring flexibility.[68] This effect is a result of the combined decrease in neuromuscular excitability (relaxation) and stretching of muscle and scar tissue.

Massage is less effective in decreasing muscular recovery time after exercise, but may be effective in reducing the amount of delayed-onset muscle soreness (when applied 2 hours after exercise) by reducing the *emigration* of neutrophils and by increasing serum cortisol levels.[69,70] Massaging muscles between exercise bouts, be it a sprinter's legs between races or a pitcher's shoulder between innings, does little to reduce muscular fatigue.[68,71]

Edema Reduction

When performed properly, massage can increase venous and lymphatic flow that assists in the removal of edema.[72] Manual or mechanical massage (see Intermit-

---

Emigration: Passage of white blood corpuscles through the walls of capillaries and veins during inflammation.

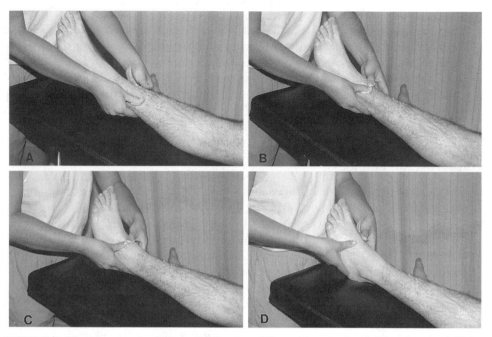

FIGURE 7–13   **Massage for Edema Reduction.** "Uncorking the bottle" involves mobilizing the proximal edema and progressively working distally.

tent Compression Pump, p 305) forces fluids within the vessels to move toward the heart.

The key to reducing edema is to first mobilize the proximal area of edema before attempting to move the distal areas (Fig. 7–13). This procedure, known as "uncorking the bottle," can be visualized as removing a traffic jam. Cars at the back of the pack cannot move forward until the car at the front of the line moves.

The step-by-step application of this method of massage is presented in the section on setup and application in this unit.

Pain Control

Pain reduction through the application of massage is no doubt the result of several different mechanisms. The benefits of massage-mediated pain reduction can last up to 24 hours after the treatment.[73]

Mechanical pain is reduced through interrupting muscle spasm and reducing edema. Chemical pain is thought to be diminished by increasing blood flow and by encouraging the removal of cellular wastes. However, simply touching the skin can also reduce the pain by activating cutaneous receptors. Gentle massage activates sensory nerves and therefore inhibits pain through the gate mechanism.[74] Massage has also been shown to activate the autonomic nervous system and *pacinian receptors,* both of which assist in hindering nociceptive impulses[72] and

Pacinian receptors: Receptors located deep in the skin that relay information regarding pressure and vibration. Within the joints, they assist in relaying proprioceptive information.

decrease H-reflex amplitude of spinal cord–injured patients, but only during the actual massage administration.[75,76] Massage has not been shown to significantly affect serum levels of endogenous opiates, such as β-endorphin, in a treatment group compared with a control group.[77] Further pain reduction may occur secondary to mediation of neural reflexes.[78]

Psychological Benefits

Despite the empirical evidence for many of the physiological benefits that are claimed to be associated with massage, support for the psychological benefits does exist. Much of this benefit extends from the one-on-one interaction required between the clinician and the patient.[74,79] This interaction reduces patient anxiety, depression, and mental stress.[63,80] Although pain reduction can be attributed to stimulation of sensory nerves and decreased spasticity within the treated area, administering massage to uninvolved areas also brings about pain relief.[81] Patient compliance in reporting for treatment sessions is greatly enhanced when massage is included as a part of the treatment regimen.[82]

Clinical Application of Massage

Setup and Application

General Considerations

1. Establish the absence of contraindications.
2. The position of the patient relative to the clinician is important to both parties. The clinician should stand in a place that requires little or no repositioning. Likewise, long strokes, such as those applied to the back or hamstrings, should be performed by taking small steps rather than by bending the back.
3. The patient should be positioned so that the muscles being massaged are in a relaxed position. If an extremity is being massaged to reduce edema, it should be elevated.
4. If a massage medium is being used, warm it slightly so that it is not uncomfortable when it is applied (i.e., not too hot or too cold).
5. When a painful area is being treated, the massage begins in a nonpainful area, works through the area of pain, and concludes on another pain-free area.
6. Drape the patient to ensure modesty.

"Classical" Massage

1. The area may be preheated with moist heat to promote relaxation of the musculature.
2. A pillow may be placed under the ankles and a small pad, such as a folded towel, placed under the abdomen to assist in the relaxation of the lumbar musculature.
3. If applicable, apply the massage medium on the body part(s) to be treated.
4. Follow the application of the medium with a light, slow effleurage.
5. Gradually build up to deeper effleurage.

6. Begin pétrissage strokes.
7. Apply deep friction massage where (and if) applicable.
8. Apply tapotement to the back and extremities (if treated).
9. Reapply pétrissage and deep effleurage.
10. End the treatment with light effleurage.

Massage for Edema Reduction

1. Elevate the body part to be treated using an incline board, pillow, or other device.
2. Cover the entire surface to be treated with a lubricating massage lotion.
3. Position yourself distal to the limb. For example, if the ankle is being massaged, stand so that you see the bottom of the foot.
4. Begin by making long, slow strokes toward the heart, starting proximal to the injured area. Every fourth or fifth stroke, move the starting point of the massage slightly distal.
5. Continue stroking longitudinally, with the starting point gradually being moved distally.
6. When the distal portion of the edematous area is reached, begin working back to the original starting point.

Termination of the Treatment

1. If a lubricant was used, remove it with a towel.
2. If appropriate for the stage of injury, encourage active ROM exercises.
3. To assist in flushing metabolic waste from the body, the patient should be encouraged to drink water after the treatment.

Duration and Frequency of Treatment

Massage for relaxation or invigoration may be given as needed. The duration of the massage ranges from a few minutes up to an hour. Massage for edema reduction is given once a day for an average duration of 5 to 10 minutes. Friction massage to tendons is performed once a day for 5 minutes or as needed.

Precaution

- Massage may increase the inflammatory response when used early in the acute or subacute stage of the injury response cycle.

Indications

- To relieve fibrosis
- To increase venous return
- To break the pain-spasm-pain cycle
- To evoke systemic relaxation
- To improve or stimulate local blood flow

Contraindications

- Sites where fractures have failed to heal
- Acute sprains or strains
- Skin conditions or lesions

SUMMARY

The modalities presented in this chapter transcend many different categories and, like most modalities, should be an adjunct to the rehabilitation progression.

Continuous passive motion, cervical traction, and biofeedback fill a gap between therapeutic modalities and therapeutic exercise. By applying mechanical forces to the body, positive stresses are introduced, serving to deter unwanted effects of the injury response process.

Massage and intermittent compression use mechanical pressure to elicit involuntary responses from the body. Massage is capable of producing local and systemic relaxation or invigoration and is also useful in reducing edema. However, massage also includes a psychological component founded in the one-on-one interaction between the clinician and patient. Intermittent compression assists in reducing the amount of edema in a limb and thus in restoring circulation. When combined with a cold fluid, this modality is useful in the immediate treatment of an injury by providing rest, ice, compression, and elevation simultaneously.

Chapter Quiz

1. All of the following effects have been attributed to continuous passive motion (CPM) **except:**
   A. Increased nutrition to the meniscus
   B. Increased nutrition of the articular cartilage
   C. Increased tensile strength of tendons and allografts
   D. Increased nutrition to the anterior cruciate ligament

2. Intermittent cervical traction can be useful in relieving the pain associated with intervertebral disk herniations. This reduction of pain occurs by reducing the bulge of the _____ through the _____.
   A. Fibrous pulposus and nucleus pulposus
   B. Annulus fibrosus and nucleus pulposus
   C. Nucleus pulposus and annulus fibrosus
   D. Nucleus pulposus and fibrous pulposus

3. When applying intermittent compression to an extremity, the pressure in the appliance should **not** exceed:
   A. The diastolic blood pressure
   B. The systolic blood pressure
   C. The difference between the diastolic and systolic blood pressure
   D. The resting heart rate

4. Electromyographic biofeedback measures:
   A. The amount of tension produced by a muscle group
   B. The amount of electrical activity with a muscle
   C. The amount of myelin activity within a muscle
   D. All of the above

5. Which of the following techniques produces the greatest amount of femoral blood flow?
   A. Pneumatic sleeve
   B. Manual calf compression
   C. Straight-leg raises
   D. Anatomic CPM

6. All of the following are indications for the use of intermittent compression **except:**
   A. Postsurgical edema
   B. Gangrene
   C. Lymphedema
   D. Venous stasis ulcers

7. Which of the following types of continuous passive motion designs provides for the **most** joint stability?
   A. Free linkage
   B. Anatomic
   C. Nonanatomic

8. The effectiveness of cervical traction is dependent on many factors, including the amount of tractive force applied. Other factors include:

    A. _____

    B. _____

    C. _____

    D. _____

9. List two reasons why separation of the vertebral column occurs at a lower percentage of the patient's body weight in the reclining position than in the sitting position.

    A. _____

    B. _____

10. Match the following massage strokes to method of delivery:

    A. Pétrissage   _____ Pounding of the skin

    B. Tapotement   _____ Kneading of the skin

    C. Effleurage   _____ Stroking of the skin

11. When applying massage to remove edema from a limb, the strokes begin _____ and are progressively worked _____.

CASE STUDY CONTINUATION

The following discussion relates to Case Study 3, found on pages 104 through 109 of Chapter 3.

Two of the modalities presented in this chapter, cervical traction and massage, would be appropriate for our patient's cervical trauma.

Massage

Soft tissue massage using effleurage and pétrissage strokes can promote relaxation of the involved muscles. Depending on the clinician's preference, the patient could be placed in the supine, prone, or seated position, with the head resting on a table to promote relaxation. The massage strokes should run parallel to the muscle fibers to help lengthen them. The patient would further benefit from massage by increased local blood flow and decreased neuromuscular excitability. Deep, localized friction massage can be used to help break up trigger points.

Cervical Traction

Cervical traction would be used only in the later stages of this patient's treatment protocol. Recall that the patient has been diagnosed as having a cervical strain and sprain. If traction were used too soon after the injury, the force may cause further damage to the cervical ligaments. Likewise, the patient does not show signs of radiating pain, decreasing the likelihood of cervical nerve root impingement.

Intermittent cervical traction, applied in two 5-minute intervals with a maximum of 25 pounds of tension, will assist in decreasing muscle spasm and pain, especially if the treatment is preceded by the application of moist heat packs. Placing the patient in the supine position lowers the amount of tension needed to elongate the muscles by decreasing motor activity in the cervical musculature.

REFERENCES

1. Muhe, E: Intermittent sequential high-pressure compression of the leg: A new method of preventing deep vein thrombosis. Am J Surg 147:781, 1984.
2. Olavi, A, Kolari, PJ, and Esa, A: Edema and lower leg perfusion in patients with posttraumatic dysfunction. Acupunct Electrother Res 16:7, 1991.
3. Rucinski, TJ, et al: The effects of intermittent compression on edema in postacute ankle sprains. J Orthop Sports Phys Ther 14:65, 1991.
4. Gilbart, MK, et al: Anterior tibial compartment pressures during intermittent sequential pneumatic compression therapy. Am J Sports Med 23:769, 1995.
5. Salter, RB: The biologic concept of continuous passive motion of synovial joints: The first 18 years of basic research. Clin Orthop 12, May, 1989.
6. McCarthy, MR, et al: The clinical use of continuous passive motion in physical therapy. J Orthop Sports Phys Ther 15:132, 1992.
7. Saringer, J: Engineering aspects of the design and construction of continuous passive motion devices for humans. In Salter, RB (ed): Continuous Passive Motion (CPM): A Biological Concept for the Healing and Regeneration of Articular Cartilage, Ligaments, and Tendons—From Origination to Research to Clinical Applications. Williams & Wilkins, Baltimore, 1993, pp 403–410.
8. Jordan, LR, Siegel, JL, and Olivo, JL: Early flexion routine: An alternative method of continuous passive motion. Clin Orthop 231, June, 1995.
9. Rosen, MA, Jackson, DW, and Atwell, A: The efficacy of continuous passive motion in the rehabilitation of anterior cruciate ligament reconstructions. Am J Sports Med 20:122, 1992.
10. Ververeli, PA, et al: Continuous passive motion after total knee arthroplasty: Analysis of costs and benefits. Clin Orthop 208, December, 1995.
11. Diehm, SL: The power of CPM: Healing through motion. Patient Care 8:34, 1989.
12. O'Donoghue, PC, et al: Clinical use of continuous passive motion in athletic training. Athletic Training 26:200, 1991.
13. Williams, JM, et al: Continuous passive motion stimulates repair of rabbit knee cartilage after matrix proteoglycan loss. Clinical Orthop 252, July, 1994.
14. Chiarello, CM, Gunderson, L, and O'Halloran, T: The effect of continuous passive motion duration and increment on range of motion in total knee arthroplasty patients. J Orthop Sports Phys Ther 25:119, 1997.
15. Gates, HS, et al: Anterior capsulotomy and continuous passive motion in the treatment of posttraumatic flexion contracture of the elbow: A prospective study. J Bone Joint Surg Am 74:1229, 1992.
16. Nadler, SF, Malanga, GA, and Zimmerman, JR: Continuous passive motion in the rehabilitation setting: A retrospective study. J Phys Med Rehabil 72:162, 1993.
17. Montgomery, F and Eliasson, M: Continuous passive motion compared to active physical therapy after knee arthroplasty: Similar hospitalization times in a randomized study of 68 patients. Acta Orthop Scand 67:7, 1996.
18. Gershuni, DH, Hargens, AR, and Danzig, LA: Regional nutrition and cellularity of the meniscus. Implications for tear and repair. Sports Med 5:322, 1988.
19. Kim, HKL, Moran, ME, and Salter, RB: The potential for regeneration of articular cartilage in defects created by chondral shaving and subchondral abrasion: An experimental investigation in rabbits. J Bone Joint Surg Am 73:1301, 1991.
20. Namba, RS, et al: Continuous passive motion versus immobilization: The effect on posttraumatic joint stiffness. Clin Orthop 218, June, 1991.

21. Von Schroeder, HP, et al: The changes in intramuscular pressure and femoral vein flow with continuous passive motion, pneumatic compression stockings, and leg manipulations. Clin Orthop 218, May, 1991.

22. Grumbine, NA, Santoro, JP, and Chinn, ES: Continuous passive motion following partial ankle joint arthroplasty. J Foot Surg 29:557, 1990.

23. Engstrom, B, Sperber, A, and Wredmark, T: Continuous passive motion in rehabilitation after anterior cruciate ligament reconstruction. Knee Surg Sports Traumatol Arthrosc 3:18, 1995

24. McCarthy, MR, et al: The effect of immediate continuous passive motion on pain during the inflammatory phase of soft tissue healing following anterior cruciate ligament reconstruction. J Orthop Sports Phys Ther 17:96, 1993.

25. Noyes, FR, Mangine, RE, and Barber, SD: The early treatment of motion complications after reconstruction of the anterior cruciate ligament. Clin Orthop 217, April, 1992.

26. Mullaji, AB and Shahane, MN: Continuous passive motion for prevention and rehabilitation of knee stiffness: A clinical evaluation. J Postgrad Med 35:204, 1989.

27. Giudice, ML: Effects of continuous passive motion and elevation on hand edema. Am J Occup Ther 44:914, 1990.

28. Dirette, D and Hinojosa, J: Effects of continuous passive motion to the edematous hands of two persons with flaccid hemiplegia. Am J Occup Ther 48:403, 1994.

29. Skyhar, MJ, et al: Nutrition of the anterior cruciate ligament: Effects of continuous passive motion. Am J Sports Med 13:415, 1985.

30. Witherow, GE, Bollen, SR, and Pinczewski, LA: The use of continuous passive motion after arthroscopically assisted anterior cruciate ligament reconstruction: Help or hindrance? Knee Surg Sports Traumatol Arthrosc 1:68, 1993.

31. Drez, D, et al: In vivo measurement of anterior tibial translation using continuous passive motion devices. Am J Sports Med 19:381, 1991.

32. McCarthy, MR, Buxton, BP, and Yates, CK: Effects of continuous passive motion on anterior laxity following ACL reconstruction with autogenous patellar tendon grafts. Journal of Sports Rehabilitation 2:171, 1993.

33. Takai, S, et al: The effects of frequency and duration of controlled passive mobilization on tendon healing. J Orthop Res 9:705, 1991.

34. Graham, G and Loomer, RL: Anterior compartment syndrome in a patient with fracture of the tibial plateau treated by continuous passive motion and anticoagulants: Report of a case. Clin Orthop 197, May, 1985.

35. Peek, CJ: A primer of biofeedback instrumentation. In Schwartz, MS (ed): Biofeedback: A Practitioner's Guide. Guilford Press, New York, 1987.

36. Coleborne, GR, Olney, SJ, and Griffin, MP: Feedback of ankle joint angle and soleus electromyography in the rehabilitation of hemiplegic gait. Arch Phys Med Rehabil 74:1100, 1993.

37. Utz, SW: The effect of instructions on cognitive strategies and performance in biofeedback. J Behav Med 17:291, 1994.

38. Segreto, J: The role of EMG awareness in EMG biofeedback learning. Biofeedback Self Regul 20:155, 1995.

39. Vander Linden, DW, Cauraugh, JH, and Greene, TA: The effect of frequency of kinetic feedback on learning an isometric force production task in nondisabled subjects. Phys Ther 73:79, 1993.

40. Draper, V: Electromyographic biofeedback and recovery of quadriceps femoris muscle function following anterior cruciate ligament reconstruction. Phys Ther 70:25, 1990.

41. Wolf, SL: Neurophysiological factors in electromyographic feedback for neuromotor disturbances. In Basmajian, JV (ed): Biofeedback: Principles and Practice for Clinicians. Williams & Wilkins, Baltimore, 1983.

42. Croce, RV: The effects of EMG biofeedback on strength acquisition. Biofeedback Self Regul 11:299, 1986.

43. Cummings, MS, Wilson, VE, and Bird, EI: Flexibility development in sprinters using EMG biofeedback and relaxation training. Biofeedback Self Regul 9:395, 1984.

44. Flor, H and Birbaumer, N: Comparison of the efficacy of electromyographic biofeedback, cognitive-behavioral therapy, and conservative medical interventions in the treatment of chronic musculoskeletal pain. J Consult Clin Psychol 61:653, 1993.

45. Newton-John, TR, Spence, SH, and Schotte, D: Cognitive-behavioural therapy versus EMG biofeedback in the treatment of chronic low back pain. Behav Res Ther 33:691, 1995.

46. Wong, AM, et al: Clinical trial of a cervical traction modality with electromyographic biofeedback. Am J Phys Med Rehabil 76:19, 1997.

47. Walker, GL: Goodley polyaxial cervical traction: A new approach to a traditional treatment. Phys Ther 66:1255, 1986.
48. LaBan, MM, Macy, JA, and Meerschaert, JR: Intermittent cervical traction: A progenitor of lumbar radicular pain. Arch Phys Med Rehabil 73:295, 1992.
49. Wong, AM, Leong, CP, and Chen, CM: The traction angle and cervical intervertebral separation. Spine 17:136, 1992.
50. Harris, PR: Cervical traction: Review of literature and treatment guidelines. Phys Ther 57:910, 1977.
51. Jette, DU, Falkel, JR, and Trombly, C: Effect of intermittent, supine cervical traction on the myoelectric activity of the upper trapezius muscle in subjects with neck pain. Phys Ther 65:1173, 1985.
52. Murphy, MJ: Effects of cervical traction on muscle activity. J Orthop Sports Phys Ther 13:220, 1991.
53. DeLacerda, FG: Effect of angle of traction pull on upper trapezius muscle activity. J Orthop Sports Phys Ther 1:205, 1980.
54. Latimer, EA, Clevenger, FW, and Osler, TM: Tear of the cervical esophagus following hyperextension from manual traction: Case report. J Trauma 31:1448, 1991.
55. Simmers, TA, Bekkenk, MW, and Vidakovic-Vukic, M: Internal jugular vein thrombosis after cervical traction. J Int Med Res 241:333, 1997.
56. Cyriax, JH: Clinical applications of massage. In Rogoff, JB (ed): Manipulation, Traction, and Massage, ed 2. Williams & Wilkins, Baltimore, 1980.
57. Goldenberg, DL: Fibromyalgia, chronic fatigue syndrome, and myofascial pain syndrome. Curr Opin Rheumatol 3:247, 1991.
58. Wolfe, F, et al: The fibromyalgia and myofascial pain syndromes: A preliminary study of tender points and trigger points in persons with fibromyalgia, myofascial pain syndrome and no disease. J Rheumatol 19:944, 1992.
59. King, JC and Goddard, MJ: Pain rehabilitation: II. Chronic pain syndrome and myofascial pain. Arch Phys Med Rehabil 75:S9, 1994.
60. Bohr, TW: Fibromyalgia syndrome and myofascial pain syndrome: Do they exist? Neurol Clin 13:365, 1995.
61. Shoemaker, JK, Tidus, PM, and Mader, R: Failure of manual massage to alter limb blood flow: Measures by Doppler ultrasound. Med Sci Sports Exer 29:610, 1997.
62. Boone, T, Cooper, R, and Thompson, WR: A physiologic evaluation of the sports massage. Athletic Training 26:51, 1991.
63. Ferrell-Torry, AT and Glick, OJ: The use of therapeutic massage as a nursing intervention to modify anxiety and the perception of cancer pain. Cancer Nurs 16:93, 1993.
64. Morelli, M, Seaborne, DE, and Sullivan, J: Changes in H-reflex amplitude during massage of triceps surae in healthy subjects. J Orthop Sports Phys Ther 12:55, 1990.
65. Sullivan, SJ, et al: Effects of massage on alpha motoneuron excitability. Phys Ther 71:555, 1991.
66. Morelli, M, Seaborne, DE, and Sullivan, SJ: H-reflex modulation during manual muscle massage of human triceps surae. Arch Phys Med Rehabil 72:915, 1991.
67. Harmer, PA: The effect of pre-performance massage on stride frequency in sprinters. Athletic Training 26:55, 1991.
68. Crosman, LJ, Chateauvert, SR, and Wesiberg, J: The effects of massage to the hamstring muscle group on range of motion. J Orthop Sports Phys Ther 6:168, 1984.
69. Smith, LL, et al: The effects of athletic massage on delayed onset muscle soreness, creatine kinase, and neutrophil count: A preliminary report. J Orthop Sports Phys Ther 19:93, 1994.
70. Tiidus, PM and Shoemaker, JK: Effleurage massage, muscle blood flow and long-term post exercise strength recovery. Int J Sports Med 16:478, 1995.
71. Cafarelli, E, et al: Vibratory massage and short-term recovery from muscular fatigue. Int J Sports Med 11:474, 1990.
72. Nalilbolff, BD and Tachiki, KII: Autonomic and skeletal muscle response to nonelectrical cutaneous stimulation. Percept Mot Skills 72:575, 1991.
73. Nixon, M, et al: Expanding the nursing repertoire: The effect of massage on post-operative pain. Australian Journal of Advanced Nursing 14:21, 1997.
74. Malkin, K: Use of massage in clinical practice. Br J Nurs 3:292, 1994.
75. Goldberg, J, Sullivan, SJ, and Seaborne, DE: The effect of two intensities of massage on H-reflex amplitude. Phys Ther 72:449, 1992.
76. Goldberg, J, et al: The effect of therapeutic massage on H-reflex amplitude in persons with a spinal cord injury. Phys Ther 74:728, 1994.

77. Day, JA, Mason, RR, and Chesrown, SE: Effect of massage on serum level of á-endorphin and á-lipotropin in healthy adults. Phys Ther 67:926, 1987.

78. Goats, GC and Keir, KA: Connective tissue massage. Br J Sports Med 25:131, 1991.

79. Ching, M: The use of touch in nursing practice. Australian Journal of Advanced Nursing 10:4, 1993.

80. Field, T, et al: Massage therapy reduces anxiety and enhances EEG pattern of alertness and math computations. Int J Neurosci 86:197, 1996.

81. Weinrich, SP and Weinrich, MC: The effect of massage on pain in cancer patients. Appl Nurs Res 3:140, 1990.

82. Ferrell, BA, et al: A randomized trial of walking versus physical methods for chronic pain management. Aging (Milano) 9:99, 1997.

83. Ramos, G and Martin, W: Effects of vertebral axial decompression on intradiscal pressure. J Neurosurg 81:350, 1994.

Answers to Chapter Quizzes

CHAPTER 1

1. B
2. B
3. A
4. A
5. D
6. C
7. B

8. B
9. C
10. A
11. A
12. C
13. A

14.

Sign	Event
Heat	Increased blood flow; increased rate of cell metabolism
Redness	Same as for heat plus histamine release
Swelling	High concentration of proteins, gamma globulins, fibrinogen; leakage of fluids into the extracellular space
Pain	Mechanical and chemical irritation of nerve endings
Loss of function	Sum of the first four signs

15. Chemotaxis
16. Edema must be passively moved through the venous and lymphatic systems. Elevation, compression, respiration, massage, muscle contractions, and respiration assist in removing edema from the extremity. Solid matter must be removed through the lymphatic system.

CHAPTER 2

1. D
2. B
3. D

7. D
8. C
9. B

4. D

5. A

6. D

10. C

11. D

12. A. Mechanical deformation

B. Chemical irritation

13. A wide range of responses is possible here. Your answer should describe methods of providing psychological comfort and distraction from the pain, as well as overt pain control methods using modalities.

CHAPTER 4

1. B

2. D

3. B

4. D

5. D

6. C

7. When metabolism is decreased, the cell's need for oxygen is reduced, increasing its ability to survive in a low-oxygen environment.

8.

Step	Effect
Rest	Prevents further physical trauma
Ice	Decreases the cell's need for oxygen
Compression	Reduces the pressure gradient, reduces hemorrhage, and limits the collection of edema
Elevation	Decreases local blood pressure and encourages venous and lymphatic return

9. Cold causes a vasoconstriction that limits the amount of warm blood entering the area. Heat application encourages blood flow, and cooled blood is constantly being delivered to the area.

10. As the percentage of the surface area being exposed to water increases, the percentage of the remaining unexposed tissues decreases. Thermoregulation must occur through this unexposed tissue.

11. A. Decreases the pressure gradient between the blood vessels and tissues, leading to a decrease in the amount of hemorrhage

B. Encourages increased lymphatic drainage

C. Causes the effects of the cold to penetrate deeper

D. Increases the joint's proprioceptive ability

12. A. If the wrap is applied too tightly, it can block venous drainage.

B. If a dry wrap is placed between skin and pack, cooling may not be sufficient.

CHAPTER 5

1. C

2. A

10. C

11. B

3. C
4. A
5. D
6. C
7. D
8. B
9. D

12. D
13. A
14. D
15. A
16. B
17. D

CHAPTER 6

1. C
2. B
3. D
4. D
5. A
6. A

7. C
8. B
9. A
10. D
11. B

12. A. Hydration
   B. Age
   C. Composition
   D. Vascularity
   E. Thickness
13. B
14. A

CHAPTER 7

1. D
2. C
3. A
4. B

5. C
6. B
7. B

8. A. Position of the neck
   B. Position of the patient
   C. Angle of pull
   D. Duration of the traction
9. A. The force of gravity is eliminated.
   B. The cervical muscles are placed in a more relaxed position.
10. B
    A
    C
11. Proximal/distal

APPENDIX A

Trigger Points and Pain Patterns

"Trigger points" are small areas of localized sensitivity and pain found in muscles and connective tissue. They may be produced by trauma, can be a result of chronic strain, or may be developed as a result of stress from daily activities or postural habits. Although the pain and sensitivity are localized, reports in the literature suggest that the discomfort may be referred to other parts of the body ("referred pain") through the autonomic nervous system.

These areas may be located by palpation, with the aid of the eraser end of a pencil, or by means of electrical currents. It has been suggested that the combination of electrical stimulation and ultrasound is beneficial in both locating and treating the involved areas. A tetanizing current within the comfortable intensity range of the patient is normally used for both location and treatment, offering "massagelike" contraction to the muscles to which it is applied.[1,2]

Illustrations are from Mettler Electronics Corporation, Anaheim, California, with permission.

REFERENCES

1. Travel, J and Rinzier, SH: The myofascial genesis of pain. Postgrad Med II(5): May, 1952.
2. Sola, AE: Myofascial trigger point pain in the neck and shoulder girdle. Northwest Medicine 54:980, 1955.

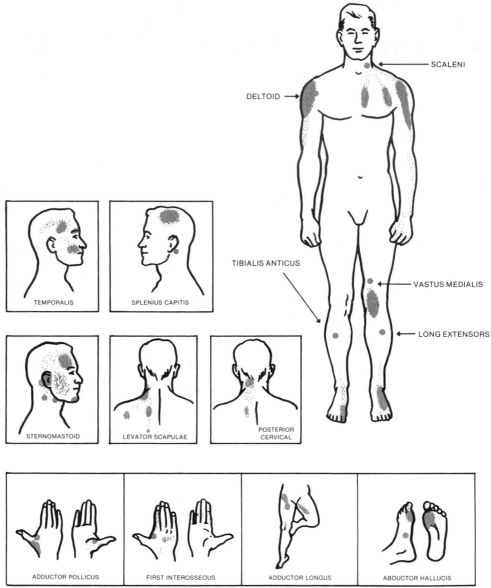

SCALENI

DELTOID

TEMPORALIS

SPLENIUS CAPITIS

STERNOMASTOID

LEVATOR SCAPULAE

POSTERIOR CERVICAL

TIBIALIS ANTICUS

VASTUS MEDIALIS

LONG EXTENSORS

ADDUCTOR POLLICUS

FIRST INTEROSSEOUS

ADDUCTOR LONGUS

ABDUCTOR HALLUCIS

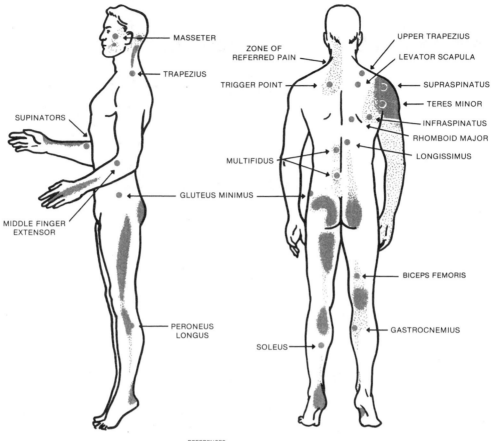

MASSETER

TRAPEZIUS

SUPINATORS

MIDDLE FINGER
EXTENSOR

PERONEUS
LONGUS

ZONE OF
REFERRED PAIN

TRIGGER POINT

MULTIFIDUS

GLUTEUS MINIMUS

SOLEUS

UPPER TRAPEZIUS

LEVATOR SCAPULA

SUPRASPINATUS

TERES MINOR

INFRASPINATUS

RHOMBOID MAJOR

LONGISSIMUS

BICEPS FEMORIS

GASTROCNEMIUS

REFERENCES:
Travel, J. and Rinzier, S.H., "The Myofascial Genesis
of Pain," POSTGRADUATE MEDICINE, Vol. II, No. 5,
May, 1952.

Sola, A. E. "Myofascial Trigger Point Pain in the Neck
and Shoulder Girdle," NORTHWEST MEDICINE, Vol.
54, pp. 980-984 September, 1955.

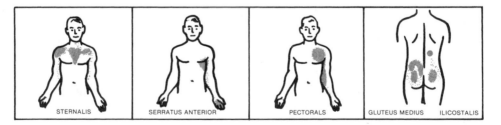

STERNALIS

SERRATUS ANTERIOR

PECTORALS

GLUTEUS MEDIUS   ILICOSTALIS

APPENDIX B

Physical Properties Governing Therapeutic Modalities

The laws of physics govern the energies used by therapeutic modalities. This appendix presents an overview of these physical properties. Modality-specific physical properties are discussed in the relevant chapters of this text.

THE ELECTROMAGNETIC SPECTRUM

Various forms of energy are constantly bombarding us: the light from the sun, the heat from a fire, and the waves emitted from radio transmitters. This energy, known as **electromagnetic radiation,** is produced by virtually every element in the universe and is characterized by the following traits:

- Transports energy through space
- Requires no transmission medium
- Travels through a vacuum at a constant rate of 300 million meters per second
- Does not have mass and is composed of pure energy

Each form of energy is ordered on the **electromagnetic spectrum** on the basis of its wavelength or frequency (Fig. B–1).

Regions of the Electromagnetic Spectrum

The energy's wavelength uniquely defines each portion of the electromagnetic spectrum. The reference measure for wavelength is the meter (Table B–1).

Ionizing Range

Energy within the ionizing range of the electromagnetic spectrum is characterized by the relative ease that atoms can release free electrons, protons, or neu-

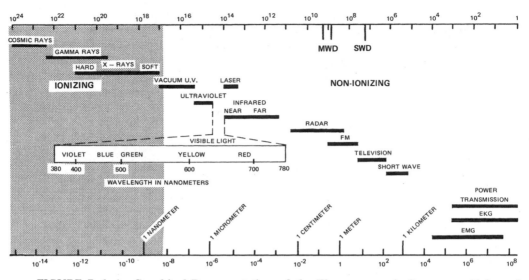

FIGURE B–1 A **Graphical Representation of the Electromagnetic Spectrum.** (Adapted from Illuminating Engineering Society of North America Lighting Handbook, New York, ed 8, 1993.)

trons. Ionizing radiation can easily penetrate the tissues and deposit its energy within the cells. If this energy is sufficiently high, the cell loses its ability to divide, eventually killing the cell.

Energy within the ionizing range is used diagnostically in x-rays (below the threshold required for cell death) and therapeutically in radiation treatment for some forms of cancer (above the threshold). Because ionizing radiation is hazardous, the total dose of exposure must be tightly monitored and controlled. Energy found in this portion of the electromagnetic spectrum is used by physicians only under closely controlled circumstances.

The Light Spectrum

This portion of the spectrum encompasses ultraviolet, visible, and infrared light energy. Electromagnetic radiation possessing a wavelength between 380 and 780 nm forms the spectrum of **visible "white" light.** White light is the combination of seven colors, each representing a different wavelength on the spectrum. These

TABLE B–1 **Units of Measure for Wavelengths Relative to the Meter (39.37 in.)**

Name	Symbol	Wavelength
Angstrom	≈	10^{-10} m
Nanometer	nm	10^{-9} m
Micrometer	μ	10^{-6} m
Millimeter	mm	10^{-3} m
Centimeter	cm	10^{-2} m
Meter	m	—
Kilometer	km	10^{3} m

seven colors, ranked from the shortest to the longest wavelength, are violet, indigo, blue, green, yellow, orange, and red.

Light energy having a wavelength greater than 780 nm is termed **infrared light** or infrared energy. Because this wavelength is greater than the upper limits of what the human eye is capable of detecting, infrared energy is invisible. Any object possessing a temperature greater than absolute zero emits infrared energy proportional to its temperature. Hotter sources transmit more infrared energy, because they possess a shorter wavelength than cooler objects.

The infrared spectrum is divided into two distinct sections. The **near infrared** is the portion of the spectrum that is closest to visible light, with wavelengths ranging between 780 and 1500 nm. The **far infrared** portion is located between 1,500 and 12,500 nm. Energy in the near infrared range is capable of producing thermal effects 5 to 10 mm deep in tissue, whereas far infrared energy results in more superficial heating of the skin (less than 2 mm deep).

Light with a wavelength shorter than visible light is ultraviolet light. Like infrared energy, **ultraviolet light** is undetectable by the human eye. Energy in the **near ultraviolet** range has wavelengths ranging between 290 and 380 nm, whereas the **far ultraviolet** range encompasses wavelengths between 180 and 290 nm. Both of these forms of ultraviolet light produce superficial chemical changes in the skin. Sunburn is an example of the effect of an overdose of ultraviolet radiation.

Many therapeutic modalities use energy within the light range of the electromagnetic spectrum. Ultraviolet light is used for the treatment of certain skin conditions. Depending on the relative temperatures involved, transfer of infrared energy is used to heat or cool the body's tissues. Medical lasers produce beams of energy in the ultraviolet, visible, and infrared light regions that can result in either tissue destruction or therapeutic effects within the tissues.

Diathermy and Electrical Currents

Electromagnetic radiation of longer wavelengths has an intensity sufficient to cause an increase in tissue temperature. Collectively known as **diathermy,** these types of electromagnetic energies create a magnetic field that is changed into heat through the process of **conversion.** The two most common types of therapeutic diathermy are microwave and shortwave diathermy.

In the range above shortwave diathermy and extending on to infinity are electrical stimulating currents. These devices use the direct flow of electrons and ions to elicit physiological changes within the tissues. It should be noted that the physical manipulations done to the electrical current do not allow for its precise location on the electromagnetic spectrum. The exception to this is uninterrupted direct current, possessing the theoretical wavelength of infinity.

PHYSICAL LAWS GOVERNING THE APPLICATION OF THERAPEUTIC MODALITIES

The efficacy of a particular treatment depends on the proper choice and application of a modality. The modality must be capable of producing the desired physiological changes at the intended tissue depth. A superficial heating agent has little positive effect on a deep-seated injury. The proper modality will not produce optimal results if it is applied incorrectly.

For physiological changes to occur, the energy applied to the body must be absorbed by the tissues. Across the electromagnetic spectrum, there is little correlation between wavelength and the ability to penetrate the body's tissues.[1] Both x-rays and radio waves penetrate the tissues despite their polar positions on the spectrum.

Cosine Law

Electromagnetic energy is most efficiently transmitted to the tissues when it strikes the body at a right angle (90°). As this angle (the angle of incidence) deviates away from 90°, the efficiency of the energy affecting the tissues is decreased by the cosine of the angle. The cosine law defines this relationship as:

$$\text{Effective energy} = \text{Energy} \times \text{Cosine of the angle of incidence}$$

With radiant energy, a difference of ± 10° from the right angle is considered within acceptable limits during treatment.[2]

Inverse Square Law

The intensity of radiant energy depends on the distance between the source and the tissues and is described by the inverse square law. The intensity of the energy striking the tissues is proportional to the square of the distance between the source of the energy and the tissues:

$$E = E_s/D^2$$

Where E = the amount of energy received by the tissue
E_s = the amount of energy produced by the source
D^2 = the square of the distance between the target and the source
Doubling the distance between the tissue and the energy decreases the intensity at the tissue by a factor of four (Fig. B–2).

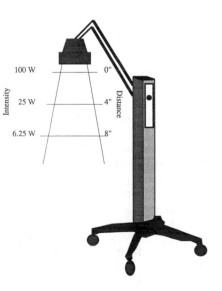

FIGURE B–2 **An Example of the Inverse-Square Law.** Each time the distance between the source of infrared energy and the tissue is doubled, the intensity of the energy delivered to the tissue is reduced by a factor of four.

Arndt-Schultz Principle

To enable energy to affect the body, it must be absorbed by the tissues at a level sufficient to stimulate a physiological response. As described by the general adaptation syndrome (see Chap. 1), if the amount of energy absorbed is too little, no reaction takes place, and if the amount of energy is too great, damage results. This concept applied to the application of therapeutic modalities is known as the **Arndt-Schultz principle** and is translated into clinical practice through the application of the proper modality at the proper intensity for the appropriate duration.

Law of Grotthus-Draper

The **law of Grotthus-Draper** describes an inverse relationship between the penetration and absorption of energy by which any energy that penetrates the body and is not absorbed by one tissue layer is passed along to the next layer. The more energy is absorbed by the superficial tissues, the less remains to be transmitted to underlying tissues.

Consider, for example, the application of moist heat to the quadriceps muscle group. Some of the energy is absorbed by the skin, decreasing the amount of energy delivered to the adipose tissue. Some of the remaining energy is absorbed by the adipose tissue, leaving only a fraction of the initial energy left to heat the muscle. This example also illustrates the fact that adipose tissue can act as an insulator, inhibiting the thermal heating of muscle. This concept applies to most therapeutic modalities, with the difference being the layer(s) in which the majority of energy loss occurs.

MEASURES

Distance Conversion

The basis of measurement in the metric system is the meter (m), a distance of 39.37 inches. The exact distance of 1 m is the wavelength associated with a specific frequency in the electromagnetic spectrum. The inch, according to history, was derived from the length of the middle phalanx of a king's index finger.

Comparison between English and SI Measures of Length

Millimeters	Centimeters	Meters	Inches	Feet	Yards
1 mm = 1.0	0.1	0.001	0.03937	0.00328	0.0011
1 cm = 10.0	1.0	0.01	0.3937	0.03281	0.0109
1 in. = 25.4	2.54	0.0254	1.0	0.0833	0.0278
1 ft = 304.8	30.48	0.3048	12.0	1.0	0.333
1 yd = 914.4	91.44	0.9144	36.0	3.0	1.0
1 m = 1000.0	100.0	1.0	39.37	3.2808	1.0936

Source: Adapted from Thomas, CL (ed): Taber's Cyclopedic Medical Dictionary, ed 18. FA Davis, Philadelphia, 1997, p 2229.

To convert English measures to meters, multiply the unit by the following conversion constants. To convert meters to the English system, divide by the constant.

English Measure	Constant
Inches	0.0254
Feet	0.3048

Weight and Mass Conversion

English Measure	Constant
Ounces	0.0283495
Pounds	0.4535924

Temperature Conversion

To convert Fahrenheit to centigrade:

$$°C = (°F - 32) \times 5/9$$

To convert centigrade to Fahrenheit:

$$°F = (°C \times 9/5) + 32$$

REFERENCES

1. Kloth, LC and Ziskin, MC: Diathermy and pulsed electromagnetic fields. In Michlovitz, SL (ed): Thermal Agents in Rehabilitation, ed 2. FA Davis, Philadelphia, 1990, pp 170–199.
2. Griffin, JE and Karselis, TC: Physical Agents for Physical Therapists, ed 3. Charles C Thomas, Springfield, IL, 1988, pp 229–263.

APPENDIX C | *Motor Points*

A motor point is the place in a muscle where the muscle is most easily excited with a minimum amount of electrical stimulation; the motor point is usually located near the center of the muscle mass, where the motor nerve enters the muscle. For each muscle, the motor point may vary from patient to patient, or even at different times for the same patient, depending on the pathology. The accompanying charts are guides to the motor points.

Illustrations are from Mettler Electronics Corporation, Anaheim, California, with permission.

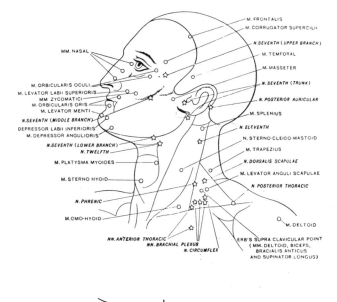

M. FRONTALIS
M. CORRUGATOR SUPERCILII
N. SEVENTH (UPPER BRANCH)
M. TEMFORAL
M. MASSETER
N. SEVENTH (TRUNK)
N. POSTERIOR AURICULAR
M. SPLENIUS
N. ELEVENTH
N. STERNO-CLEIDO-MASTOID
M. TRAPEZIUS
N. DORSALIS SCAPULAE
M. LEVATOR ANGULI SCAPULAE
N POSTERIOR THORACIC
M. DELTOID
ERB'S SUPRA CLAVICULAR POINT
(MM. DELTOID, BICEPS,
BRACIALIS ANTICUS
AND SUPINATOR LONGUS)

MM. NASAL
M. ORBICULARIS OCULI
M. LEVATOR LABII SUPERIORIS
MM ZYCOMATICI
M. ORBICULARIS ORIS
M. LEVATOR MENTI
N. SEVENTH (MIDDLE BRANCH)
DEPRESSOR LABII INFERIORIS
M. DEPRESSOR ANGULIORIS
N. SEVENTH (LOWER BRANCH)
N. TWELFTH
M. PLATYSMA MYOIDES
M. STERNO HYOID
N. PHRENIC
M. OMO-HYOID

NN. ANTERIOR THORACIC
NN. BRACHIAL PLEXUS
N. CIRCUMFLEX

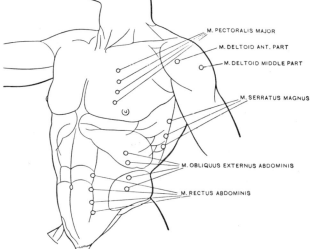

M. PECTORALIS MAJOR
M. DELTOID ANT. PART
M. DELTOID MIDDLE PART
M. SERRATUS MAGNUS
M. OBLIQUUS EXTERNUS ABDOMINIS
M. RECTUS ABDOMINIS

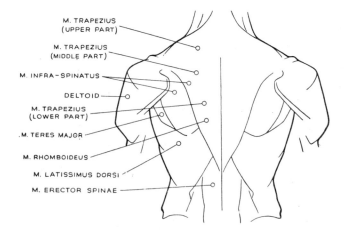

M. TRAPEZIUS
(UPPER PART)
M. TRAPEZIUS
(MIDDLE PART)
M. INFRA-SPINATUS
DELTOID
M. TRAPEZIUS
(LOWER PART)
.M. TERES MAJOR
M. RHOMBOIDEUS
M. LATISSIMUS DORSI
M. ERECTOR SPINAE

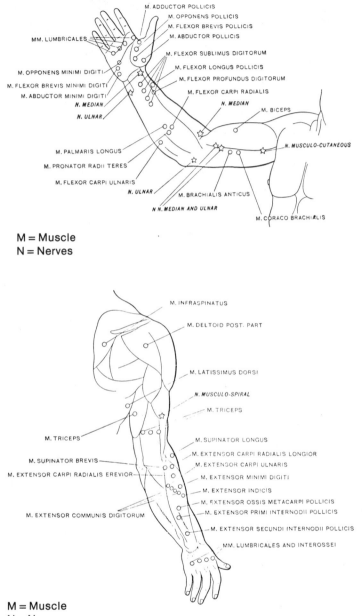

M. ADDUCTOR POLLICIS
M. OPPONENS POLLICIS
M. FLEXOR BREVIS POLLICIS
M. ABDUCTOR POLLICIS
MM. LUMBRICALES
M. FLEXOR SUBLIMUS DIGITORUM
M. OPPONENS MINIMI DIGITI
M. FLEXOR LONGUS POLLICIS
M. FLEXOR BREVIS MINIMI DIGITI
M. FLEXOR PROFUNDUS DIGITORUM
M. ABDUCTOR MINIMI DIGITI
M. FLEXOR CARPI RADIALIS
N. MEDIAN
N. MEDIAN
M. BICEPS
N. ULNAR
M. PALMARIS LONGUS
N. MUSCULO-CUTANEOUS
M. PRONATOR RADII TERES
M. FLEXOR CARPI ULNARIS
N. ULNAR
M. BRACHIALIS ANTICUS
N N. MEDIAN AND ULNAR
M. CORACO BRACHIALIS

M = Muscle
N = Nerves

M. INFRASPINATUS
M. DELTOID POST. PART
M. LATISSIMUS DORSI
N. MUSCULO-SPIRAL
M. TRICEPS
M. TRICEPS
M. SUPINATOR LONGUS
M. SUPINATOR BREVIS
M. EXTENSOR CARPI RADIALIS LONGIOR
M. EXTENSOR CARPI RADIALIS EREVIOR
M. EXTENSOR CARPI ULNARIS
M. EXTENSOR MINIMI DIGITI
M. EXTENSOR INDICIS
M. EXTENSOR OSSIS METACARPI POLLICIS
M. EXTENSOR PRIMI INTERNODII POLLICIS
M. EXTENSOR COMMUNIS DIGITORUM
M. EXTENSOR SECUNDI INTERNODII POLLICIS
MM. LUMBRICALES AND INTEROSSEI

M = Muscle
N = Nerves

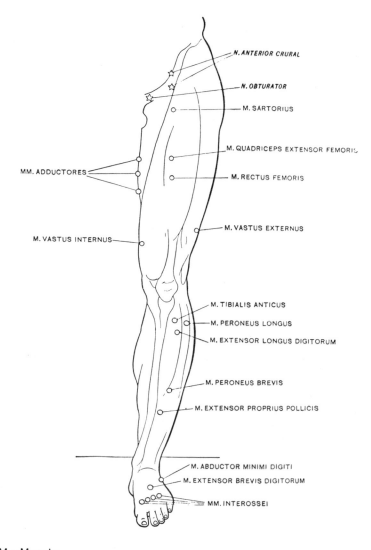

N. ANTERIOR CRURAL

N. OBTURATOR

M. SARTORIUS

M. QUADRICEPS EXTENSOR FEMORIS

MM. ADDUCTORES

M. RECTUS FEMORIS

M. VASTUS EXTERNUS

M. VASTUS INTERNUS

M. TIBIALIS ANTICUS

M. PERONEUS LONGUS

M. EXTENSOR LONGUS DIGITORUM

M. PERONEUS BREVIS

M. EXTENSOR PROPRIUS POLLICIS

M. ABDUCTOR MINIMI DIGITI

M. EXTENSOR BREVIS DIGITORUM

MM. INTEROSSEI

M = Muscle
N = Nerve

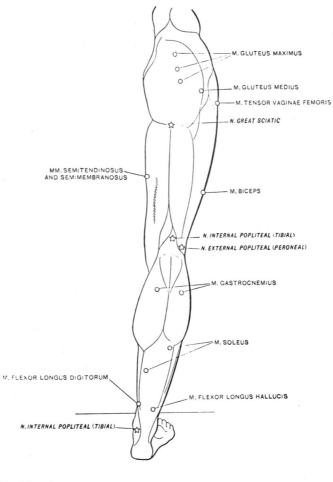

M. GLUTEUS MAXIMUS

M. GLUTEUS MEDIUS

M. TENSOR VAGINAE FEMORIS

N. GREAT SCIATIC

MM. SEMITENDINOSUS
AND SEMIMEMBRANOSUS

M. BICEPS

N. INTERNAL POPLITEAL (TIBIAL)
N. EXTERNAL POPLITEAL (PERONEAL)

M. GASTROCNEMIUS

M. SOLEUS

M. FLEXOR LONGUS DIGITORUM

M. FLEXOR LONGUS HALLUCIS

N. INTERNAL POPLITEAL (TIBIAL)

M = Muscle
N = Nerve

Medical Shorthand

The following is an abbreviated list of commonly accepted shorthand that may be used when documenting treatments. An excellent resource on medical notetaking and record keeping is *Writing SOAP Notes*, edition 2, by Ginge Kettenbach (FA Davis, Philadelphia, 1995).

THERAPEUTIC MODALITIES AND/OR TREATMENTS

CWP	Cold whirlpool
EMS	Electrical muscle stimulation
ES	Electrical stimulation
HP	Hot pack
HVGS	High-voltage electrogalvanic stimulation
HWP	Hot whirlpool
ICE	Ice, compression, elevation
MENS	Microcurrent electrical neuromuscular stimulation
MWD	Microwave diathermy
RICE	Rest, ice, compression, elevation
SWD	Shortwave diathermy
TENS	Transcutaneous electrical nerve stimulation
US	Ultrasound
UV	Ultraviolet
WP	Whirlpool

DOSAGE AND/OR MEDICATION

Meds	Medication
od	Once daily
pc	After meals
PRN	Whenever necessary
q	Every
qd	Every day
qh	Every hour

qid	Four times a day
qn	Every night
tid	Three times a day
W/cm^2	Watts per square centimeter

RANGE OF MOTION AND EXERCISE

ADL	Activities of daily living
AROM	Active range of motion
BR	Bedrest
CWI	Crutch walking exercise
FWB	Full weight-bearing
NWB	Non–weight-bearing
PWB	Partial weight-bearing
PNF	Proprioceptive neuromuscular facilitation
PREs	Progressive resistance exercises
PROM	Passive range of motion
ROM	Range of motion
ROT	Rotate, rotational
RROM	Resistive range of motion
SLR	Straight-leg raise

MEASUREMENTS AND TIME

+, pos	Positive
−, neg	Negative
<	Less than
=	Equals
>	Greater than
cm	Centimeter
F	Fair
ft	Foot/feet
G	Good
h, hr	Hour
hs	At bedtime
H&P	History and physical
in.	Inch
lb	Pounds
min	Minutes
mo	Month
N	Normal
P	Poor
sec	Seconds
SOS	When necessary, if necessary
stat	Immediately
UNK	Unknown
wk	Week

wt	Weight
WNL	Within normal limits
×	Number of times performed
y/o	Years old
yr	Year

BODY AREA

Ⓛ	Left
Ⓡ	Right
ACJ	Acromioclavicular joint
ACL	Anterior cruciate ligament
AIIS	Anterior inferior iliac spine
AP	Anterior-posterior
ASIS	Anterior superior iliac spine
ATF	Anterior Talofibular ligament
CF	Calcaneofibular ligament
CV	Cardiovascular
DIP	Distal interphalangeal joint
GH	Glenohumeral joint
LCL	Lateral collateral ligament
LE	Lower extremity
MCL	Medial collateral ligament
PCL	Posterior cruciate ligament
PIP	Proximal interphalangeal joint
PSIS	Posterior superior iliac spine
PTF	Posterior talofibular ligament
SCJ	Sternoclavicular joint
UE	Upper extremity

PERSONNEL

DO	Doctor of osteopathy
MD	Medical doctor
PT	Physical therapist/physical therapy
Pt, pt	Patient

GENERAL NOTE TAKING

$\bar{p}$	After
~	Approximately
$\bar{a}$, a	Before
Δ	Change
↓	Down, decreasing
♀	Female
♂	Male

1°	Primary
2°	Secondary
↑	Up, increasing
c̄	With
s̄	Without
c/o	Complains of
CC	Chief complaint
D/C	Discontinue
Dx	Diagnosis
eval	Evaluation
Hx, hx	History
M&R	Measure and record
PH	Past history
postop	After surgery
preop	Before surgery
RO, r/o	Rule out
re:	Regarding, relating, pertaining
Rx	Treatment, prescription
Sx	Symptoms
vo	Verbal orders

Book Glossary

Absolute refractory period: The period after a nerve's depolarization during which a subsequent depolarization cannot occur, used for recharging the electrical potential.

Absolute zero: Theoretically, the lowest possible temperature, equal to $-273°C$ or $-460°F$. At this point, all atomic and molecular motion ceases.

Absorption: The process of a medium collecting thermal energy and changing it to kinetic energy.

Acclimatization: The process of becoming physiologically adapted to an environment.

Accommodation: The decrease in a nerve's action potential frequency over time when exposed to an unchanging depolarization stimulus.

Acoustical interface: A surface where two materials of different densities meet.

Acoustical spectrum: Energy transmitted through mechanical waves.

Acoustical streaming: The unidirectional flow of fluids within the tissues caused by the application of therapeutic ultrasound.

Actin: A contractile muscle protein.

Action potential: The change in the electrical potential of a nerve or muscle fiber when stimulated.

Activities of daily living: Fundamental skills required for a certain lifestyle, including mobility, self-care, and grooming.

Acupuncture points: Points on the skin theorized to control systemic functions. These points lie along 12 main channels, 8 secondary channels, and a network of sub-channels.

Acute: Of recent onset. The period after an injury when the local inflammatory response is still active.

A-delta fibers: A type of nerve that transmits painful information that is often interpreted by the brain as burning or stinging pain.

Adenosine triphosphastase: An important source of energy for intracellular metabolism.

Aerobic: Requiring the presence of oxygen.

Afferent: Carrying impulses toward a central structure, for example, the brain.

Alarm stage: The first stage in the general adaptation syndrome in which the body readies its defensive systems.

Allograft: A replacement or augmentation of a biological structure with a synthetic one.

Alternating current: The uninterrupted flow of electrons marked by a change in the direction and magnitude of the movement.

Amino acids: Building blocks of protein.

Amperage: The rate of flow of an electrical current. One ampere is equal to the rate of flow of 1 coulomb per second.

Amplitude: The maximum departure of a wave from the baseline.

Amplitude ramp: The gradual rise or fall in a pulse train's amplitude.

Anaerobic: Able to survive in the absence of oxygen. Anaerobic systems derive their energy through the breakdown of adenosine triphosphate (ATP) into adenosine diphosphate (ADP).

Analgesia: Absence of the sense of pain.

Analgesic: A pain-reducing substance.

Analog: A readout on a continuously variable scale. A clock with hands is a type of analog display.

Anesthesia: A loss of, or decrease in, sensation.

Angstrom (Å): A distance equal to 10^{-10} m or one-billionth of a meter.

Annulus fibrosus: The dense, inflexible outer layers of an intervertebral disk.

Anode: The positive pole of an electrical circuit. It has a low concentration of electrons and is the opposite of the cathode.

Antalgic gait: A gait resulting from pain on weight bearing. The stance phase of gait is shortened on the affected side.

Antibiotic: A substance that inhibits the growth of, or kills, microorganisms.

Arndt-Schultz principle: A principle stating that for energy to affect the body, it must be absorbed by the tissues at a level sufficient to stimulate a physiological response.

Arteriole: A small artery leading to a capillary at its distal end.

Arthroplasty: Surgical reconstruction or replacement of an articular joint.

Asymmetrical: Lacking symmetry (e.g., two halves of unequal size and/or shape).

Attenuation: The decrease in a wave's intensity resulting from the absorption, reflection, and refraction of energy.

Average current: The average amplitude of a current. When the current can be represented by a sine wave, the average current is calculated by multiplying the amplitude by 0.637.

Axon: The stem of a nerve.

Axonotmesis: Damage to nerve tissue without physical severing of the nerve.

Bacterium (plural Bacteria): A microscopic organism.

Basement membrane: Extracellular material that separates the base of epithelial cells from connective tissue.

Battery: The unwanted touching of one person by another.

Beam nonuniformity ratio (BNR): The ratio between the highest intensity in an ultrasonic beam and the output reported on the meter.

Beat pattern: The frequency formed when two electrical circuits of two different frequencies are mixed.

β-endorphin: A neurohormone similar to morphine.

Bilateral: On both sides of the body.

Biphasic current: A pulsed current possessing two phases, each of which occurs on opposite sides of the electrical baseline. The bidirectional flow of electrons that is marked by discrete periods of noncurrent flow.

Bipolar stimulation: Electrical stimulation using electrodes of approximately equal surface area from each lead. The resulting current density under the electrodes from each lead is approximately equal.

Breach of duty: A departure from the implied duty based on the reasonable and prudent doctrine.

Calorie: The amount of energy needed to raise the temperature of 1 g of water by 1°C.

Capacitance: The frequency-dependent ability to store a charge. The symbol for capacitance is (C) and is expressed in farads (F).

Capillary filtration pressure: The pressure that moves the contents of a capillary outward to the tissues.

Cardinal signs of inflammation: Heat, redness, swelling, pain, and loss of function in the area; used as a gauge in determining the extent and stage of the injury response process.

Carotid sinus: An enlargement of the carotid artery near the branch of the internal carotid artery, located distal to the inferior arch of the mandible. Baroreceptors at this site monitor and assist in the regulation of blood pressure.

Catalyst: A substance that accelerates a chemical reaction.

Cathode: The negative pole of an electrical circuit. It has a high concentration of electrons and carries the opposite charge to the anode.

Cavitation: The formation of microscopic bubbles during the application of therapeutic ultrasound.

C fiber: A type of nerve that transmits painful information that is often interpreted by the brain as throbbing or aching.

Change of state: Transformation from one physical state to another (e.g., ice to water).

Channel (electrical): An electrical circuit consisting of two poles that operate independently of other circuits.

Chassis: The framework to which electrical components are attached.

Chemosensitive receptors: Nerves that are excited by the presence of certain chemical substances.

Chemotaxis: Movement of living protoplasm toward or away from a chemical stimulus.

Chronic: Continuing for a long period; with injury, extending past the primary hemorrhage and inflammation cycle.

Circuit, closed: A complete pathway that allows electrons to flow to and from the electrical source.

Circuit, open: An incomplete pathway that does not allow electrons to flow to or from the electrical source.

Circumferential compression: Compression applied in a manner that provides even pressure around the circumference of the body part.

Coagulation: The process of blood clotting.

Cold-induced vasodilation: An unsubstantiated theory suggesting that cold application results in a net increase in the cross-sectional diameter of blood vessels.

Collagen: A protein-based connective tissue.

Collagenase: A substance that causes collagen to break down.

Collateral compression: A form of compression that provides pressure on only two sides of the body part

Collimated: Possessing a beam of parallel rays or waves that form a column of energy.

Commission: Response to a situation in a manner that is not reasonable and prudent.

Compartment syndrome: A condition in which nerves, blood vessels, or tendons are constricted within a confined space (e.g., the anterior compartment of the lower leg).

Compression (mechanical): An external force applied to the body (e.g., an elastic wrap) that serves to decrease the pressure gradient between the blood vessels and tissue.

Compression (ultrasonic): A decrease in the size of a cell during high-pressure peaks.

Conduction: The transfer of heat from a high temperature to a low temperature between two objects that are touching each other.

Conductive properties: The ability of a tissue to transfer heat (from a high temperature to a low temperature) or electrical energy.

Conductor (electrical): A material having the ability to transmit electricity. Conductors have many free electrons and provide relatively little resistance to electrical flow. Within the body, tissues having a high water content are considered conductors.

Connective tissue: Tissue that supports and connects other tissue types.

Consensual touching: A situation in which the person being touched has agreed to be touched. Consensual agreements negate the charge of battery.

Constructive interference: Two waves that, perfectly synchronized, combine to produce a single wave of greater amplitude.

Continuous interference: Two waves that are slightly out of phase interacting to produce a single wave whose amplitude and/or frequency varies.

Contracture: A condition resulting from the loss of a tissue's ability to lengthen.

Contraindicate: To make inadvisable.

Contralateral: Pertaining to the opposite side of the body. The left side is contralateral to the right.

Convection: The cooling of one object and the subsequent heating of another by the circulation of a fluid, usually water, or air.

Convergent: Two or more input routes reduced to a single route.

Conversion: Transformation of high-frequency electrical energy into heat.

Cortisol: A cortisonelike substance produced in the body.

Cosine law: A law stating that, as an angle deviates away from 90°, the effective energy is reduced by the multiple of the cosine of the angle: Effective energy = Energy × Cosine of the angle. A deviation of ±10° is considered within acceptable limits for therapeutic treatments.

Coulomb: The amount of charge produced by 6.25×10^{18} electrons (negative charge) or protons (positive charge).

Coulomb's law: A law stating that opposite charges attract and like charges repel each other.

Counterirritant: A substance causing irritation of superficial sensory nerves to reduce the transmission of pain from underlying nerves.

Crepitus: A grinding or crunching sound or sensation.

Cryokinetics: A treatment technique that involves moving the injured body part while it is being treated with cold, thus decreasing pain while increasing range of motion.

Cryotherapy: The application of therapeutic cold to living tissues.

Cyanosis (cyanotic): A blue-gray discoloration of the skin caused by a lack of oxygen.

Degassed water: Water that has been allowed to sit undisturbed for 4 to 24 hours, allowing gaseous bubbles to escape.

Degeneration (muscular): The decrease in size and strength of a muscle that occurs secondary to atrophy.

Delayed-onset muscle soreness: Residual muscle soreness, caused secondary to damage of the muscle cells, that appears within 24 hours after heavy muscular activity, particularly with eccentric muscle actions.

Dementia: The progressive loss of cognitive and intellectual functions without impairment of perception or consciousness. Symptoms include disorientation, memory impairment, impaired judgment, and impaired intellectual ability.

Dendrite: Synaptic connections of a nerve arising from a body.

Denervation: Lack of the proper nerve supply or nerve function to, for example, an area or muscle group.

Dependent position: An arrangement in which the body part is placed lower than the heart, increasing the intravascular pressure.

Dermal ulcer: A slowly healing or nonhealing break in the skin.

Dermatome: A segmental skin area supplied by a single nerve root.

Destructive interference: Two waves that are exactly out of phase, interacting to cancel each other out.

Diagnosis: A physician's determination of the nature and scope of an injury or illness.

Dialysis: An external device that is used to assist or replace the kidney's function of filtering blood.

Diastolic blood pressure: The lowest level of pressure in the arteries. For example, when a blood pressure reading is given as 120/80, 80 represents the diastolic value.

Diathermy: A classification of therapeutic modality that uses high-frequency electrical energy to heat subcutaneous tissues.

Dipole: A pair of equal and opposite charges separated by a distance.

Direct current: The uninterrupted, one-directional flow of electrons.

Divergence: The spreading of a beam or wave.

Doctrine: A statement of fundamental government policy.

Due care: An established responsibility for an individual to respond to a given situation in a certain manner.

Duty cycle: The ration between the pulse duration and the pulse interval: Duty cycle = Pulse duration/(Pulse duration + Pulse interval) × 100.

Dynamometer: A device used for measuring muscular strength.

Ecchymosis: A blue-black discoloration of the skin caused by movement of blood into the tissues. In the later stages, the color may appear as a greenish-brown or yellow.

Edema: An excessive accumulation of serous fluids.

Effective radiating area (ERA): The portion of an ultrasonic transducer's (sound head) surface that emits ultrasonic energy.

Efferent: Carrying impulses away from a central structure. Nerves leaving the central nervous system are efferent nerves.

Efficacy: The ability of a modality or treatment regimen to produce the intended effects.

Effleurage: Massage using long, deep strokes.

Electromagnetic field: The lines of force created by positive and negative poles.

Electromagnetic radiation: Energy found on the electromagnetic spectrum capable of traveling near the speed of light and exhibiting both electrical and magnetic properties.

Electromagnetic spectrum: A continuum ordered by the wavelength or frequency of the energy produced.

Electromyogram: A recording of the electrical charges associated with the contraction of a muscle.

Electron: A negatively charged atomic particle.

Electro-osmotic: Pertaining to the movement of ions as a result of electrical charges. Positive ions move away from the positive pole toward the negative pole; negative ions move away from the negative pole toward the positive pole.

Electrostatic field: A field created by static electricity.

Emigration: Passage of white blood corpuscles through the walls of capillaries and veins during inflammation.

Endogenous opiates: Pain-inhibiting substances produced in the brain. These include endorphins and enkephalins.

Endorphin: A morphinelike neurohormone produced from β-lipotropin in the pituitary.

Endorphins are thought to increase the pain threshold by binding to receptor sites.

Endothelial cells: Flat cells lining the blood and lymphatic vessels and the heart.

Enkephalin: A substance released by the body that reduces the perception of pain by bonding to pain receptor sites.

Epicritic pain: The aching or throbbing sensation that follows protopathic pain. Transmitted along C fibers, epicritic pain is also referred to as "second pain."

Epiphyseal plates: Growth plates of bones.

Epithelial tissue: Tissue that forms the outer skin and lines the body's cavities. This type of tissue has a high potential to regenerate.

Ergometer: A device used to measure the amount of work performed by the legs or arms.

Evaporation: The change from a liquid to a gas state.

Exhaustion stage: The third and final stage in the general adaptation syndrome; the stage when cell death occurs.

External fixation: A fracture-setting technique incorporating the use of metal rods that extend through the skin and are attached to a device outside the body.

Extracellular: Outside the cell membrane.

Extravasation: To exude from or pass out of a vessel into the tissues, said of blood, lymph, or urine.

Exudate: Fluid that collects in a cavity and has a high concentration of cells, protein, and other solid matter.

Far infrared: The portion of the light spectrum location between 1,500 and 12,500 nm.

Far ultraviolet: The portion of the light spectrum located between 180 and 290 nm.

Farad: A measure of the storage capability of capacitors. One farad stores a charge of 1 coulomb when 1 V is applied.

Fibrin: A filamentous protein formed by the action of thrombin on fibrinogen.

Fibrinogen: A protein present in the blood plasma, essential for the clotting of blood.

Fibrinolysis: Pathological breaking up of fibrin.

Fibromyalgia: Chronic inflammation of a muscle or connective tissue.

Fibrosis: An abnormally large formation of inelastic fibrous tissue.

First-order neurons: Sensory nerves that course outside the central nervous system and have their bodies in a dorsal root ganglion.

Flux: A residual electromagnetic field created by two unlike charges.

Focal compression: Applying direct pressure to soft tissue surrounded by prominent structures.

Foramen: An opening (e.g., in a bone) to allow the passage of blood vessels or nerves.

Free radical: A highly reactive molecule having an odd number of electrodes. Free radical production plays an important role in the progression of an ischemic injury.

Frequency: The number of times an event occurs in 1 second; measured in hertz (cycles per second) or pulses per second.

Galvanic current: A low-voltage direct current.

Galvanic effect: The migration of ions as the result of the application of a galvanic current.

Gamma globulin: An infection-fighting blood protein.

General adaptation syndrome: A theory stating that the body has a common mechanism for adapting to stress. The three stages of this response are alarm, resistance, and exhaustion.

Golgi tendon organ: A sensory nerve ending found in tendons and aponeuroses.

Granulation tissue: Delicate tissue composed of fibroblasts, collagen, and capillaries formed during the revascularization phase of wound healing.

Granuloma: A hard mass of fibrous tissue.

Gross negligence: Total failure to provide what would normally be deemed proper in a given situation.

Grotthus-Draper, Law of: A law stating that there is an inverse relationship between the amount of penetration and absorption. The more energy that is absorbed by the superficial tissues, the less that remains to be transmitted to underlying tissues.

Ground: An electrical connection that provides a path for leaked current to return safely to the earth.

Ground fault: A disruption in the electrical circuity where the current exits from the normal path.

Ground-fault interrupter: An interrupter that discontinues the current flow when a ground fault is detected.

Ground substance: Material occupying the intercellular spaces in bone, fibrous connective tissue, cartilage, or bone (also known as matrix).

Growth factors: Substances that stimulate the production of specific types of cells.

Habituation: A function of the central nervous system that filters out nonmeaningful information.

Half-layer value: The depth, measured in cm, at which 50 percent of the ultrasonic energy has been absorbed by the tissues.

Hemarthrosis: Blood in a joint.

Hematoma: A mass of blood confined to a limited area, resulting from the subcutaneous leakage of blood.

Hemorrhage: Bleeding from veins, arteries, or capillaries.

Henry: A measure of inductance (H). One henry induces an electromagnetic force of 1 V when the current changes at a rate of 1 A per second.

Heparin: An inflammatory mediator produced by the mast cells of the liver. It inhibits the clotting process by preventing the transformation of prothrombin into thrombin.

Hertz (Hz): The number of cycles per second.

High frequency (electrical stimulation): An electrical current having a frequency greater than 100,000 cps.

High TENS: The application of transcutaneous electrical nerve stimulation possessing high-frequency, short-duration pulses and applied at the sensory level.

Histamine: A blood-thinning chemical released from damaged tissue during the inflammatory process.

Homeostasis: State of equilibrium in the body and its systems that provides a stable internal environment.

Hunting response: A vascular response to cold application marked by a series of vasoconstrictions and vasodilations. This response has been shown to occur only in limited body areas.

Hydrocortisone: An antiinflammatory drug that closely resembles cortisol.

Hydrostatic: Relating to the pressure of liquids in equilibrium or to the pressure they exert.

Hydrostatic pressure: The pressure of blood within the capillary.

Hyperalgesia, primary: Pain resulting from a lowering of the nerve's threshold.

Hyperalgesia, secondary: The spreading of pain caused by chemical mediators being released into the painful tissues.

Hyperemia: A red discoloration of the skin caused by increased blood flow. The skin turns white when pressure is applied.

Hypermobile: An abnormally large amount of motion.

Hypersensitive: Abnormally increased sensitivity; a condition in which there is an exaggerated response by the body to a stimulus.

Hyperthermia: Increased core temperature.

Hypertrophic: Increased size.

Hypertrophy: To develop an increase in bulk, for example, in the cross-sectional area of muscle.

Hypomobile: An abnormal limitation of normal motion.

Hyporeflexia: Diminished function of the reflexes.

Hypothalamus: The body's thermoregulatory center.

Hypothermia: Decreased core temperature.

Hypoxia: Lack of an adequate supply of oxygen.

Immediate treatment: Used in the initial management of orthopedic injuries. Immediate treatment is composed of four components: rest, ice, compression, and elevation.

Impedance: The resistance to flow of an alternating current resulting from inductance and capacitance.

Impedance plethysmography: A determination of blood flow based on the amount of electrical resistance in the area.

Inductance: The degree to which a varying current can induce voltage, expressed in henries (H).

Infection: A disease state produced by the invasion of a contaminating organism.

Inflammation: Tissue reaction to injury.

Inflammatory response, acute: The stage of the body's response to injury that attempts to isolate and localize the trauma.

Inflammatory response, maturation phase: The stage of injury response during which the body attempts to restore the orientation and function of the injured tissues.

Inflammatory response, proliferation phase: The stage of injury response during which the body prepares to rebuild the damaged tissues.

Infrapatellar: The distal portion of the patella including the patellar tendon.

Infrared light: Electromagnetic energy possessing a wavelength between 770 and 12,500 nm. Infrared light is invisible to the human eye.

Injury potential: Disruption of a tissue's normal electrical balance as a result of injury.

Innervate: Normal and sufficient nerve supply to a muscle, body area, and so on.

Interferon gamma: A group of proteins released by white blood cells and fibroblasts when devouring the unwanted tissues. The gamma classification is also referred to as "angry macrophages" because of their heightened phagocytic activity.

Interneuron: A neuron connecting two nerves.

Interpulse interval: The elapsed time between the conclusion of one pulse and the start of the next.

Interstitial: Between the tissues.

Intra-articular: Within a joint.

Intracellular: Within the membrane of a cell.

Intrapulse interval: The period within a discrete pulse when the current is not flowing. The duration of the intrapulse interval cannot exceed the duration of the interpulse interval.

Intrauterine device (IUD): A plastic or metal coil inserted within the uterus to prevent pregnancy.

Inverse square law: A law stating that the intensity of the energy striking the tissues is proportional to the square of the distance between the source of the energy and the tissues: Energy received = Energy at the source ÷ Distance from the source squared.

Ion: An atom, or group of atoms, with a net charge other than zero.

Iontophoresis: Introduction of ions into the body through the use of an electrical current.

Ischemia: Local and temporary deficiency of blood supply caused by obstruction of circulation to a part.

Isoelectric point: The point at which positive and negative electrical points are equal. The electrical baseline of zero.

Isometric contractions: Muscle contraction without appreciable joint motion.

Isotonic contractions: Muscle contraction through a range of motion against a constant resistance.

Joule: Basic unit of work in the International System of Units. One joule equals 0.74 foot-pounds of work. Joules = Coulombs × Volts.

Keloid: A nodular, firm, movable, and tender mass of dense, irregularly distributed collagen scar tissue in the dermis and subcutaneous tissue. Common in the African-American population, keloid scarring tends to occur after trauma or surgery.

Keratin: A dry, fibrous protein that replaces cytoplasm in the cells of the stratum corneum.

Kinetic energy: The energy possessed by an object by virtue of its motion.

Kinins: A group of polypeptides that dilate arterioles, serve as strong chemotactics, and produce pain. They are primarily involved in the inflammatory process in the early stages of vascular response.

Lactic acid: A cellular waste product produced by muscular contraction or cell metabolism. A fatiguing carbohydrate.

Laminectomy: Surgical removal of the lamina from a vertebra.

Legal guardian: An individual who is legally responsible for the care of an infant or minor.

Leukocytes: White blood cells that serve as scavengers.

Leukotrienes: Fatty acids that cause smooth muscle contraction, increase vascular permeability, and attract neutrophils.

Liable cells: Cells located in the skin, intestinal tract, and blood possessing good regenerative abilities.

Lipid: A broad category of fatlike substances.

Lordosis: The forward curvature of the cervical and lumbar spine.

Low frequency (electrical stimulation): An electrical current having a frequency of less than 1000 cps.

Low TENS: The application of transcutaneous electrical nerve stimulation using low-frequency, long-duration pulses, applied at a motor-level intensity.

Luminous infrared: See Near infrared.

Lymphatic return: A return process similar to that of the venous network but specializing in the removal of interstitial fluids.

Lymphedema: Swelling of the lymph nodes caused by blockage of the vessels.

Macrophage: A cell having the ability to devour particles; a phagocyte.

Magnetic resonance image (MRI): A view of the body's internal structures obtained through the use of magnetic and radio fields.

Malfeasance: The performance of an unlawful or improper act.

Malpractice: Negligence on the part of a professional person serving in the line of duty.

Malunion fracture: The faulty or incorrect healing of bone.

Margination: A state in which platelets and leukocytes, normally flowing in the bloodstream, begin to tumble along the walls of the vessel.

Master points: Points that, according to the theory of acupuncture, connect skin areas to deeper energy channels. Stimulating master points results in systemic changes.

McGill Pain Questionnaire: One of many pain rating scales, a method using pictures, scales, and words to describe the location, type, and magnitude of pain.

Mechanosensitive receptors: Nerve endings that are sensitive to mechanical pressure.

Medial glide: The American Academy of Orthopedic Surgeons' (AAOSs') evaluation technique of patellar mobility identifying two quadrants as normal.

Mediators: Chemicals that act through indirect means.

Medium: A material used to promote the transfer of energy. An object or substance that permits the transmission of energy through it.

Medium frequency (electrical stimulation): An electrical current having a frequency of 1,000 to 100,000 cps.

Meningitis: Inflammation of the membranes of the brain or spinal cord.

Meniscectomy: The surgical removal of the knee's meniscal cartilage.

Meridians: In acupuncture, primary pathways through which the body's energy flows.

Metabolism: The sum of physical and chemical reactions taking place within the body.

Metabolite: A by-product of metabolism.

Mho: The measure of a material's electrical conductance; the mathematical reciprocal of electrical resistance.

Microcoulomb: The charge produced by 10^{-6} electrons.

Microstreaming: During ultrasound application, the localized flow of fluids resulting from cavitation.

Misfeasance: The improper performance of an otherwise lawful act.

Modality: The application of a form of energy to the body that elicits an involuntary response.

Modulate: To regulate or adjust.

Modulation: Regulation or adjustment.

Monocyte: A white blood cell that matures to become a macrophage.

Monophasic current: The unidirectional flow of electrons that is interrupted by discrete periods of noncurrent flow.

Monopolar stimulation: The application of electrical stimulation in which the current density under one set of electrodes (the active electrodes) is much greater than that under the other electrode (the dispersive electrode). All of the effects of the treatment should be experienced only under the active electrodes.

Motor nerve: A nerve that provides impulses to muscles.

Motor point: An area on the skin used to stimulate motor nerves.

Motor unit: A group of skeletal muscle fibers that are innervated by a single motor nerve.

Motor-level stimulation: Electrical stimulation applied at an output intensity that produces a visible muscle contraction without activating pain fibers.

Mottling: A blotchy discoloration of the skin.

Muscle, cardiac: Muscle associated with the heart and responsible for the pumping of blood.

Muscle guarding: A voluntary or subconscious contraction of a muscle to protect an injured area.

Muscle, skeletal: Responsible for the movement of the body's joints.

Muscle, smooth: Contractile tissue that is associated with the body's hollow organs. Smooth muscle is not under voluntary control.

Muscle spindle: An organ located within the muscular tissue that detects the rate and magnitude of a muscle contraction.

Muscular tissue: Tissue comprised of smooth (found in the internal organs) cardiac and skeletal muscle; has the ability to actively shorten and passively lengthen.

Myelin: A fatty layer around nerves.

Myelinated: Having a fatlike outer coating (myelin) that serves as insulation for nerves.

Myocardial: Pertaining to the middle layer of the heart walls.

Myofibroblasts: Fibroblasts that have contractile properties.

Myosin: Noncontractile muscle protein.

Myositis: Inflammation of muscular tissue.

Myositis ossificans: Ossification or deposition of bone in muscle fascia, resulting in pain and swelling.

Nanometer: One-billionth (10^{-9}) of a meter.

Nanosecond: One billionth (10^{-9}) of a second.

Near field: The portion of an ultrasonic beam that is close to the sound head.

Near infrared: The range of infrared light that is closest to visible light, with wavelengths ranging between 770 and 1500 nm on the electromagnetic spectrum. Also known as luminous infrared.

Near ultraviolet: The range of light having wavelengths between 290 and 390 nm on the electromagnetic spectrum. This is the portion of the ultraviolet spectrum that is located the closest to visible light.

Necrosin: Increases the permeability of a cell membrane.

Necrosis: Cell death.

Negligence: Departure from the standard of care or duty. See also Omission and Commission.

Neoplasm: Abnormal tissue such as a tumor that grows at the expense of healthy organisms.

Neoprene: A synthetic rubber material.

Nervous tissue: Tissue possessing the ability to conduct electrochemical impulses.

Neurapraxia: A temporary loss of function in a peripheral nerve.

Neurological: Pertaining to the nervous system.

Neutron: An electrically neutral particle found in the center of an atom.

Nociceptive stimulus: Impulse giving rise to the sensation of pain.

Nociceptors: Nerves that transmit pain impulses.

Nonfeasance: Failure to act when there is a duty to act.

Nonunion fracture: Fracture that fails to heal spontaneously within a normal time frame.

Normative data: Information that can be used to describe a specific population.

Noxious: Harmful, injurious.

Noxious-level stimulation: Application of electrical stimulation that produces pain; caused by activation of C fibers.

Noxious-level TENS: Brief, intense electrical stimulation (above the threshold of pain) that is thought to activate the release of endogenous opiates.

Nucleus pulposus: The gelatinous middle of an intervertebral disk.

Numbness: Lack of sensation in a body part.

Occiput: The posterior base of the skull.

Occupational Safety and Health Administration (OSHA): A federal agency responsible for ensuring safe working conditions. This agency has enforcement powers and is capable of levying fines against employers.

Ohm: Unit of electrical resistance required to develop 0.24 calories of heat when 1 A of current is applied for 1 second.

Ohm's law: A law stating that current is directly proportional to resistance: Amperage = Voltage/Resistance ($I = V/R$).

Omission: Failure to respond to a situation in which actions are necessary to limit or reduce harm.

Ordinary negligence: Failure to act as a reasonable and prudent person would act under similar circumstances.

Organelle: A specialized portion of a cell that performs a specific function, such as the mitochondria and the Golgi apparatus.

Orthotics: The use of orthopedic devices for correcting deformity or malalignment.

Osteoarthritis: Degeneration of a joint's articular surface.

Osteoblast: A cell involved in the formation of new bone.

Osteoclast: A cell that absorbs and removes unwanted bone.

Osteogenesis: Healing of fracture sites through the formation of callus, followed by the deposition of collagen and bone salts.

Osteomyelitis: Inflammation of the bone marrow and adjacent bone.

Osteoporosis: A porous condition resulting in thinning of bone. Most commonly seen (but not exclusively) in postmenopausal women.

Outcome measures: Data that are used to evaluate the efficacy of a treatment program or protocol.

Overload principle: A principle stating that for strength gains to occur, the body must be subjected to more stress than it is accustomed to. This is accomplished by increasing the load, frequency, or duration of exercise.

Pacinian receptors: Receptors located deep in the skin that relay information regarding pressure and vibration. Within the joints, they assist in relaying proprioceptive information.

Pain threshold: The level of noxious stimulus required to alert the individual to possible tissue damage.

Pain tolerance: The amount of time an individual can endure pain.

Pallor: Lack of color in the skin.

Parallel circuit: An electrical circuit in which electrons have more than one route to follow.

Pathology: Deviations from the normal that characterize disease or injury.

Pavementing: Adherence of platelets to the vessel walls in multiple layers to form a patch over the injury site.

Peak-to-peak value: The sum of a pulse's maximum deviation above and below the baseline.

Penetration: Depth at which energy absorption takes place.

Periosteal pain: A deep-seated ache resulting from overly intense application of ultrasonic energy that irritates the bone's periosteum.

Peripatellar: Around the patella.

Peripheral vascular disease: A syndrome describing an insufficiency of arteries and/or veins for maintaining proper circulation (also known as PVD).

pH: (potential of hydrogen) A measure of acidity or alkalinity (bases). A neutral solution has a pH of 7. Acids have a pH of less than 7; bases have a pH greater than 7.

Phagocytosis: The ingestion and digestion of bacteria and particles by phagocytes.

Phase: Individual sections of a single pulse that remain on one side of the baseline for a period.

Phase duration: The amount of time for a single phase to complete its route. During monopolar application, the terms "phase duration" and "pulse duration" are equivalent. The phase duration must be of sufficient duration to cause depolarization.

Phonophoresis: The introduction of medication into the body through the use of ultrasonic energy.

Phosphocreatine system: A compound that is important in muscle metabolism.

Photon: A unit of light energy that has zero mass, no electrical charge, and an indefinite life span.

Piezoelectric crystal: A crystal that produces positive and negative electrical charges when it is compressed or expanded.

Pitting edema: An exudate-rich form of edema characterized by being easily indented by pressure (hence, "pitting").

Placebo: A substance of no objective curative value given to a patient to satisfy a need for treatment or used as a control treatment in an experimental study. Interestingly, this word means "I shall please" in Latin.

Platelet: A free-flowing cell fragment in the bloodstream.

Polymodal: Capable of being depolarized by different types of stimuli.

Polymorph: A type of white blood cell; a granulocyte.

Power (electrical): See Watt.

Precedent: A previous ruling that serves as a guide in future legal action.

Precursor: A substance that is formed before changing into its final state or substance.

Pronation: An inward flattening and tilting of the foot, resulting in the lowering of the medial longitudinal arch.

Propagation: Transmission through a medium.

Prothrombin: A chemical found in the blood that reacts with an enzyme to produce thrombin.

Proton: A positively charged atomic particle.

Protopathic pain: The stinging and burning sensation experienced immediately after trauma resulting from the activation of A-delta fibers. Protopathic pain is also referred to as "first pain."

Psychogenic: Pain of mental rather than physical origin.

Pulsatile current: See Pulsed current.

Pulse charge: The number of coulombs contained in one electrical pulse.

Pulse duration: The amount of time from the initial nonzero charge to the return to a zero charge, including the intrapulse interval.

Pulse frequency: The number of electrical pulses that occur in a 1-second period.

Pulse period: The period of time between the initiation of a pulse and the initiation of the subsequent pulse, including the phase duration(s), intrapulse interval, and interpulse interval.

Pulse width: See Pulse duration.

Pulsed current: A flow of electrons marked by discrete periods of nonelectron flow.

Quadripolar stimulation: Electrical stimulation applied with two channels.

Radiant energy: Heat that is gained or lost through radiation.

Radiation: The transfer of electromagnetic energy that does not require the presence of a medium.

Range of motion: The distance, measured in degrees, that a limb moves in one plane (e.g., flexion-extension, adduction-abduction).

Raynaud's phenomenon: A vascular reaction to cold application or stress that results in a white, red, or blue discoloration of the extremities. The fingers and toes are the first to be affected.

Rebound vasoconstriction: A reflex constriction of blood vessels caused by prolonged exposure to extreme temperatures.

Reflection: The return of waves from an object.

Refraction: The bending of a wave as it passes through an object.

Regeneration (tissue): Restoration of damaged tissues with cells of the same type and function as the damaged cells.

Replacement (tissue): Replacement of damaged tissues by cells of a different type from the original.

Resistance stage: The second stage in the general adaptation syndrome. During this stage, the body adapts to the stresses placed on it.

Resistor (electrical): A material that has few free electrons and opposes the flow of electricity. Within the body, tissues having a low water content are considered resistors.

Resonating: Vibrating.

Respondeat superior: See Vicarious liability.

Reticular formation: A diffuse network of cells and fibers located in the brain stem. The reticular formation influences alertness, waking, sleeping, and certain reflexes.

Retinaculum: A fibrous membrane that holds an organ or body part in place.

Rheobase: The minimum amount of voltage under the negative pole that is required for depolarization when a direct current is applied to living tissues.

Root-mean-square value: A conversion of the electrical power delivered by an alternating current into the equivalent direct current power, calculated by multiplying the peak value by 0.707.

Salicylates: A family of analgesic compounds that includes aspirin.

Satellite cell: Spindle-shaped cell that assists in the repair of skeletal muscle.

Sclerotome: A portion of bone that is supplied by a spinal nerve root.

Second-order neuron: A nerve having its body located in the spinal cord. It connects second- and third-order neurons (nerves having their bodies in the thalamus and extending into the cerebral cortex).

Secondary hypoxic injury: Cell death resulting from a lack of oxygen.

Sedation: The result of calming nerve endings.

Sedative: An agent that causes sedation.

Self-treatment: Treatment or rehabilitation performed by the patient without direct supervision, including home treatment programs.

Sensitization: The process of being made sensitive to a specific substance.

Sensory-level stimulation: Electrical stimulation applied at an intensity at which sensory nerves are stimulated without also producing a muscle contraction.

Sequential compression: Compression of an extremity characterized by a distal to proximal flow.

Series circuit: A circuit in which the current has only one path to follow.

Serotonin: A substance that causes local vasodilation and increases permeability of the capillaries.

Silica: A finely ground form of sand capable of holding water.

Somatic: Pertaining to the body.

Somatic receptive field: Area to which a stimulus is applied to obtain the optimum response.

Specific heat: The ratio of a substance's thermal capacity to that of water, which has a thermal capacity of 1. The specific heats of the three states of water are: ice 0.50, water 1, and steam 0.48.

Spondylolisthesis: Forward slippage of the lower lumbar vertebrae on the vertebrae above.

Sprain: A stretching or tearing of ligaments.

Stable cells: Cells possessing some ability to regenerate.

Stable cavitation: The gentle expansion and contraction of bubbles formed during ultrasound application.

Standard of practice: The criteria against which an individual's performance is measured.

Standing orders: A "blanket prescription" from a physician describing how injuries are to be managed when the physician is not present.

Standing wave: A single-frequency wave formed by the collision of two waves of equal frequency and speed traveling in opposite directions. The energy with a standing wave cannot be transmitted from one area to another and is focused in a confined area.

States of matter: The three forms of physical matter: solid, liquid, and gas. Using water as example, we see the three states of matter as ice, water, and steam.

Statute of limitations: A legal time limit allowed for the filing of a lawsuit.

Strain: A stretching or tearing of tendons or muscles.

Stratum corneum: The outermost, nonliving portion of the epidermis.

Stress: A force that disrupts the normal homeostasis of a system.

Subacute: Between the acute and chronic stages of the inflammatory stages.

Subcutaneous: Beneath the skin.

Subjective: Symptoms stated by the patient that are not externally apparent, such as pain. Personal beliefs and attitudes may alter subjective symptoms.

Substance P: A neurotransmitter thought to be responsible for the transmission of pain-producing impulses.

Summation: An overlap of muscle contractions that is caused by electrical stimulation.

Synapse: The junction at which two nerves communicate.

Synapse, chemical: The junction between two nerves that is characterized by a synaptic cleft. Chemical neurotransmitters carry the impulse from one nerve to the next.

Synapse, electrical: The junction between two nerves that is characterized by a gap junction. The nervous impulse is transferred directly to the subsequent nerve.

Synapse, excitatory: The release of the neurotransmitter tends to activate the postsynaptic nerve.

Synapse, inhibitory: The release of the neurotransmitter increases the nerve's resting potential, decreasing the probability that the nervous impulse will be propagated.

Synovium: Membrane lining the capsule of a joint.

Systemic: Affecting the body as a whole.

T cell: A transmission cell that connects sensory nerves to the central nervous system. Not to be confused with T cells found in the immune system.

Temporal average intensity: The average amount of power delivered to the body during pulsed ultrasound.

Tensile strength: The ability of a structure to withstand a pulling force along its length. Resistance to tear.

Tetany: Total contraction of a muscle achieved through the recruitment and contraction of all motor units.

Thalamus: Gray matter located at the base of the brain.

Therapeutic: Having healing properties.

Thermal capacity: The number of heat units required to raise a unit of mass by 1°C.

Thermolysis: Chemical decomposition caused by heating.

Thermotherapy: The application of therapeutic heat to living tissues.

Third-order neuron: A nerve having its body located in the thalamus and extending into the cerebral cortex.

Thoracic duct: A central collection point for the lymphatic system. The contents of the thoracic duct are routed into the left subclavian vein where it returns to the blood system.

Thrombin: An enzyme formed in the blood of a damaged area.

Thrombophlebitis: Inflammation of the veins.

Tissue hydrostatic pressure: The pressure that moves fluids from the tissues into the capillaries.

Tonic contraction: Prolonged contraction of a muscle.

Transcutaneous: Through the skin.

Transdermally (transdermal): Introduction of medication to the subcutaneous tissues through unbroken skin.

Transducer: A device that converts one form of energy to another.

Transfer: Assisted patient mobility, such as when moving from a wheelchair to a bed.

Transient cavitation: See Unstable cavitation.

Translation: Sliding or gliding of opposing articular surfaces.

Trigger point: A localized area of spasm within a muscle.

Turf burn: A deep abrasion caused by friction between the skin and artificial playing surfaces.

Twitch contraction: Repeated muscle contraction characterized by the fibers returning to their original length subsequent to the next contraction. Twitch contractions are distinguishable from each other.

Type I muscle fibers: Muscle fibers that generate a relatively low level of force but can sustain contractions for a long period. Geared to aerobic activity, these muscle fibers are also referred to as tonic or slow-twitch fibers.

Type II muscle fibers: Muscle fibers that generate a large amount of force in a short time. Geared to anaerobic activity, they are also referred to as phasic or fast-twitch fibers.

Ultraviolet light: Energy on the electromagnetic spectrum having a wavelength between 180 and 390 nm. Ultraviolet light is invisible to the human eye.

Universal precautions: A series of steps, established by OSHA, that individuals should take to avoid accidental exposure to blood-borne pathogens.

Unstable cavitation: The violent oscillation of bubbles during ultrasound application at too high an intensity.

Upper motor neuron lesion: A spinal cord lesion resulting in paralysis, loss of voluntary movement, spasticity, sensory loss, and pathological reflexes.

Valence shell: An imaginary shell in which the electrons responsible for chemical reactivity orbit around the nucleus of an atom.

Vasoconstriction: Reduction in a blood vessel's diameter, resulting in a decrease in blood flow.

Vasodilation: Increase in a blood vessel's diameter, resulting in an increase in blood flow.

Venous stasis ulcer: Ischemic necrosis and ulceration of tissue, especially that overlying bony prominences caused by prolonged pressure. Also referred to as decubitus ulcers or "bedsores."

Venule: A small vein exiting from a capillary.

Vicarious liability: Liability of employers for the acts of their employees.

Visceral: Pertaining to organs enclosed by the abdominal cavity.

Viscosity: The resistance of a fluid to flow.

Visible light: Electromagnetic energy possessing a wavelength between 390 and 760 nm. Visible light is a combination of violet, indigo, blue, green, yellow, orange, and red.

Voltage: A measure of the potential for electrons to flow.

Volumetric measurement: Determination of the size of a body part by measuring the amount of water it displaces.

Wallerian degeneration: Gradual physiological breakdown of a nerve axon that has been severed from its body.

Watt: A unit of electrical power. For an electrical current: Watts = Voltage × Amperage.

Weaning: Decreasing dependence on a substance or device by gradually reducing its use.

White light: See Visible light.

X-ray: An electromagnetic wave 0.05 to 100 Å in length that is able to penetrate most solid matter.

Index

Page numbers followed by f indicate figures; page numbers followed by t indicate tables; page numbers followed by b indicate boxed material.

MPQ. *See* McGill Pain Questionnaire
MRI. *See* Magnetic resonance imaging
Multimodality(ies), electrical stimulation, 214–215, 214f
Muscle(s)
  cardiac, 7
    defined, 374
  function of, cold effects on, 116
  skeletal, 7
    defined, 374
  smooth, 7
    defined, 374
Muscle contractions
  electrical stimulation in, 206–208, 206t, 208f
  skeletal, 19
    in venous return, 19, 20f
Muscle fibers
  type I, 7
    defined, 379
  type II, 7, 209
    defined, 379
Muscle guarding, defined, 15, 374
Muscle soreness, delayed-onset, defined, 231, 370
Muscle spasm
  cervical traction effects on, 325–326
  cold effects on, 116
  heat effects on, 125
  in injury response process, 22
Muscle spindle, defined, 374
Muscular degeneration, defined, 370
Muscular tissue, 7
  defined, 374–375
Myelin, defined, 375
Myelinated, defined, 375
Myocardial, defined, 3, 375
Myofascial release, 332–333, 334f
Myofibroblast(s), defined, 27, 375
Myosin, defined, 22, 375
Myositis, defined, 375
Myositis ossificans, defined, 375

Nanosecond, defined, 183, 375
Near field, defined, 274, 375
Near infrared, defined, 375
Near ultraviolet, defined, 375
Necrosin, defined, 375
Necrosis, defined, 375
Negligence, 97–98, 99t
  defined, 375
  gross, defined, 371
  negligent care of facilities, 98, 99t
  negligent delivery of treatment, 98
  ordinary, defined, 375
Neoplasm(s), defined, 375
Neoprene, defined, 138, 375
Neoprene toe cap, 136, 138f
Neospinothalamic tract (NSTT), 44

Nerve(s)
  motor
    defined, 7, 374
    type I, 209
  stimulation of, 202–203, 203b, 204f
Nerve endings
  chemical irritation of, 37–38
  mechanical deformation of, 37
Nerve fibers, terminating in laminae, 41, 41t
Nerve impulses, propagation of, 7, 8b
Nerve transmission, 7, 9f
Nervous tissue, 7–10, 8b, 9f, 10t
  defined, 375
Neurapraxia, defined, 117, 375
Neurological, defined, 375
Neuromuscular electrical stimulation (NMES), 244–249
  biophysical effects of, 218, 218t, 245–246, 246t
  contraindications to, 249
  described, 244–245, 244f
  duration and frequency of treatment with, 248
  effects associated with, 246t
  electrical parameters used in, 245t
  electrode placement in, 246–247
  indications for, 249
  instrumentation in, 247
  precautions with, 248
  setup and application of, 248
  using high-voltage pulsed stimulation units, 218t
Neuromuscular stimulation, interferential stimulation in, 239
Neuron(s)
  first-order, defined, 41, 371
  in laminae, 42
  nociceptive-specific, 42
  postsynaptic, 7, 9f
  presynaptic, 7, 9f
  second-order, defined, 42, 377
  third-order, defined, 378
  wide—dynamic-range, 42
Neurotransmitters, site and functions of, 9, 10t
Neutron, defined, 375
NMES. *See* Neuromuscular electric stimulation
Nociception, chemical initiation of, 39f
Nociceptive stimulus, defined, 37, 375
Nociceptive-specific (NS) neurons, 42
Nociceptor(s), 36
  chemosensitive, 38
  defined, 375
  mechanosensitive, 38
Nonexcitable tissues, 193b
Nonfeasance, defined, 375
Nonunion fracture, defined, 212, 375
Norepinephrine, site and functions of, 10t
Normative data, defined, 375
Note taking, shorthand terms for, 365–366
Noxious, defined, 10, 37, 375
Noxious-level stimulation, defined, 375
Noxious-level TENS, 230
  defined, 375